/2020/

/2020/

ONE CITY, SEVEN PEOPLE, AND THE YEAR EVERYTHING CHANGED

Eric Klinenberg

ALFRED A. KNOPF   NEW YORK   2024

THIS IS A BORZOI BOOK
PUBLISHED BY ALFRED A. KNOPF

Copyright © 2024 by Eric Klinenberg

All rights reserved.
Published in the United States by Alfred A. Knopf,
a division of Penguin Random House LLC, New York,
and distributed in Canada by
Penguin Random House Canada Limited, Toronto.

www.aaknopf.com

Knopf, Borzoi Books, and the colophon are
registered trademarks of Penguin Random House LLC.

Grateful acknowledgment is made to Metropolitan Transportation Authority for
permission to reprint "TRAVELS FAR" by Tracy K. Smith, copyright © 2020 by
Tracy K. Smith, commissioned by Metropolitan Transportation Authority for
TRAVELS FAR: A Memorial Honoring Our MTA Colleagues Lost to COVID-19.

Library of Congress Cataloging-in-Publication Data
Names: Klinenberg, Eric, author.
Title: 2020 : One city, seven people, and the year
everything changed / Eric Klinenberg.
Other titles: Twenty twenty.
Description: First United States edition. |
New York : Alfred A. Knopf, 2024. | Includes index.
Identifiers: LCCN 2023016554 (print) | LCCN 2023016555 (ebook) |
ISBN 9780593319482 (hardcover) | ISBN 9780593319499 (ebook).
Subjects: LCSH: Social history—21st century. | Presidents—United
States—Election—2020. | COVID-19 Pandemic, 2020—Influence |
Equality—History—21st century.
Classification: LCC HN18.3 .K56 2023 (print) | LCC HN18.3 (ebook) |
DDC 306—dc23/eng/20230523
LC record available at https://lccn.loc.gov/2023016554
LC ebook record available at https://lccn.loc.gov/2023016555

Front-of-jacket photograph by Robert Hamada
Jacket design by John Gall

Manufactured in the United States of America
First Edition

For Lila, Cyrus, and Kate.
My family, my pod.

CONTENTS

/2020/

MANHATTAN
May Lee

BROOKLYN
Enuma Menkiti
Brandon English

STATEN ISLAND
Daniel Presti

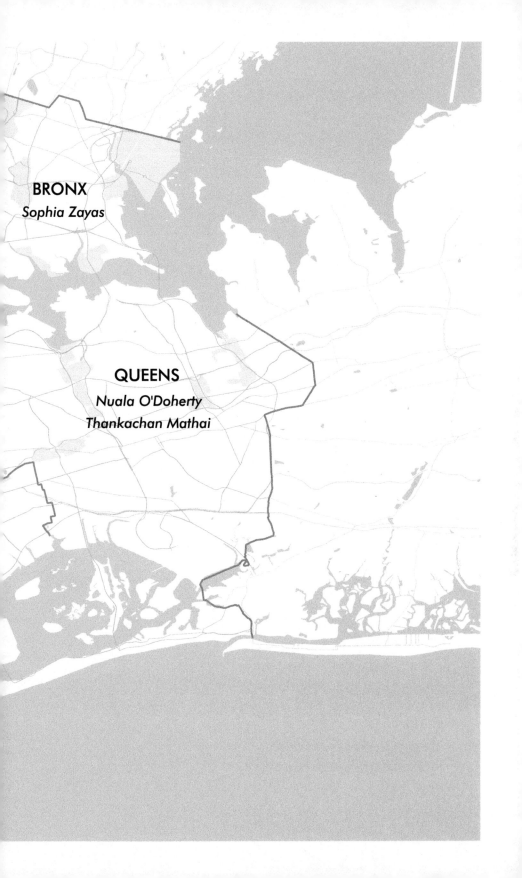

BRONX
Sophia Zayas

QUEENS
Nuala O'Doherty
Thankachan Mathai

Prologue

BREATHE

"Breathing isn't just about staying alive. It's about living. It's how you inhabit a place. Where you live. Where you work. Where you eat. You take in the air, bring the world in. You exhale, give something back. Breathing is our fundamental chemistry. It's where all our connections begin. And that, for me, was the thing that made COVID so difficult, so scary. It was like, suddenly, whenever I left home, I was afraid to take a breath."

Benjamin Bier is a cardiologist and critical care physician in New York City. He was thirty-one years old, in his fellowship at Mount Sinai Hospital at the start of 2020, when the main thing we need to stay alive became the thing most likely to kill us. In January and February, everyone in the medical community was talking about the new coronavirus that had just emerged in China and begun circulating through societies across the planet. "One of my co-fellows was from Italy, and they had friends in the Milan health system. They were texting reports from the hospitals to us. Horrible. The doctors were saying, 'This is like nothing we've ever seen before.' I'll never forget that sinking feeling in my gut."

COVID-19's arrival in New York City seemed inevitable.* On

---

* COVID-19 is the proper acronym for Coronavirus Disease 2019, and COVID is the popular colloquialism. I use the terms interchangeably in this book.

March 1, the first confirmed case was announced. "I was working in the Cardiac Intensive Care Unit, my primary clinical focus. In early March, I was talking to the nursing team. They said, 'We're going to be the first place the patients go. The ICU is going to be a COVID ward. We're going to get hit hard.'" Bier admired the way that Mount Sinai's leaders were planning for the surge in patients. Retrofitting patient rooms with better air filtration systems. Procuring personal protective equipment. Putting extra beds in the ICU. "We were like, 'All right, we think we're ready.' We knew it was going to be bad. We just didn't know how bad it was going to be."

The truth is, no one did. Usually, people turn to medical science in hope of answers. There's the right way to treat something and the wrong way. We want our doctors to know the difference, to have the data. We want facts. With COVID-19, though, there was mainly uncertainty. Was the virus transmitted through droplets or aerosols? Could children be vulnerable? Would intubation help or hurt? In this context, routine decisions about how to live became fraught and consequential. Bier's friends were asking whether they should leave the city. He and his wife, who had recently gone through a series of brutal treatments for a rare lymphoma and was now immunocompromised, started talking about whether she should go, too. The hospital, they feared, was about to become dangerous. Bier—young, healthy, and an expert at keeping the heart beating—would be at the center of everything, taking it all in.

Bier's supervisor knew about his family situation and wanted to help. They gave him a week in March to quarantine at home and then move his wife to his parents' house in Massachusetts, where she would have more fresh air, space, and support. After that, Bier drove back to New York and returned to the hospital. "I was scared," he told me. "A long time before, they had fitted us for N95s. You go into this room and they put a hood on you and like spray some stuff to make sure that you can't smell it. Usually, no one takes it seriously because you never need it. But with COVID, it was like, okay, this is not a drill." At the ICU, a nurse handed Bier a new mask. "I remember holding my breath before I put it on, and then checking all the seals like they taught us, because I didn't want to breathe the air of the ICU. And I realized that I was going to be in that thing for the rest of the day. This is how I'm going to work here. This is how I'm going to breathe."

It wasn't just the day, though, nor even the month. The outbreak became the pandemic, and the pandemic became an enduring reality. Bier worked in the hospital for all of it, and the mask, he said, became "my guard against any exposure, the thing that made me okay." Of course, he took it off when it was appropriate. "I drove a lot in the first months of the pandemic," he recounted. "And my car became this safe space. It was amazing, actually. There was no traffic, no one on the roads. So I'd drive to the hospital and I'd just feel free." But his wife returned home after the first surge subsided and he still had to be careful. In most places—at work, in stores, anytime he was around other people, really—Bier kept his mask on, snug and secure. "It's weird," he said, "but it became my habitat, the only place I really felt comfortable."

I met Bier in the fall of 2021, at the first large indoor gathering he had attended since the pandemic started, a Yom Kippur service in Brooklyn. Yom Kippur is the holiest day on the Jewish calendar. It's the day of atonement, when Jews ask forgiveness and repent for their sins. It's the day of remembering and mourning for the dead. It's also the day when the Book of Life, the sacred text where God writes the names of every person whose deeds merit another year on earth, is sealed. I don't know many of the prayers that Jews say on this day, but there is one, *Unetaneh Tokef,* whose words I've been able to recite since childhood: "On Rosh Hashanah it is inscribed, and on Yom Kippur it is sealed—how many shall pass away and how many shall be born, who shall live and who shall die, who in good time, and who by an untimely death, who by water and who by fire, who by sword and who by wild beast, who by famine and who by thirst, who by earthquake and who by plague . . ." In the service, the prayer continued beyond these lines, but this is where my mind lost focus, where I couldn't help but think about the millions of people who had died of COVID since 2020 started, and of the millions more whose names would not be inscribed in the Book of Life that day.

Thinking about millions of people means thinking about statistics, however, and the truth is that most of us, myself included, have trouble making sense of loss at this scale. Instead, I found myself wondering about those closer to me. My elderly parents and relatives, whose fate concerned me. My wife's uncle, who had died of COVID-19 a few months before, and her mother, who lived alone, and had grown relatively isolated during the pandemic even though she was just a few blocks away. My colleagues, some of whom perished in the early days of the pandemic. My children, whose lives were reduced and interrupted, whose dreams were now haunted, whose futures would be altered in ways we could not yet understand. I also knew that we were fortunate. The ones with good health care, with food on the table, with steady income, with savings, with love and support. Who shall live and who shall die? I could not say. But I knew it would be shaped by whether, and how, a person was protected or exposed.[1]

Despite his job, Bier had found a way to keep himself and his wife safe through the pandemic. "I always felt protected because I had this sealed bubble around my face," he told me. "I know people hated the mask, but I wound up liking it, because it allowed me to be human again." But the mask could not keep out his anxiety about the virus and the situation it had created, in the hospital, the city, and beyond, and both the virus and the situation kept evolving, sparking new emergencies, inducing new traumas, testing everyone, each in their own way.

For Bier, the trauma of 2020 came not only from working in a place where death suffused the environment, but also from the sense that his world had narrowed, that he and his family had gotten through it by locking themselves in a chamber, holding their breath. Bier had moved to New York City because he wanted to breathe in everything. The people. The street life. The food, the music, the theater, the works. The pandemic had changed his relationship to all of that. His life was different. The fundamental chemistry was off.

It's not just breathing. The story of what happened in 2020, and in the pandemic years that followed, goes deeper, with more expansive consequences, than conventional accounts acknowledge. Today, across the planet, people inhabit their world differently than they did before the plague hit. But what changed, where, and how, is not yet fully apparent. Like Bier, most of us have been busy trying to get through the crisis. We've lacked the time and space to consider what we have lived through, or to ask why things turned out the way they did. For many, thinking back about what happened in that fateful year feels overwhelming. Our private conversations, and our public ones, too, have been shaped by what sociologists call "the will not to know."

Fixing our chemistry requires breaking these habits and facing up to tough questions about the social life of the pandemic that we have thus far avoided. Why, in some places, did face masks become loaded objects that triggered cultural, political, and physical conflict, while in others they were used widely, with little controversy or debate? What made some neighborhoods so much more vulnerable to COVID-19 than others, and why did some that looked destined to suffer wind up relatively safe? How did some nations manage to build trust in government, science, and fellow citizens during 2020, while others went in the opposite direction? How, exactly, did race and class matter in the pandemic? What could members of communities do to help each other survive?

We need our day of reckoning. First, we must return to 2020, and take a closer look at what we lived through.

That January, I was teaching a sociology course at New York University. One of the key themes was the cognitive challenge of dealing with threats that are dire, yet distant. The human nervous system is designed to take swift action when danger is imminent. But when the threat feels far off, our brains refocus and the to-do list comes out. The danger gets deprioritized, a problem to be dealt with on another day.

This has been a perennial problem for a number of social issues. Consider global warming. No matter how much we recognize the threat presented by increasing temperatures, rising sea levels, and dangerous storms, other issues—crime, housing, education, unemployment, immigration, inflation—usually feel more pressing. Climate change is scary, but it's rarely a crisis we experience in the place where policy decisions are made: the here and now.

When my class met for the first time, I introduced students to this problem, called the "tragedy of cognition." I asked them to raise their hand if they had heard about the new coronavirus that had just emerged in China. Only a few knew what it was, and one of them was a Chinese student who had arrived in New York City that month. I then asked the students to raise their hand if the virus was one of the things that they worried about most. None did. Some actually laughed.

I understood their reaction. I've spent my career doing research on crises and disasters, but I didn't see this one coming. Not even when it was at my door.

On March 9, 2020, I was scheduled to fly to Cleveland and give a public lecture at a big civic celebration. For months, I had been looking forward to speaking in a crowded theater downtown and signing books for hundreds of people. Now, I was full of apprehension. The week before, COVID-19 officially arrived in New York City. New cases were being reported daily. I sent an email to the lead organizer in Cleveland: "Do you think we should discuss the situation there?" I asked. He offered me the option of postponing. But in the end, I decided to go.

LaGuardia Airport was empty, and my plane was, too. No one was wearing a mask, though the flight attendant offered me a sanitary wipe. By the time we landed, the landscape had shifted. The stock market was crashing, on its way toward losing nearly 8 percent of its value that day. Ohio was reporting its first three confirmed cases of COVID, with public health restrictions sure to follow. The streets were empty. "We're giving you an upgrade," the hotel receptionist told me. "You'll be one of our only guests."

More than half of the people who had tickets for the lecture stayed home that night, but the theater was still buzzing. "You might not be aware of this, but this was not the best day to travel by plane," I announced, to a roomful of nervous laughter. "There was a big part of me that said, 'You should not get on an airplane today!' And there was another big part of me that said, 'If you miss this, you're going to regret it for the rest of your life.'" It was the last night I would spend in public that year.

The next morning, March 10, I returned to New York City. My wife was also on the road that day, and her mother had stayed at our apartment with the kids. On my way back from the airport, she called me: our thirteen-year-old son had a fever. On Lexington Avenue, I passed a pedestrian wearing a gas mask. On Fifth Avenue, a woman donned a face shield and gloves. When I arrived home, I found my son on the couch, distraught and exhausted. My mother-in-law, in her mid-seventies and all too aware of the dangerous new virus, looked equally distressed.

"Do you think I have COVID?" my son asked.

There were no tests available, no way to know the real answer. Like everyone else, we were left to wonder. Should we isolate our child in a room of his own or hug and hold him? Establish distance or deepen the connection? How were we to care for each other? Would our instinct to keep each other close make the situation worse?

The next morning, NYU shuttered its classrooms and moved all courses online. Our children's school was next. Then the soccer club. Gymnastics, piano lessons, basketball games, and birthday parties were called off. The city, famous for its constant thrum of activity, was grinding to a halt. We packed up our car, rounded up our kids and the puppy, and drove to a house some fifty miles outside of Manhattan.

That night, our son's fever nudged higher. He had a headache. Stomach pains. He was so tired that he could not get off the couch. Grandma was feeling ill. Soon, my wife started coughing. "It's just allergies," she insisted. "Postnasal drip." And, wait. Was that a scratch in my throat?

There was no way we were going to the hospital, not with all the COVID cases there, with the medical staff in moon suits and the long lines of sick people waiting to get tested and the patients dying alone in their rooms. We were not going to a pediatrician, since they had no tests to administer and no knowledge of how to treat the disease. Instead, I did what I often do to harness my anxiety and figure out what's happening. I sat down and wrote.

The essay, which was published in *The New York Times*, conveyed my fear that America's deep divisions would make the pandemic more devastating than it needed to be. Social distancing, I acknowledged, appeared vital to slowing the spread of the coronavirus. But it was clearly a crude and costly public health strategy. What if, rather than social distancing, we responded to the threat by building social solidarity, acknowledging our interdependence and linked fate, and doing whatever we could to protect each other?

I knew it was a far-fetched suggestion. At the outset of 2020, the U.S. was politically divided and fragmented. People fought not only over their opinions, but also over basic facts. The nation may well have been founded on ideals of liberty, justice, and prosperity, but for decades Americans had been losing their sense of shared purpose. The country was polarized, segregated, and unequal. Distrust—of government, media, scientists, and fellow citizens—was rampant. Any appeal for public health or the common good would have to overcome these social chasms. But sometimes crises are switching points for states and societies. Was America capable of turning in a new direction? If not, how would we survive?

When that terrible week finally ended, it felt as though our family had come through relatively unscathed. In fact, the upheavals—which would shake nearly every household and every national government—were only beginning. Before long, we would endure a spate of mental health problems, move our children to a new school, cancel treasured family events, and recoil as neighbors acted out. For all of us, it seemed, the first week of horror became a month. The month became a year. And the year, 2020, became a period of world historical significance, a time—like 1492, 1776, 1918, 1939, or 1968—that history will never forget.

The events of 2020 would do considerably more damage, and induce far more sweeping changes, than anyone anticipated. The coronavirus, we now know, was only the primary cause. The deeper threat came from us.

Societies have a way of revealing themselves during crises. Who we are. What we value. How much we trust each other and our government. Whether we cooperate or sink into conflict. Whose lives matter. Who we're willing to leave in harm's way.

Consider the contrast between how Japan and the U.S.

responded when two ships, each operated by Princess Cruises and owned by the British-American conglomerate Carnival Corporation & PLC, rammed directly into a viral emergency during the first months of 2020. One, the *Diamond Princess*, was traveling on the East China Sea when authorities in Hong Kong discovered that at least one of its 3,700 passengers and crewmembers had COVID. The other, the *Grand Princess*, was carrying some 3,600 people on waters near Mexico when medical officials learned that they had an outbreak on board, too. The *Diamond Princess* returned to its point of origin, the Yokohama Port in Japan, where the national government took responsibility; the *Grand Princess* headed for its point of origin, the San Francisco Bay, where U.S. officials had a strikingly different response.

When the *Diamond Princess* docked near Tokyo, Japanese officials went on board to assess the situation, hoping to find that the virus was no longer spreading on board. Instead, ten passengers tested positive and the government announced that they would enforce a two-week quarantine, giving epidemiologists and medical scientists time to investigate. It was not an easy decision. Being detained in a small room is always difficult and sometimes dangerous. But Japanese leaders were far more concerned about the risk that allowing people to leave the ship would result in widespread transmission of the virus within the nation, and that repatriating foreigners would leave them responsible for its global spread. With no good options, Japan erred on the side of caution, choosing the plan that seemed best for public health.

Japan's approach to the crisis was hardly perfect. The first stage of the quarantine was chaotic, with people circulating between zones that should have been isolated. Its strategic approach to confinement and disembarkation shifted, sometimes without sufficient explanation, leaving passengers and their families anxious and confused. Crewmembers had some personal protective equipment, but were exposed to unsanitary conditions. So were government officials and health workers who went on the ship. At least one Japanese person who was released onto land after testing negative wound up testing positive after traveling home by train. Fourteen people who were infected on the *Diamond Princess* ultimately died.[2]

On balance, however, Japan's response was humane and helpful—to Japanese citizens, to foreign passengers, and to the global scientific community as well. They provided hospital care for 712 passengers and crew who contracted COVID-19 on the *Diamond Princess*, and offered mental health support for those suffering from stress, anxiety, and insomnia on the ship. They distributed some two thousand iPhones and set up Wi-Fi routers to improve communications options for those under quarantine. They offered medical attention to everyone with a chronic illness. They dramatically reduced the spread of the disease for those stuck on board, and contained the outbreak before it got worse.[3]

What's more, Japanese scientists and officials used the unfolding situation to advance their understanding of effective disease control with the new virus, and to help officials in other nations develop better policies, too.[4] Through their experience with the *Diamond Princess*, for instance, they began to suspect that asymptomatic people might be sources of contagion, which meant it was important to test extensively and trace the behavior of positive cases.[5] They learned about the high risk of transmission for people sharing indoor spaces, which suggested that aerosols might be playing a role in spreading disease and that improving air circulation could be a powerful mitigation measure. They learned about the heightened danger of severe illness among the elderly and sick. They learned how quickly symptoms could progress in those who were hospitalized, which helped administrators prepare for surges in intensive care units. Crucially, they learned about the danger of super-spreader events, in which small numbers of infected people, including some who cared for the sick, could spread the disease to others in their networks—a threat that endangered residents of nursing homes, where deaths would soon spike in nations that did not actively prevent such circulation. All of these lessons shaped Japan's public health strategy for the remainder of the crisis. They help explain why Japan became one of the safest countries in the world during the first stages of the pandemic, and particularly in 2020, when its mortality rate was just slightly above what it is in a typical year.

The United States treated the health crisis on the *Grand Princess* with decidedly less forethought, generosity, and care. When officials discovered the outbreak, Vice President Mike Pence held a press conference announcing that twenty-one passengers and crew had tested positive, and reporting that the ship was in international waters, heading back to the U.S. This was news to other passengers on the *Grand Princess*, who had not yet been informed of the situation. Pence promised that the ship would be docked as soon as possible at a noncommercial port, and that everyone on board would be tested and quarantined before being released.[6]

That same day, at a press conference in the U.S. Centers for Disease Control and Prevention (CDC) headquarters, President Donald Trump opposed any prospective medical response that involved allowing people with COVID, including American citizens on the *Grand Princess*, onto U.S. soil. His concern, it seemed, was adding any new cases to the nation's statistics. "I would rather have people stay [on board] . . . because I like the numbers being where they are," the president said. "I don't need to have the numbers double because of one ship that wasn't our fault."[7]

For the next two days, the *Grand Princess* remained at sea, with passengers and crew unsure about where they were headed and how they would be treated when they arrived. President Trump tweeted that the government had "a perfectly coordinated and fine tuned plan at the White House for our attack on CoronaVirus."[8] His own cabinet members said the very opposite, however. On national television, the surgeon general acknowledged that the government didn't yet have a plan.

The Trump administration had already come under attack for putting American passengers with COVID-19 on the same repatriation flight as those who had tested negative. They also neglected to disclose this to the passengers, who were irate when they found out. This decision, said Michael Osterholm, the director of the University of Minnesota's Center for Infectious Disease Research and Policy, was "one of the cruelest human experiments I've seen in my entire career."[9]

Quarantined in their rooms without any reliable information about what would happen, passengers on the *Grand Princess* also felt like the subjects of a cruel human experiment. The government finally allowed the ship to dock in California—not in San Francisco, the affluent jewel of a city where it was originally scheduled to make anchor, but in Black, brown, and working-class Oakland. "There's a feeling, particularly among people of color in this city, that things keep happening to us and not for us," the activist Cat Brooks told *The Guardian*. "When something like this happens, that allows for a breeding ground of hysteria and mistrust."[10]

Passengers with COVID-19 were sent, with very little information, to quarantine in hotels or military bases in California, Texas, and Georgia.[11] At Travis Air Force Base, more than eight hundred people refused to be examined. Some denounced the government for its interventions into their personal lives and dramatic efforts to exert control. Others insisted that they had a right to return home. "You are NOT required to be tested. It will be your choice," said a notice posted at Travis.[12] Although early results from those who consented to testing turned up many new infections, America's policies prevented officials from assessing exactly how many people were sick, and how many remained a threat to spread the disease.[13] The process ended in disarray and a slew of lawsuits.

How many people returned home while still contagious, and what happened to those in their communities, no one will ever know. Neither will we know whether the U.S., which became one of the deadliest places on the planet during 2020, could have staved off disaster had it responded to the crisis on the *Grand Princess* like Japan responded to its sister ship. After all, the differences in how nations acted in their early encounters with the virus—particularly their efforts to stop transmission, understand the situation, and develop emergency health policies—proved deeply consequential. They set entire populations on diverging paths, and shaped the course of their pandemic experience for years to come.

We need virology to understand the particular features of the novel coronavirus, SARS-CoV-2, that made COVID-19 so deadly. We need economics to explain why some financial remedies proved so much more effective than others. Social factors, some of which played out on the sidewalks and streets, others in statehouses and corporate suites, played a pivotal role in determining who lived and who died, who prospered and who famished, who came out depressed and depleted and who found new strength. We need a social autopsy—an examination of the social, political, and institutional organs that broke down during 2020—to identify the underlying conditions and acute shocks that shaped these patterns. We also need to recover the human stories that convey how a range of ordinary people experienced the pandemic. That is what this book provides.

It also offers something more important. "2020" refers not only to a year of great transformations, but to the capacity to see with clarity and acuity. For the last two decades, my work had been motivated by the idea that crises generate extraordinary opportunities—for politicians and corporations, whose interest in exploiting disasters to advance their own agenda is now well documented, but also for society as a whole. Extreme events can make visible a range of conditions that are always present but difficult to perceive. Reckoning with the traumas they induce requires asking hard questions about the nature of our experiences and taking a long, deep look inside ourselves to register what we endured. No matter how many places shut down during the early stages of the pandemic, 2020 was also the year that the world cracked open. My job, here, is to shine a light on the things so many of us have denied, avoided, or failed to see.

There was nothing inevitable about the way that COVID spread through a nation or a neighborhood. There were, however, strong social forces shaping every aspect of the crisis, from the flow of vital goods and reliable information to the provision of medical care and support. Some places were exposed to all kinds of danger while others were well protected. Some neighbors banded together to look after one another; others took up arms and prepared for a fight. New York City, with 8.5 million residents dispersed in some 250 neighborhoods across five boroughs, experienced everything, intensely and unequally, at once. By March, it had become the global hot spot for the coronavirus, and in 2020, it recorded more COVID-19 cases and fatalities than any city in the world.

Ultimately COVID-19 would reach nearly every town, city,

and community, and each would experience the plague in its own distinctive way. Given the scale and duration of the pandemic, there was no single place where an observer could register every variation of the COVID experience. But it's hard to imagine a vantage point more advantageous than New York City, where remarkable diversity and glaring disparities afforded a wide perspective. In most respects, being stuck in New York during the outbreak of COVID-19 was a terrible misfortune. For my research, it was a blessing.

Early in the pandemic, when New York City was officially on "pause" but its hospitals and health clinics were near desperation, I began tracking the striking variation in conditions across the five boroughs: Brooklyn, the Bronx, Manhattan, Queens, and Staten Island. There was social drama everywhere, and I decided to conduct in-depth interviews with a person in every borough whose experiences represented larger patterns in their community. (See Appendix: A Note on the Research.) An elementary school principal whose community was among the first to understand the threat; a political appointee in the Bronx whose job was to help local hospitals get the resources they needed and keep her constituents alive; a bar owner in Staten Island who was struggling to make ends meet; a retired district attorney in Queens who started a mutual aid network; a couple in Brooklyn who did essential work and needed someone to take care of their young kids.

Later, I added two other people: the child of an "essential worker" who caught COVID-19 and died while working in the city's public transit system during the first weeks of the pandemic, and an artist who became active in Black Lives Matter protests. Both were involved in problems that were central to 2020: how to mourn and memorialize a person who perished while serving a society intent on staying open, and how to address the racial violence that makes contemporary life so much more brutal than it needs to be. Together, these seven biographical stories from different parts of the city offer insight on the pandemic experience that no statistics or big datasets afford. Moreover, they provide something for which narratives are distinctly suited: a chance to see how people found meaning and purpose when their lives, and those of their loved ones, were on the line.

I also did research on a larger scale, trying to solve puzzles about the pandemic experience that begged for deeper sociological investigation. In the U.S., for instance, it is common to hear that social distance and isolation explain why America experienced so much conflict during the pandemic, with spikes in violence and antisocial behavior (from vehicular manslaughter to altercations on airplanes) giving rise to a de-pacification of daily life. As it happens, sociologists have a theory for why there are spikes in destructive behavior during times of crisis. It's based in the work of Émile Durkheim, and it concerns social disintegration, the collapse of a shared moral order, and the phenomenon that he calls "anomie." Society, Durkheim argued, has a profound influence on both individual development and collective life. It provides our core ideas about what it means to be a person; it establishes the norms, values, beliefs, and routines that make us who we are; it organizes us into cultural groups and moral communities; it binds us into relationships and sets civic obligations; it animates our passions and interests, but it also regulates them, redirecting our egocentric tendencies toward the pursuit of common goals. Sometimes, however, during periods of rapid social change—an economic transformation, a retreat from religion, mass urbanization, a plague—society buckles. The social structures that usually hold us in place suddenly seem flimsy. Authorities appear unreliable, neighbors unworthy of trust. Instead of convening, people hunker down at home and avoid interactions. Mutual obligations weaken. We act out, driven by our private needs and desires. When there's anomie, narcissism trumps solidarity. The social glue comes undone.[14]

There's ample reason to explain the outburst of antisocial behavior in America during 2020 as a direct result of pandemic anomie. The mystery, however, is that Durkheim's theory of social disintegration during a period of upheaval fails to explain what happened in nearly every country outside of the U.S. They, too, experienced a spike in generalized anxiety when the pandemic started. Their lockdowns were extensive. Their social gatherings were restricted. Their borders were sealed. Their offices were closed. Yet no other society experienced a record increase in homicides. None saw a surge in fatal car accidents. And, of course, none had skyrocketing gun sales, either. In 2020, nations around the world experienced an upheaval of historic proportions, with a variety of social problems, but nothing like what happened in the United States. Why?

What made the U.S. so exceptionally explosive during the crisis, and what helped other countries, such as Japan, hold together, is a question whose significance transcends the pandemic, and whose relevance extends far beyond 2020. We need to see and understand ourselves more clearly, because today, in the wake of the pandemic, and for the first time in recent history, everything is up for grabs. In the coming years, nations around the world will face fundamental questions about their principles and ambitions. Will we choose democracy or despotism? How will we balance individual liberties with our pursuit of the common good? What will we do about the mounting climate emergency? How can we achieve racial justice? Will we be capable of dealing with the next threat, or are we spiraling, inexorably, toward something far more catastrophic than what we have just been through?

If the pandemic taught us one thing, it is the urgency of heading off another tragedy of cognition, of finding the determination to tackle the dire but seemingly distant threats we face at this very moment, before it's too late.

CHAPTER 1

"It Was a Battle"

MAY LEE

The calendar broke the wrong way in 2020. In lucky years, January 1 came late in the week, a Thursday or Friday, and the school holiday extended through the weekend. A few more days to relax. This year, it hit on a Wednesday, and the New York City Department of Education decided that winter vacation, which began, stingily, on December 24, would end on January 2. It was a cold start for the 150,000 people employed in the nation's largest public school system, with an enrollment of nearly 1.1 million kids, more than 100,000 of whom are homeless. But that's how some years go.

May Lee, the principal of P.S. 42, an elementary school in Manhattan's Chinatown, wasn't thrilled to get back to the office so quickly, but she recognized the upside. At fifty-nine, Lee had been working at P.S. 42 for more than twenty-five years, first as a teacher, then as assistant principal, and now as the person in charge. Before that, she was a student there, as were her brother, her husband, and the youngest of her four children, a girl she adopted from Ethiopia because her family had more love to give. Lee, who's from a family of Chinese immigrants, describes herself as "argumentative and contrarian," as well as a "fighter" who is "totally committed to my families [her term for everyone with a student at P.S. 42] and my kids." She has wavy black hair, sometimes with blond streaks, multiple piercings, and "Grace" tattooed across her neck. "My mother was very liberal and very aggressive," Lee told me, in an accent that's pure New York City. "She taught me not to take any bullshit from anyone. She taught me to be fierce."

A child of the Lower East Side, Lee grew up a few blocks away from the hulking brick building where, each school day, roughly 550 students climb five concrete steps, enter three oversized double doors, and scatter across some sixty classrooms in one of America's densest urban areas. She still lives there, in a large, multigenerational house on Forsyth Street that she, her husband, and her brother's family purchased with their parents in 1999.[1] They share food, space, child care, feelings . . . everything, really. In Chinatown, thousands of immigrant families cram together with friends, coworkers, and relatives in small apartments, several people to a room, adults rotating in and out with each day's restaurant or factory shift. "One apartment will house three families," Lee said. "A lot of my families, they have, like, three families in one apartment. They share one kitchen, one bathroom. The kids' world is the bunk bed."

As a principal, and as a longtime Chinatown resident, Lee is all too aware of how situations like this can get during school holidays. It starts nicely: a special meal, a movie, a video call with friends and relatives in China, a trip to the library or park. Then the second day of vacation arrives. The adults go back to work. The grandparents need some rest. The kids demand televisions or phones or video games and there aren't enough to go around. People start to bicker. The apartment gets impossibly noisy. Then come the dishes, and the break is only just beginning. Everyone needs a vacation in December, but by January 2, everyone needs the kids to get out of the apartment, too. Fortunately, the city offers a release.

P.S. 42 is a release for every family with a student there, and for all the unrelated people who live with them, too. The school is fundamentally there to educate young people, and P.S. 42 does that so well that it ranks near the top of the city's performance standards, even though some 60 percent of its students come from poor families and 70 percent have parents who know little or no English. "But there is so much more that brings the kids here," Lee told me. The majority of P.S. 42 students rely on the school for breakfast, lunch, and an after-school snack. They get free music classes, soccer instruction, books, arts and crafts, and internet access. For years, Lee arranged for the YMCA to provide swimming lessons, because who else was going to do it? "I'll do anything to give these children the same experiences as my own kids," she told me. "I tell the teachers that we are all public servants. For a lot of our families, the teacher is the sun, moon, and God. Our job is to take care of them."

The new year began without much drama. The weather was mild, so comfortable that, in the month's second weekend, it caused some distress. High 60s? In January? That must be a bad omen. But it also meant the streets were booming with activity. The playgrounds were full. Restaurants were crowded. New York City was alive. Soon, though, Lee started hearing about a more immediate source of anxiety that was upsetting her families, more than 80 percent of whom were of Asian descent, and mainly Chinese. Their relatives in China were sending dire warnings about a deadly new virus that had started to spread in Wuhan, Hubei Province, a crowded city with some 11 million residents, and a major national transportation hub. That last detail mattered, because January 10 marked the beginning of the Lunar New Year Spring Festival, which the Chinese celebrate by traveling to visit friends, relatives, and tourist destinations throughout the country. The government expected that, collectively, Chinese people would take roughly three billion trips during the forty-day holiday, making it the world's largest annual migration event. At first, Lee recalled, it was hard to know what to make of the stories, what was rumor and what was fact. There wasn't much official news coming out of China, and what the government did say couldn't necessarily be trusted. She remembered 2003, when Chinese health agencies covered up an outbreak of SARS, the respiratory disease caused by a new coronavirus that killed nearly one of every ten people who contracted it, and more than half of those aged sixty and above. Back then, Chinese leaders spent months insisting that there were hardly any cases and that the situation was "under control." Only later did they acknowledge that there were more than five thousand cases in China alone, and that the government had failed to prevent it from spreading to other countries.[2] When the truth came out, national officials tried to save face by firing the minister of health and the mayor of Beijing. But it didn't help restore China's reputation in the international community, nor among Chinese Americans in places like New York City. For them, the lesson was straightforward: When you hear about a lethal virus, listen to the government, but act as if the situation is worse than they acknowledge. Protect yourself and your family. Only trust your family and friends.

On December 31, 2019, the Chinese government issued its first official report of a pneumonia of unknown etiology to the World Health Organization (WHO), acknowledging dozens of cases in Wuhan. Today, scientists believe that a novel coronavirus began infecting people in China sometime in October or, more likely, November 2019, with a spike in the number of patients admitted to Wuhan area hospitals for "flu-like symptoms" throughout December.[3] By December 15, we now know, the use of the words "Feidian" (Chinese for SARS) and "pneumonia" was rising sharply on the Chinese social media app, WeChat.[4] In January, as other nations began to report their first cases, too, these terms would be replaced by a new one: COVID-19.

The distance between Wuhan and New York City is approximately 7,497 miles, but it only takes a second for a WeChat message to travel between friends and relatives in the two cities. May Lee doesn't recall her families discussing the possibility of SARS or a new coronavirus in December, but by late January the anxiety was palpable, and by February it had disrupted daily life in the school. "My families are all on WeChat," Lee explained. "They were getting day-by-day details from their own families, who were suffering in China, and they were also getting a lot of crazy news. They were saying that it's really bad in China, and it's gonna get really bad here. They knew better. And they were stocking up on Lysol, tissues, masks, gloves. They were prepping! Packing up instant noodles. You name it. And they kept pressuring me to hold a meeting. They wanted to know what we were going to do."

Lee looked for guidance from the city government, from the state, the White House, the news media. They had nothing to offer. "I remember people saying, 'Oh, this thing might happen but we're going to get it under control,'" she told me. Her families weren't buying it, and they certainly weren't going to wait for political officials here to figure things out on their own. "They started taking their kids out of school," Lee explained. "At first it was my Asian families, but then my non-Asian families got really upset, too. We had a teacher coming back from Asia. We had families that got stranded there. And the non-Asian families just didn't have much information. They were freaking out!"

In late February, a group of parents began pushing Lee to close P.S. 42 altogether. "They knew what was going on in China, and they were like, 'Why are you keeping it open?' I had to tell them that it's not my decision. It's the Department of Education." As more families pulled their kids out of school, Lee got worried about her attendance figures. By chance, the city was in the midst of its annual quality review at P.S. 42, with an in-person inspection scheduled for mid-March. In typical years, attendance was one thing that Lee didn't have to worry about. Now a crisis was brewing, and not just for the school. "Attendance is really important for middle school admissions in New York City," she explained. If her fourth graders had too many absences, the best public schools would automatically turn them down. To prevent that, she had to make sure that parents who kept their kids at home reported them as sick, rather than just disappearing. But then she'd have to explain to the Department of Education why so many of her students weren't showing up.

By March, Lee said, "I knew the shit was going to hit the fan." She was torn between trying to support the families that were afraid of their kids catching COVID and bringing it home with them, and keeping the school intact for the quality review. "We had some kids who were really sick," she recalled. "They probably had COVID, but no one knew because there was no testing at that point." There were rumors of parents getting sick, aunts and uncles, too. "It made me realize, you know, we were probably going to wind up shutting down the schools." Yet just then, Lee saw Mayor Bill de Blasio on television. "He was saying, 'Don't worry! Go to theaters. Go to restaurants. Go to movies.'" She was skeptical. Restaurants? Theaters? Her families were wearing surgical masks and stockpiling food.

They were also encountering hostility in public, some of it violent, all of it driven by racial animus. Americans were getting anxious about the dangerous new virus, and a growing number were blaming Chinese people, including Chinese Americans, for spreading it. Prominent conservatives, including the hosts of leading conservative news programs and high-ranking officials in the Trump administration, were actively promoting this idea. On March 7, Secretary of State Mike Pompeo went on Fox News and warned about a diplomatic crisis related to the "China virus." The next day, Congressman Paul Gosar, an Arizona Republican who championed extreme right positions, announced that he would quarantine after being exposed to the "Wuhan virus."[5] By mid-March, President Trump himself would deploy this rhetoric, defying the World Health Organization's calls to avoid association of the virus with a people or place, a practice that, in 2020 as in previous outbreaks, was certain to generate stigma, discrimination, and racist attacks. On Twitter, in rallies, and at press conferences, Trump routinely referred to COVID-19 as the "Chinese virus" or "China virus," encouraging everyone in his orbit to do the same.

"We've always had to deal with racism in Chinatown," Lee told me. "Young people come to the bars here at night and scream all kinds of insults to our elderly. Groups of homeless men yell anti-Asian slurs because they think it's funny." Sometimes the hatred gets physical. For years, Asians on the Lower East Side were targeted for stabbings and assaults, and their kids were regularly subjected to bigotry and spite. FBI data suggest that anti-Asian hate crimes declined precipitously in the first two decades of the twenty-first century.[6] In New York, as in the rest of the United States, March 2020 marked a turning point. Once Americans began associating COVID-19 with Chinese people, anti-Asian violence spiked.

Lee's first encounter with hostility related to the virus came before that, in February, when she walked into a magazine store on Mulberry Street on her way to work. "I go there every morning," she told me. "But this day a Black woman working at a construction site comes and goes, 'Oh fuck, they're everywhere.' At first, I couldn't figure out what she was mumbling about, but then I realized: It was me!" She had picked the wrong target. "I started chasing her around the store, taking videos with my phone. She can't run away from me! I got the name of the construction company and I told them: I have video of being verbally assaulted by one of your workers. If she doesn't want to be around Asian people, she shouldn't be in Chinatown! Either you remove her from the site or I post this."

By the time she got to P.S. 42 that morning, Lee realized that the incident had implications beyond the one worker, or her own sense of outrage. She had to consider what it meant for the school community as well. "I told my family, and I told the other principals that I was just verbally assaulted here, at the newspaper stack! And here's my dilemma: How do I protect my Asian children—how do I protect my non-Asian children who happen to be with a group of Asian children—if they're out in the neighborhood? How do I keep my community safe?" She decided, for the first time in her career, to stop all school trips, everything that required transit or groups going far from the building. It was a big deal, Lee explained. Trips had always been a key part of the P.S. 42 experience. But the environment, even on the Lower East Side of New York City, felt toxic and unstable. If they went out there, Lee said, "I can't protect the human beings that are under my watch."

In the second week of March, school districts in other parts of the United States were coming to the same conclusion—not because of racist violence, but because they knew the virus was spreading quickly, and they feared that schools would become super-spreaders of the deadly disease. In Washington State, where, on January 21, the U.S. recorded its first COVID-19 case, the Northshore district shifted to online education for its 24,000 students on March 5. On March 12, the state's largest school district, Seattle, ordered all its public schools closed as well. It was not an easy decision, since local officials understood just how much local families depend on public schools, and that shutting them down would have ripple effects in every family, and throughout the city's economy, too. Perversely, it would also deepen inequality, in a city already riven between the haves and have-nots. "We know that closing our schools will impact our most vulnerable families and we recognize that working families depend on the consistency and predictability of supports and services our schools offer," the public affairs office wrote. But they determined that the closure was "an effective way to disrupt widespread infection," and, therefore, a "necessary action."[7]

New York officials had resisted school closures, even as cases in the city soared. As mayor, Bill de Blasio's greatest achievement was establishing universal access to pre-K for all New York City families, which he championed not only for its educational benefits but also for the way it improved lives of low-income, working parents. On March 12, the same day Seattle initiated its system-wide shutdown, de Blasio announced that New York City would do the opposite. "We are going to do our damnedest to keep the schools open," he stated. "It is where our children are safe in the day, and many parents have no alternative. It's where our kids—a lot of kids get their meals. It is the pivot for a lot of people we need to get to work that their kids have a place to be. A lot of them have no other choice."[8]

It only took a few more days for the city to recognize that this choice was not a real option. On Sunday, March 15, de Blasio conceded that keeping schools open was unsafe and untenable, and declared that they would begin shutting down the next day, remaining closed until at least April 20, perhaps later. "This is not something in a million years I could have imagined having to do," he said, in a press conference where one reporter described him as "visibly distraught."[9] School cafeterias would remain open for a few more days, so that the 700,000 children who relied on free or subsidized meals could continue getting them. After that, the mayor said, the city would find "alternative sites" for food service, but no one knew exactly where they would be or how it would work.

There was another thing for which no one could say how, or even whether, it would work: education. Beginning March 23, all students were expected to be taught remotely, at home, in conditions that were likely crowded and chaotic, by teachers who were also at home, many with their own children and family members, in similarly cramped and stressful states.

There were, of course, problems that everyone could anticipate: home internet access, for instance. In spring 2020, more than 500,000 city households lacked broadband connections, and relied entirely on cellular service to get online.[10] Naturally, families without wireless internet access were concentrated in the city's poorest neighborhoods, places where, even in the best of times, schools struggled to serve children well. Lee and her colleagues at P.S. 42 were committed to teaching their students, no matter the circumstances. But on the Lower East Side, nearly 40 percent of all households had no broadband service, laptops were scarce, and no one was stepping up to bridge the digital divide.[11] "We were in deep doo," Lee told me. "It was a hot mess."

In February, the U.S. Centers for Disease Control and Prevention (CDC) had warned school districts to prepare for the possibility of remote education, and the leaders of two major teachers' unions had called on the Trump administration to issue specific guidance for how schools should prepare for system-wide closures. "You should ask your children's schools about their plans for school dismissals or school closures," said Nancy Messonnier, a director at the Centers for Disease Control. "Ask about plans for teleschool."[12] But the federal government, as per the president's orders, insisted that COVID-19 was a problem for each state to handle on its own. Betsy DeVos, the secretary of education, offered so little help that, on March 10, more than twenty U.S. senators issued an open letter demanding answers to fourteen questions about what her agency was doing to help students and families affected by the pandemic.[13] She did not respond.

New York City's local government was more communicative than the U.S. Department of Education, but it, too, did little to prepare school leaders, teachers, and families for the shutdown. Richard Carranza, a champion of racial integration whom de Blasio had hired as the school system chancellor to push a social justice agenda, had been facing intense criticism from teachers and families since the outbreak penetrated the system.

Around March 7, Michael Mulgrew, president of the United Federation of Teachers, began pushing for the city to close all public schools because of concerns about faculty and community health. As Mulgrew saw it, each day of delay meant countless new cases, and each case amplified the risk of exponential spread. How much risk was uncertain, however, in part because the New York City Department of Education had been instructing schools not to report positive cases among staff members to the NYC Department of Health and Mental Hygiene, or even to teachers and families. An investigation of internal emails by *The City* uncovered "a pattern of Department of Education officials playing down the threat of COVID-19 in the days before the schools shuttered, during the week teachers were required to come in for training, and even after the start of remote learning."[14]

Lee didn't know about this pattern in the weeks before the shutdown. But she was certain that the closure was coming, and that if anyone was going to get her faculty and students ready for the crisis, it was her. Before she could take that on, however, she had to deal with a more immediate crisis. Lee's husband, a delivery driver, came home one day with a fever and shortness of breath. "It was horrible, scary. He never gets sick," she said. "Suddenly he couldn't breathe, couldn't taste, couldn't smell." The family moved him to a separate bedroom and kept him there, quarantined, for three weeks, leaving only to get him tested, and then carrying him back up to the room. "We fed him like he was an inmate," Lee recalled. "Slid his food under the door." At the time, there were no good treatments for COVID patients. In Manhattan, and everywhere else in the city, hospitals were turning into mortuaries. People with dire illness were avoiding them, for fear of dying alone in an intensive care unit. The most terrifying thing anyone could imagine was winding up in that situation. You didn't even want to think about it, but how could you avoid it? Miraculously, her husband recovered, and no one else in the family got sick. His return felt like a victory, like clearing a level of a video war game. A moment of optimism. A burst of relief. Then on to the next battle.

At school, that meant fighting to get her students equipped for the looming shutdown. Some people were talking about the need for new technology. Laptops. Tablets. An app called Zoom that Lee had never heard of, and another, Google Classroom, that sounded like a sick joke. As Lee saw it, the most important thing was to get her families the basic supplies that wealthier communities take for granted: Pencils. Crayons. Erasers. Books. Moreover, she wanted her kids to get hard copies of their lessons and assignments, and she instructed her staff to rush to the copy machines and printer banks, praying that the cursed machines wouldn't break. "We cranked out printing like you wouldn't believe," Lee recalled. "We made packets for each student to take home, and each kid got books from our library that they were told to keep." The NYC Department of Education allowed school staff to work in the school buildings during the first week of the shutdown, and nearly everyone on the P.S. 42 staff returned to help. By the time they finished, they had printed materials for about six weeks of instruction, and a bag for each student. "We set up a system where families could meet us in the yard and pick up the packets," Lee said. "A lot of families came, but a lot of families were too scared." This is where having a big house with children and other family members proved especially helpful. "They live very privileged lives," Lee explained. "And I told them the least they could do with that privilege was help me do some deliveries." When the school shutdown got extended (and extended, and extended again), that wound up becoming a bigger job than she anticipated.

The packets would not last forever. By late March, New York City's caseload and death counts were soaring, and it was hard to believe that schools would reopen in late April, or even in May and June. She recognized that public schools were unlikely to reopen for the remainder of the academic year, which meant everyone at P.S. 42 would need to get online, and stay there, for the next four months of classes. For $269 million, the city purchased 300,000 iPads, equipped with learning apps and an unlimited cellular data plan, and promised to deliver them, "on loan," to everyone in need. To get one, though, families would have to fill out paperwork attesting to their eligibility and sharing a mailing address with the system. This, Lee said, created a mini-crisis in her community. "The forms were in English and Spanish, so a lot of my families couldn't even read them. They didn't know what to do. This wasn't a micro-aggression. My God! It was a macro-aggression. I was furious. It was all a bunch of crap."

Lee assembled a team to fill out the forms for students who needed equipment. Even that proved difficult, and not only because of the language barrier. First, Lee discovered that several families were afraid of sharing their home address with the distributor, because they were undocumented, or because they were living in an illegal sublet, or because they feared they were ineligible and would be punished for cheating the system. Then her team figured out another problem: most of her families lived in apartment buildings with no one working the front door, and many refused to answer the buzzer for strangers. When delivery services came, they tended to leave packages in the entryway, unattended, and sometimes they simply left them on the landing outside. This compounded everyone's anxiety about borrowing an expensive machine from the city. What would happen if it got stolen? Would they have to cover the bill?

It took a few weeks, but eventually Lee and her team figured out a solution. They used Lee's address for every student whose family was nervous about putting their own on the application, and offered the phone number of the assistant principal in case the district or the delivery service had concerns about the request. The orders were not fulfilled in time to get every student a device for the spring term. Some kids disappeared. Others logged in occasionally, often using a parent's phone. But by the end of spring, Lee was deluged with iPads. "Hundreds of them," she said. Once again, Lee enlisted her children to help her deliver the goods. "That's how we spent the summer," she told me. "We'd organize a route and tell the families when we were coming. We'd ask them to come down about ten minutes before we were supposed to get there, or to look out the window if they had a doorbell. We'd spend the day delivering boxes. All the way to September, all summer long."

Getting the iPads delivered to her families was Lee's first technological challenge; teaching them to use it was next. P.S. 42 is an elementary school, which means the kids range in age from four to eleven, and only a handful had older siblings or parents who could figure out how to use the Remote Learning Portal, which featured software from companies like Google and Microsoft. Lee asked her teachers to schedule a video call with each family and guide them through the system. "We had to figure out which dialect each family spoke, and then make sure we had a teacher who could communicate with them," Lee explained. "Sometimes we'd walk to an apartment and the grandma would come down, with gloves on, so we could show her how it works." Then there were the routine problems: Slow connections. Kids who couldn't log on. Kids who weren't supervised. Kids who couldn't focus. Kids who wouldn't turn their cameras on. Kids who didn't show up.

Kids were not the only ones struggling with remote education. Teachers and staff were also having a hard time with the transition, sometimes because of technology, but more often because their homes weren't designed for classroom instruction, and certainly not for teaching when their own children were cooped up there, too. Many were coping with anxiety related to the pandemic, or with the virus itself. By early May, hundreds of city education workers had contracted COVID-19; at least seventy-four had died.[15] P.S. 42 had not lost any teachers, but many were unable to work and needed medical accommodations. Occasionally, they missed class, too. Lee could feel the turbulence in her community. To stabilize things, she decided to do a daily read-along for all the children, and she promised her families that she would be there, on the screen, every morning. "I did it every day from March to June," she told me. It quickly became sacred, a ritual consecrating her pact with the families. For a time, it was beautiful, Lee said. But eventually, she confessed, those extra hours in front of the screen became a burden. She was exhausted, stressed, sometimes sleepless. Human. "Maybe I'm being too honest, but it got horrible," she said, laughing at herself and the absurdity of the situation. "Like, I'm never doing that again!"

Other responsibilities felt more urgent. From the beginning of the shutdown, Lee had worried about how her children and their parents would stave off hunger. In ordinary times, the school offers two meals and a snack every weekday. What would happen when the cafeteria closed? How many parents would see their salaries disappear or diminish as the economy contracted?

Local officials shared her concerns. On March 23, the day New York City began remote education, the city opened 439 food hubs where families could pick up "grab and go" meals—breakfast, lunch, and dinner—five days a week.[16] At first, Lee told me, P.S. 42 was not included in the list of food hubs. "I went right to the Department of Education and said, 'How dare you?'" she remembered. "They pointed to another school where they were opening, and I was like, 'You don't understand. My families do not cross Allen Street. And a lot of my kids rely on grandparents, who can't walk all the way over there. What do you want them to do?'"

"It was a battle," Lee explained, and though that's unmistakable, it's hard not to notice that she takes pleasure in the tale, if not in the fight itself. After three decades of working in the public education system that educated her, and the rest of her family as well, Lee understands both how much it can deliver and how much it requires you to fight. She's good at it, always has been. As a P.S. 42 student, nearly fifty years ago, she didn't just graduate, she earned a place at Hunter College High School, the gem of the entire city system. Now, as a principal "at the end of my career," she wasn't going to let her families lose their access to school meals. "I put my foot down," she said, conveying just the slightest sense of accomplishment, a modest administrator's flex. "And now we're a feeding site."

It didn't take long to see that the feeding sites, which served approximately 560,000 meals across the city in the first week of remote classes, were woefully inadequate for the situation. The problem wasn't only that this number, vast as it is, represents only a fraction of the meals that schools serve poor children during ordinary times. It was also that poor students lived in families where everyone was at risk of going hungry. On what grounds could their parents, grandparents, and other members of their households be left out? As the pandemic progressed, the city expanded access to the food program, using federal and state emergency funds for the effort. P.S. 42 set up an adjacent space where anyone could pick up food, no questions asked. "The mornings are supposed to be for families, the afternoons for adults," Lee told me. "But I stopped them from questioning people. I mean, nobody waits on line for school lunch—which is pretty disgusting, right?—unless they're hungry. And there's a line every day."

As the weather warmed, and New York City enjoyed a sharp downturn in COVID cases, Lee found herself dealing with a different kind of backup. In August, both the governor and the mayor declared that public schools would be open in the fall, and roughly three quarters of those surveyed by the New York City system indicated their intent to return in-person, rather than online. "We're the only major school district in America, the only major urban district, planning for in-person classes this fall," de Blasio boasted.[17] But critics, including parents and educators, worried that the schools, with their outdated ventilation systems, small bathrooms, and crowded cafeterias, were not fit for a safe return. "I don't believe schools are ready and I've been very clear on that," said City Councilman Mark Treyger, a former teacher who chaired the city's education committee. "Schools do not have enough money, time or space to operationalize safety plans."

Lee was determined to get P.S. 42 ready for her staff and students. The problem was that neither the city nor the state was offering much help. "They just wanted to open," she complained. "They didn't give us time for anything, didn't give us any guidance. They were making these blanket announcements about the things we were going to do in the schools. How were we supposed to do all of them? We were all in the dark."

In Chinatown, Lee had bonded with the principals of three other schools and formed something like a support group. "We call ourselves the Joy Luck Club," she told me. "We talk all the time, and none of us were getting any guidance." The city had pledged that each classroom would have a new air filter, that all desks would be six feet apart, that teachers could do hybrid instruction. "It was all baloney," Lee said. "My building is over a hundred years old. I have no air filtration system. It's dusty. So I got my own air purifiers. I got my filters out of my own school budget. I bought each teacher a Plexiglass shield so they would be more comfortable teaching in person. All I know is we had to make it work. Every single principal had to figure it out on their own."

There was another thing that Lee had to figure out that August, something more personal and dire. Years before, doctors had found a precancerous growth on her left breast and told her to check in regularly. No one wanted to visit the doctor in 2020. (In the U.S., visits to physicians for both routine checkups and non-COVID emergency care plummeted during the pandemic.[18]) But Lee went anyway, and just before summer ended, she was diagnosed with Stage 2 breast cancer and prescribed a round of chemotherapy. "Thank God it was not Stage 3 or 4," she exclaimed. "I lost a good friend to Stage 4 colon cancer, and oh my God, it was fast."

The diagnosis and treatment protocol gave Lee a reason to remain at home that fall. She now had an underlying condition that made her more vulnerable to dangerous symptoms from Covid, and a lot of pain to endure as well. That's not how she saw it, though. "I mean, there were a few times when I couldn't go to school because of the timing," Lee explained. "But going into school was never an issue for me. I really feel safe in the building." Work, for Lee, is a vocation. She tells her teachers that they're all doing public service, but at a personal level, in her bones and tissues, going to school makes Lee feel better than anything else.

She got P.S. 42 ready to open in the fall of 2020, and about one third of her families signed up to send their students back on the first day of classes, September 11. The educators' unions were not yet on board, however, and Mayor de Blasio, facing the threat of a teachers strike due to concerns about occupational safety, pushed the start back ten days.[19] The academic year was rocky, with a fall surge forcing the city to shut down the system in November, and disruptions continuing throughout the winter and spring.

"I'm extremely optimistic," Lee told me when I asked about how P.S. 42 would fare as the city made another push to reopen. "Next fall I know we'll be here five days. I'm not worried, because at this point, I know that we could do anything." She paused, drew a breath, and flashed a defiant smile. "Bring it on."

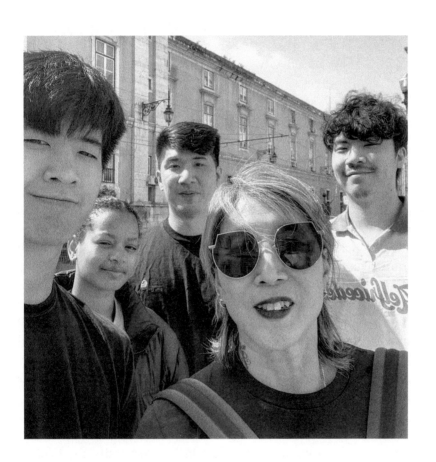

CHAPTER 2

Initial Response

We will never know exactly when the novel coronavirus SARS-CoV-2 spilled over into the human population, nor when the first person developed the disease we now call COVID-19. Some scientists claim that the initial case emerged in the province of Hubei, China, during November 2019.[1] Officials in Wuhan dated the first cases on December 8, 2019.[2] An influential paper in *Science* suggests that these patients did not develop COVID-19 until later in December, which would make the first diagnosed patient a female vendor at the Huanan Seafood Wholesale Market, where live mammals, reptiles, poultry, and fish are sold. Her illness began on December 10.[3]

What's clear, however, is that by the end of December, dozens of people in and around Wuhan had been diagnosed with a pneumonia of unknown origin. On December 30, the Wuhan Municipal Health Commission issued two internal notices to local hospitals, warning about a spike in respiratory illnesses that were apparently linked to the Huanan Market.[4] But the government's message was designed to hide as much as to reveal, since it contained an order that prohibited any member of the health system to disclose information about the disease without authorization.[5] The next day, December 31, the Chinese government informed the World Health Organization about a cluster of pneumonia cases, and on January 1, 2020, local officials closed the market, due to concerns that the virus was being transmitted from animals to people. As worrisome as that sounded, it was better than the alternative: that transmission was human-to-human, which would mean it might soon spread beyond anyone's control.

On January 5, 2020, the WHO published its first "Disease Outbreak News" item on the new virus. The article notes that there are "44 cases of pneumonia clustered in space and time," and that a "reported link to a wholesale fish and live animal market could indicate an exposure link to animals." The "WHO is closely monitoring the situation and is in close contact with national authorities in China," it explains. Based on current information, though, "WHO advises against the application of any travel or trade restrictions on China."[6]

On January 7, Chinese scientists traced the pneumonia to a novel coronavirus that was similar to but distinct from the viruses that produced an outbreak of severe acute respiratory syndrome, or SARS, in 2003, and Middle East Respiratory Syndrome, MERS, in 2012. On January 11, a consortium of researchers in China publicly shared the genetic sequence of COVID-19. "Scientists worried about China's lack of transparency about a month-old outbreak of pneumonia in the city of Wuhan breathed a sigh of relief today," an article in *Science* reported, quoting a tweet from Jeremy Farrar, head of the Wellcome Trust, in London: "Sharing of data good for public health."[7]

That same day, Wuhan authorities confirmed the first death from the virus, a sixty-one-year-old man who had frequented the Huanan Market. On January 13, Thailand announced that a visitor from Wuhan had been admitted to a local hospital with symptoms of COVID-19, the first recorded case outside of China. Japan confirmed its first case on January 16: a resident of Kanagawa Prefecture who had recently returned from Wuhan.[8] The first U.S. case, a thirty-five-year-old man in Snohomish County, Washington, was reported less than one week later, on January 20; as was the first case in South Korea (January 20) and Taiwan (January 21).[9] The following week, COVID-19 arrived in Australia and Canada (January 25), and by the end of the month it reached the United Kingdom as well.[10]

. . .

Once it left China, the SARS-CoV-2 coronavirus and COVID-19 arrived in different countries at roughly the same moment, yet the initial responses of nation-states—their reactions from January to April 2020—varied dramatically, in timing and in substance.[11] These variations mattered in ways that we've yet to account for, protecting or imperiling entire societies, and setting the context for the next several years. The immediate, if not reflexive, responses in different countries deserve attention not only because they influenced the course of the health crisis; they also illuminate something important about the character of particular states and societies. By looking closely at their distinctive ways of reacting to a common hazard, we learn how nations work, what their leaders value, and what kinds of challenges their citizens face. Both structural features of a government, such as the power of the president, and conjunctural factors, such as which person or party is in office when the threat appears, shape a government's approach to health emergencies. (The White House would surely have acted differently if Hillary Clinton had been president in 2020, yet Republican governors would likely have rejected federal guidelines and pursued their own policies, too.) But the way nation-states act in decisive moments, including when a pandemic begins, reveals what they are willing to do to protect life.

Didier Fassin, an eminent medical anthropologist at Princeton's Institute for Advanced Study, argues that the distinctive feature of the global reaction to COVID was "the primacy of the saving of lives over all other considerations." For the first time in history, states in every part of the world asked citizens to make extraordinary personal sacrifices so that people around them would be more likely to survive. "There was, first, a partial suspension of civil liberties and individual rights: freedom of movement, of meeting, of protest, sometimes of expression; the right to education, work, private life, asylum protection, intimacy with loved ones at the end of life, and honoring of the dead at funerals." Second, Fassin explains, there was "a temporary cessation of much of the economy, with predictable deleterious effects."[12] Small businesses collapsed. Jobs disappeared. Public debt soared.

Equities markets tanked. What justified asking the young to give up the fleeting pleasures of youth? What legitimated the assertion of power by government officials? Public health—and specifically the health of the oldest and most frail people in the community.

Public health has always been a hybrid and hotly contested field, constituted by scientists and medical workers whose approach to policymaking is largely driven by epidemiological research, and by political officials who often consider other factors, from economics to international relations, the lobbying efforts of influential industries and professional organizations, and naturally, their own popularity and status. The balance of power within a country's public health field varies over time, but is typically determined by the ideological commitments of the dominant political party, the priorities and interests of its leaders, and the relative strength of corporate firms (pharmaceuticals, for instance), labor unions, and scientific organizations in the nation's political system. During a crisis, the public health response is often shaped by those who have what a research team led by Harvard science studies scholar Sheila Jasanoff calls "epistemic authority"—i.e., "the knowledge and evidence used to make public decisions, and on what basis."[13]

There's another key factor that shapes national public health systems: whether they recognize and respect the public that they are set up to protect. Jasanoff and her collaborators call this the nature of the "social compact." Each nation has its own social compact, and some—as varying national rates of poverty, homelessness, and medical care suggest—offer citizens considerably more protection than others. In practice, nations have different social compacts with different groups of residents. They can be more or less generous to the old, more or less punitive to convicted criminals, more or less inclusive to immigrants, more or less discriminatory toward nondominant ethnic or racial groups. Public health systems generally turn on the answer to a few core questions: Do they guarantee health care as a human right or let the market allocate who has access? Do they make vital information available to scientists, doctors, and hospital administrators? How, and to what extent, do they inform citizens about risks, threats, and vulnerabilities? Do they encourage fact-based reporting and open debate or restrict it? Do they communicate what they know, what they don't know, and what they are learning? Do they care about earning their constituents' trust?

Trust is an especially difficult problem for public health agencies, partly because in the twenty-first century some areas of medical science have become the objects of fierce ideological battles, and partly because in some cases, including the emergence of a novel infectious disease, doctors and health officials may need to make consequential decisions without all the time or data, or data over time, that they would ideally want. During the first year of the pandemic, for example, public health experts issued a number of recommendations based on knowledge that turned out to be partial or incorrect, and then changed their advice. At first, some epidemiologists thought the coronavirus did not spread through the air. One infamous tweet, which the WHO put out on March 28, 2020, read: "FACT: #COVID19 is NOT airborne. The #coronavirus is mainly transmitted through droplets generated when an infected person coughs, sneezes or speaks."[14] Soon, they discovered that the virus was indeed carried by aerosols; their "FACT" was not even a fact. Initially, global and national health agencies said that masks were unnecessary for civilians; later, they called them essential. Reversals like these are all but inevitable when there's a new pathogen, because science is a competitive but collective effort to establish facts and develop theories, and scientific findings—which we sometimes refer to as "the truth"—evolve over time. Science advances through the discovery of errors, with corrections getting us closer to truth. The act of knowing, as the philosopher of science Gaston Bachelard argued, is never complete.[15]

It was common, in the pandemic, to hear journalists and officials distinguish between the actions of governments or societies that "believed in science" or were "anti-science." But this distinction mischaracterizes the situation. People who trust science when, for instance, they board an airplane, use a microwave oven, take Tylenol, or have knee surgery, may well be skeptical about the long-term safety of a new vaccine or the effectiveness of an antiviral medication. Some may well cite previous cases when a vaccine had unanticipated side effects, when a prescription drug did more harm than good, or when a supposedly disinterested medical researcher was being funded by a pharmaceutical company and failed to disclose it.

In the U.S. and Europe, a growing number of conservatives say they distrust "government scientists," especially when they advocate public health interventions, while a growing number of progressives distrust industry scientists, especially when they are touting a profitable new product.[16] "Science," moreover, is not a unified actor or institution that speaks with one voice. There are different fields within science, examining different problems, and sometimes their findings lead to suggestions that conflict. Consider the case of children's health and wellbeing. The science of disease prevention tells policymakers that closing schools during an infectious disease outbreak is an excellent way to protect students, families, and teachers. But the science of education and economic mobility tells policymakers that closing schools is dangerous, increasing the risk of learning loss and widening inequality, as poor children are left behind. Policy decisions involve trade-offs. During a pandemic, the stakes of those decisions are enormous.

Since the pandemic started, policy analysts have focused their attention on how the structure of nations' public health systems affected their responses. In some countries, including China, public health is centralized with a top-down authority that dictates policies and programs down to the local level. In others, such as the U.S., it's federalized, with local authorities allowed to make their own decisions on a range of policy issues. The disorganized, incoherent, and generally weak performance of the American public health system during the first year of the pandemic led some experts to extol the virtues of systems like China's, and ask if decentralization, or perhaps even democratic governance, is a liability when disaster strikes.[17] But as the Harvard political scientist Danielle Allen has noted, Australia and Germany also have federal systems that delegate control to local states, and both nations proved remarkably adept at handling COVID-19.[18] What's more, there are considerable downsides to strong centralized government planning—most notably, the monumental cost of getting things wrong. In China, for instance, the government was so confident about its capacity to control the outbreak with lockdowns and quarantines that it failed to develop alternative measures, particularly effective vaccines. This would prove disastrous as the virus evolved and the pandemic persisted far longer than authorities expected.

The variations in how nations initially responded to the threat of a highly infectious, potentially lethal disease cannot be explained by what were, in 2020, the prevailing ways of measuring "pandemic preparedness." Consider the Global Health Security Index (GHSI), "the first comprehensive assessment and benchmarking of health security and related capabilities across the 195 countries that make up the States Parties to the International Health Regulations." A collaborative project of the Nuclear Threat Initiative and the Johns Hopkins Center for Health Security, with funding from the Gates Foundation and an impressive panel of international experts offering advice, the GHSI was explicitly designed to measure national capacity to address "infectious disease outbreaks that can lead to international epidemics and pandemics."[19] In 2019, the highest rated nations in the index were the United States and the United Kingdom, ranked first and second, respectively. Sweden ranked seventh; South Korea ranked ninth; Germany, fourteenth; New Zealand, thirty-fifth; and China, fifty-first.

No one would rank national performance in the COVID-19 pandemic this way. The countries with the lowest mortality levels, including nations such as Taiwan, South Korea, New Zealand, and Australia, reacted swiftly, taking what the medical anthropologist Andrew Lakoff calls a vigilant, "precautionary" approach, based on careful monitoring, intense surveillance, and continuous reassessments of the unfolding crisis. "A principle of precaution in the face of an incalculable threat [like a new pathogen] enjoins against risk-taking," Lakoff argues. "It seeks to keep the dangerous event from occurring."[20]

Countries where the public health approach worked poorly used more risky or incoherent approaches, and in some cases they were reckless. The U.S. and Great Britain entered the pandemic with the highest rankings in the GHSI index, but both the U.S. and Great Britain wound up among the deadliest places to be in 2020 and 2021. President Donald Trump and Prime Minister Boris Johnson ignored the recommendations of established epidemiologists and public health leaders, choosing instead to take advice from behavioral economists and political advisers who prioritized keeping the economy "open." Both governments wound up adopting high-risk approaches to pandemic management, including the theoretically plausible but ultimately disastrous strategy of letting the virus circulate freely in (at least) younger and healthier populations, so that the society could reach "herd immunity." China's approach was altogether different. When the virus first emerged in Wuhan, the fate of the world was in its hands, and its reflexive response was to clench them into a fist, controlling and concealing as much as it could until the ill-fated plan collapsed.

Fassin rightly claims that the global response to COVID was inspired by "the recognition of life as a supreme good." But in some nations, life is more supreme than in others, and in most nations, some people's lives matter hardly at all. Rarely are the politics of public health as visible as they were in the first stages of the pandemic, and comparing the responses of two different sets of states and societies—the "Two Chinas," China and the Republic of China (Taiwan), and three of the largest countries in the "Anglosphere," Australia, the U.K., and the U.S.—is a powerful way to see how the value of life and the values of its leaders lash up when everything is at stake.[21]

CHINA

"The year 2020 opened with a piece of news about eight individuals being punished for spreading 'untruthful information,'" writes Guobin Yang, a Chinese American sociologist at the University of Pennsylvania and author of a scholarly book about the first months of the coronavirus outbreak, *The Wuhan Lockdown*.[22] One of the detained individuals was Dr. Li Wenliang, an ophthalmologist who used the internet to tell fellow doctors about cases of a pneumonia of unknown origin in Wuhan that resembled SARS. In a matter of weeks, Dr. Li would be dead from COVID-19, and soon after that he would become an international hero, a whistleblower who tried to warn the world about the dangerous new disease. At the beginning of 2020, however, he was an outlaw and a pariah, associated with bloggers and civilians who were accused of spreading rumors and fake news. According to the Xinhua News Agency, the official state press agency of the People's Republic of China, all of the pneumonia cases Li worried about could be traced to the Huanan Market in Wuhan. None had spread from human to human, and no medical workers had become infected.[23] The only way Li could return to work was by signing a confession admitting he had made false statements and disturbed the public order.[24]

The first six weeks of China's response to the new coronavirus involved a mad scramble to control information and maintain order, achieved through the suppression of medical reporting and the aggressive sanctioning of those, like Dr. Li, who wanted other health care providers to know. Independent analysts disagree about the extent to which Beijing was aware of the emerging health crisis in December 2019 and January 2020. An assessment by U.S. intelligence agencies reports that Wuhan officials hid information from national leaders for weeks, fearing the repercussions.[25]

Katherine Mason, an anthropologist at Brown University who has studied China's public health reforms after the SARS epidemic, argues that outside observers usually overestimate the Chinese government's capacity to obtain or disseminate vital information about medical situations. The nation's "fragmented authoritarianism" works because every official in the system feels pressure to please those above them, and there are countless reasons for health workers not to raise dire concerns about a problem that may not be real. "Transparency is hard, and transparency has costs," Mason writes. "Proper reporting . . . has very little benefit to the person at the local level and may have immediate repercussions for them personally and professionally because no low-level official wants their institution or city to be the source of a major outbreak."[26]

Mason's work helps to show that what looks like malfeasance by local officials is, in fact, a symptom of problems that saturate the Chinese political system. "China's failures in the early stages of the crisis, and in the overseas propaganda campaign it later mounted, were baked into the [Chinese Communist Party] system," a report from Australia's Lowy Institute concludes. "The entire system, beset with fear, uncertainty, cover-ups, bad faith, and indecision at multiple levels, misfired until the top tier finally realized the gravity of the situation. The result was that the virus spread beyond Wuhan, into the rest of the country, and then the world—further, and faster, than it ever should have."[27]

The decisions that Chinese leaders made had massive implications for everyone on the planet, and to this day, scientists wonder what might have happened had China handled things differently. Why was maintaining public order so important in Wuhan? Or in China more generally? Why censor doctors, scientists, and civilians who had good reason to raise concerns about a dangerous new infectious disease that, like all infectious diseases, would become harder to contain every day they delayed?

The answer is layered. At the level of international relations, there's a long-standing history of nations and people associated with them being stigmatized, punished, and cut off from the global economy once they're identified as the source of an infectious disease. One journalistic report recalls an illustrative case from fall 1994 when "a plague outbreak struck the Indian port city of Surat. Hysteria erupted, and countries quickly banned travel to India. Tourists abandoned their vacations. Airlines canceled flights. The United Arab Emirates banned Indian cargo, while Russia demanded quarantines on shipments."[28] In *Epidemics and Society*, Yale historian Frank Snowden explains that although the death toll was limited, just seven hundred cases and fifty-six deaths, news about the situation "unleashed an almost biblical exodus of hundreds of thousands of people from the industrial city" and "cost India an estimated $1.8 billion in lost trade and tourism." India is hardly the only country to pay dearly for its association with a contagious disease. Consider Zaire (now the Democratic Republic of the Congo), where international anxiety about Ebola hemorrhagic fever has undermined economic development and increased insecurity ever since the outbreak of 1995.

Snowden points to a headline in the Sydney, Australia, newspaper *The Daily Telegraph,* "Out of the Jungle a Monster Comes," as an example of the rhetoric that so often damages a place where a lethal pathogen originates, whipping up racist hatred and tarnishing an entire nation or region.[29]

Sometimes racism and prejudice lead to misattribution of a disease altogether. "In the early 1980s, the public was informed by health officials that AIDS had probably emerged from Haiti," writes the medical anthropologist Paul Farmer. "Result: more poverty, a yet steeper slope of inequality and vulnerability to disease, including AIDS. The label 'AIDS vector' was also damaging to the million or so Haitians living elsewhere in the Americas."[30]

In early 2020, international health and development agencies as well as nation-states worried that warnings about a "Chinese virus" could lead to costly travel and trade restrictions as well as ethnic and racial discrimination on a global scale. China, after all, had faced significant criticism for maintaining "wet markets," which sell live mammals, reptiles, poultry, and fish, despite the risk of introducing new pathogens such as SARS into the human population.[31] Government leaders could not help but fear that China would be held responsible, and that the economic consequences could be severe.

Factors specific to Wuhan and the Chinese national cultural economy were also important, as was the nature of the Chinese political system, in which local officials must always worry about mistakes that anger Beijing and jeopardize their careers. January is a special time for the city and the region. Wuhan, with a population of 11 million, is a major transit hub for China, and it is especially busy during the holiday season. Every January, the city hosts a series of large festivals and public gatherings in the weeks leading up to the most important national holiday, Lunar New Year. Corporations, universities, government agencies, and residential communities organize gala events and celebrations throughout the area. "A public announcement about an epidemic outbreak would halt all those festive activities," Yang writes, "and could potentially trigger chaos and public panic."[32] In 2020, Wuhan would also hold two major political congresses: one between January 6 and 10, and the other between Janu-

ary 11 and 17. Yang reports that local media are typically prohibited from negative coverage during the two congresses; their
mandate, which comes from Beijing through the local government and into the newsroom, is to sustain a tone of "positive
energy" and promote China's image of success. Local media outlets "made no mention of the epidemic" during this crucial time,
he argues, and instead Wuhan carried on as if nothing unusual
was happening—until January 23, that is, when the government
suddenly locked down the entire city.[33]

China's effort to block information about the virus was made
considerably easier by the United States government, which,
under President Trump's regime of "America First" policies, had
cut two thirds of staff on the CDC's infectious disease surveillance program in Beijing, and closed the Chinese bureaus of the
National Science Foundation and the United States Agency for
International Development, which had been helping to monitor
and respond to outbreaks.[34] On January 3, Robert Redfield, the
CDC director, contacted George Fu Gao, the head of the Chinese Center for Disease Control and Prevention, and offered to
send a team of American scientists. Gao said he was not authorized to approve the offer, and when the CDC made a formal
pitch to the Chinese national government, they were effectively
refused.[35] Meanwhile, the number of severe COVID-19 cases in
China rose rapidly, infecting health workers and others who had
spent no time in the Huanan Market. But China insisted that
there was no evidence of human-to-human transmission, and the
World Health Organization accepted this claim. On January 14,
the WHO tweeted: "Preliminary investigations conducted by
the Chinese authorities have found no clear evidence of human-
to-human transmission of the novel #coronavirus (2019-nCoV)
identified in #Wuhan, #China."[36]

China maintained this position until January 19, 2020, when
it issued a late-night announcement acknowledging a spike in new
cases that were definitively spread from person to person. President Xi Jinping, who had been silent during the first six weeks of
the outbreak, made his first public statement: "The recent outbreak of novel coronavirus pneumonia in Wuhan and other places
must be taken seriously. Party committees, governments and rel-

evant departments at all levels should put people's lives and health first."[37] Since this statement, China has insisted that protecting life and prioritizing health had always been its top priority, even in the initial weeks of the outbreak. By now, journalists and scholars have established the depth of this misrepresentation—even after January 19, since China allowed holiday celebrations in Wuhan and travel in and out of Hubei Province to continue for days after it publicly recognized that the coronavirus was transmitted from human to human.

Some scientists have attempted to calculate the human toll of China's attempts to suppress information about the new virus and its delayed public health response. Roughly five million residents of Wuhan traveled outside the city during January, mainly to other towns in Hubei Province but also to large cities in China and around the world.[38] According to a study published in *Nature:* "if interventions in China had been implemented one week, two weeks or three weeks earlier than they actually were, the number of cases of COVID-19 could have been reduced by 66% (IQR 50–82%), 86% (81–90%) or 95% (93–97%), respectively."[39] Such dramatic reductions in the first stage of the outbreak might have turned the global catastrophe into a far more manageable event.

If China's initial acts of denial and suppression failed the world, its subsequent national public health campaign—long lockdowns, extensive tracing, mask mandates, extensive quarantines and isolation, and the threat of severe punishment for anyone who violated the rules—prevented the spread of disease within the country when medical doctors did not know how to treat it, and protected countless lives. The costs of these efforts were considerable. First, they came at great expense to the quality of China's public life, and generated formidable social and psychological problems in people's private lives, too. Second, they failed to protect Chinese citizens from contracting severe disease when the coronavirus evolved and residents, desperate to return to the public realm but lacking access to effective vaccines, demanded release from their confinement. China's strategy postponed the crisis that hit so much of the world in 2020, but it could not stave off disaster altogether, as the world found out in 2022, when infections in China surged.

Even during 2020, scientists and officials in other nations found it impossible to judge just how well China had fared in the initial outbreak. The government had withheld vital information from international health agencies, foreign governments, and dissidents at home, leaving everyone unsure about the number of cases and fatalities it had experienced. Facing criticism about its response to the coronavirus, the Chinese government launched a new public relations campaign, "rebranding itself as the unequivocal leader in the global fight against the virus," as *The New York Times* reported, while "accusing countries like the United States and South Korea of acting sluggishly to contain the spread."[40] It was a hard sell for every nation dealing with the repercussions of China's early blunders, but it was particularly upsetting for its neighbors, whose proximity made disaster an especially urgent matter.

TAIWAN

Taiwan, officially the Republic of China, is a densely inhabited island nation of 23.5 million people that's separated from China by the roughly one-hundred-mile-wide Taiwan Strait and by a fiercely contested political decree. China considers Taiwan part of its sovereign territory, and there is ongoing tension around whether, if not when, it will attempt to reassert control. Taiwan's independence was on full display in January 2020. Not only did it hold a democratic election for president, as it had done regularly since 1996, in which it elected a female legal scholar, Tsai Ing-wen, to her second term in office; it also mounted a sweeping, aggressive, and highly publicized initial response to the threat of a new coronavirus, one that would soon rank among the world's most effective public health campaigns.

In fact, Taiwan's efforts began on December 31, 2019, the day that China first reported cases of a pneumonia of unknown origin to the WHO. That day, Taiwan's Central Epidemic Command

Center (CECC) held a press conference in which leaders publicly explained what they had learned about the virus spreading in Wuhan. Although they urged citizens "to refrain from sharing unsubstantiated information and hearsay,"[41] they did not issue a gag order or threaten to punish those who speculated about the risks. Instead, their press event effectively created a public sphere for processing the unfolding situation. So did their initial public health measure, screening passengers who arrived from Wuhan for symptoms of fever and pneumonia. Taiwan implemented this measure on December 31 as well, citing lessons learned from the SARS epidemic in 2003.[42]

Along with Singapore, Hong Kong, Vietnam, and Canada, Taiwan is one of several nation-states whose direct experience with the SARS epidemic triggered dramatic changes to the public health system, particularly its emergency infectious disease programs. In April 2003, when the WHO identified 3,947 probable cases and 229 deaths worldwide, Taiwan had only 29 suspected cases and no deaths. Initially, health officials believed they had successfully contained the crisis, but a new cluster that began in a Taipei hospital sparked a chain of transmission resulting in 684 cases and 81 deaths in less than six weeks.[43] Fortunately, SARS proved less contagious than scientists initially feared and never became a national or international catastrophe. But Taiwanese officials recognized that they had averted a disaster because of good luck, not good policy, and launched an ambitious project to shore up their national health infrastructure, communications strategies, and local response programs. They created the CECC, with a commander whose job involved coordinating the work of government agencies, private organizations, and civic actors; they opened the National Health Command Center in 2005, and began running regular drills based on simulations of SARS-like events.[44] Fifteen years later, on January 5, 2020, the CECC announced that all medical institutions should be on alert for illnesses related to what was likely a dangerous coronavirus, and public servants used immigration and customs records to alert everyone in Taiwan who had been in Wuhan in the prior two weeks to monitor themselves for symptoms.[45] It was the first time Taiwan's system was activated.

The cross-agency response ramped up quickly, forming a National Epidemic Prevention Team that integrated public and private sector institutions in a series of shared projects, from testing and tracing to the production of PPE.[46] Immediately, Taiwan increased the pace of mask production, using government funds and military personnel, and developed plans for mask rationing and distribution through local pharmacies.[47] On January 12, just one day after China released the full genomic sequence of the new coronavirus, Taiwan Centers for Disease Control announced they had created a rapid, reliable, four-hour test kit, and were quickly working to increase the scale and speed of their testing operation.[48] On January 21, Taiwan diagnosed its first case of COVID-19 in a woman who had just arrived from Wuhan, and, though not formally a party to the WHO, it immediately reported the case to the organization. By Lunar New Year, January 26, Taiwan had suspended all tour groups to China and issued a strict travel advisory for Hubei Province, a dramatic restriction of travel during the holiday period, and announced that it had issued a fine of NT$300,000 (almost $10,000 U.S.) to a resident who failed to report symptoms of illness after returning from Wuhan.[49] When, on January 28, health officials identified the first domestically transmitted case of COVID-19, the government warned that further restrictions, including school closures, were inevitable.[50]

As a democratic society, Taiwan could not impose such an imposing and ambitious public health campaign without cooperation from private corporations, local officials, civic groups, and members of minority political parties. None of this could be taken for granted. As the Brookings Institution has reported, Taiwan was struggling with low levels of public trust in the years before the pandemic, with political polarization fueled by disinformation campaigns online and the specter of Chinese aggression looming over the country.[51] In addition to its investments in public health and infectious disease management, Taiwan had appointed Audrey Tang as "digital minister" in 2018, and assigned her the job of building trust by making government decision-making more open and transparent. Tang implemented a variety of new programs, from livestreaming public forums and increasing opportunities for civic participation to real-time campaigns, staffed by "citizen hackers" and social media companies, to refute and combat disinformation before it gains wide circulation. These efforts did not eliminate "fake news" or ideological divisions, but they improved the situation and helped restore trust when the country needed it most.

Taiwan's initial response to COVID-19 was stunningly effective. Its close proximity and deep cultural and economic ties to China placed the nation at such great risk of a coronavirus outbreak that, in January 2020, when scientists at Johns Hopkins University modeled the spread of the new coronavirus, they ranked Taiwan second in "country importation risk."[52] One month after its first COVID-19 patient, however, Taiwan had just twenty-two cases, only five of which had been transmitted on the island.[53] Its case numbers and COVID-mortality rates remained among the world's lowest throughout the pandemic, showing, as an article in the *International Political Science Review* puts it, "how liberal democracies can control and counteract COVID-19 without resorting to authoritarian methods of containment."[54]

Like most countries, Taiwan was unable to control COVID forever. After months of maintaining zero community-spread cases, the country experienced a short but lethal outbreak during May and June 2021, with roughly fourteen thousand reported cases and seven hundred deaths.[55] The government responded quickly, requiring masks of everyone in public areas, quarantines for those exposed to the virus, and contact tracing for those who fell ill. Citizens complied with the mandates. The media endorsed them. By July, the nation had flattened the curve.

As of October 2021, according to reports from the British research group the Economics Observatory, Taiwan "ranked lowest in total number of COVID-19 cases and second lowest in deaths per 100,000 population among comparable OECD countries."[56] Taiwan remained at that level for the following year as well, and in February 2023, its overall Covid mortality rate, 72 per 100,000, was only slightly higher than the two most successful countries, Japan (56 per 100,000) and South Korea (66 per 100,000), and nearly five times lower than the U.S. (339 per 100,000).[57] Realism, it turns out, is a surprisingly powerful foundation for a policy response.

AUSTRALIA

Australia's initial response to COVID-19 was also marked by a high level of scientific realism—perhaps a surprisingly high level, given that, at the very moment that the outbreak began, its conservative government was downplaying the impact of global warming in a historic series of devastating bushfires. Prime Minister Scott Morrison had already earned his reputation as one of the world's most influential skeptics of climate science, casting doubt on widely accepted findings about the relationship between fossil fuel emissions and ecological risk and resisting the transition to renewable energy. In November 2019, his deputy prime minister, Michael McCormack, dismissed climate activists who insisted that warming trends were turning Australia into a tinder box as "inner-city raving lunatics."[58] On this global health issue, at least, the nation's political leadership showed little interest in governing based on science.

Infectious disease control was another matter. Like Taiwan, Australia had been shaken by the SARS epidemic of 2003. The country has deep connections to China's economy and culture, with more than one million Chinese-Australian residents and more than 1.4 million Chinese tourists arriving each year. Although it had only six probable SARS cases, Australia's health leaders understood this as an accident of fortune, and committed to act quickly and aggressively when the next pathogen arrived. It helped that the nation has a history of strong public health programs, including a universal health care system and a series of successful campaigns to curb dangerous behaviors, from bans on public smoking to gun control. Officials were prepared to impose strict policies to limit the spread of a new disease, and they believed Australian citizens would support them as well.

Despite its origins as a nation of outlaws and its reputation as a country of free-spirited libertarians, Australians embraced these reforms. "Our whole history is one of reliance on the state, heightened regulation and mass compliance," argues the *Sydney Morning Herald* columnist Waleed Aly. "So, we were the first nation to make seatbelts compulsory in cars. We're one of extremely few to make bicycle helmets compulsory. We were early adopters of

mandatory breath tests for motorists. . . . We might despise politicians, but we ultimately like government for the very simple
reason that the modern nation-state of Australia could never have
existed without it."[59]

Border control has always been a major concern in Australia, and on February 1, Prime Minister Morrison defied WHO
recommendations by establishing the nation's first travel ban,
this one for foreigners who had been on mainland China during the previous two weeks.[60] The ban would be extended until
it was expanded, in dramatic fashion, on March 19, when Morrison announced that Australia would close its borders to everyone except citizens, residents, and essential health workers.[61]
The travel restriction remained in place until February 21, 2022,
when vaccinated tourists were finally allowed to visit. The long
duration was not the only unusual feature of Australia's border
controls; at various times in the pandemic, Australia's six separate
states limited entry to nonresidents, lest they carry the virus from
one part of the country to another.

Australia is a federation, with a tradition of autonomy at the
local and state level and considerably less centralized power than
the governments of, say, China or Taiwan. During a pandemic,
federalism can be a strength or a liability, depending on how
states communicate, cooperate, and learn from each other, and
whether national leaders can effectively distribute resources and
coordinate a response.

When, in late February, Morrison declared that "we believe
the risk of a global pandemic is very much upon us," Australia's
national government acted decisively, warning of a crisis that
"could last up to ten months," force some 40 percent of workers
to stay home, cut the gross domestic product by 10 percent, and
require closures of schools and public spaces. Australia deployed
army personnel to a mask factory, where they helped ramp up
production, and enlisted 130 private companies to help manufacture PPE.[62] It invested in rapid COVID tests, quickly becoming a
global leader in identifying and isolating positive cases, and made
plans for tracing as well. But Australia's most important early
policy innovation was the creation, on March 13, of a National
Cabinet for managing the disease outbreak, made up of the prime

minister as well as the first ministers and chiefs from every state and territory. This body was unusual for Australia. Members of the National Cabinet belonged to different political parties and governed territories with unique population profiles, living conditions, and levels of exposure to the disease. The goal was to set up a space for genuine collaboration, where leaders could assess new data and scientific research, information that would help the country balance national policy priorities with local preferences and needs. There was a benefit to "broad consistency without uniformity," the University of Melbourne legal scholar Cheryl Saunders argued, because it "left room for innovation by particular states and territories, in the manner of testing, in ways of supporting health workers, in approaches to distance learning, and in supporting livelihoods, to take only a few examples."[63]

The National Cabinet met regularly during the pandemic, including three times in March 2020 alone. Crucially, its main source of advice and support was the Australian Health Protection Principal Committee (AHPPC), which was composed of the chief health officers from every state and territory, and chaired by the Australian chief medical officer. The AHPPC played a key role in shaping Australia's initial response to the coronavirus. Early border controls, along with mandatory quarantines for travelers and isolation for positive cases, limited the penetration of COVID-19. But by March 23, Australia had recorded two thousand cases and eight deaths, and the AHPCC recommended "a strong general statement be made by Governments on the need to limit all unnecessary personal interactions, for people to stay at home when not engaged in employment, necessary shopping or individual outdoor exercise."[64] More specific policy changes followed. Weddings were limited to five attendees, including the couple and officiant, and funerals were capped at ten. Beauty salons and restaurants in malls were closed altogether, and in-person dining in pubs and restaurants was prohibited. Most citizens were blocked from leaving the country. School closures, which were determined by state governments, became widespread.[65]

Some of the government's policies proved controversial. On March 26, with the nation's cases topping three thousand, Morrison deployed the Australian Defence Force to ensure compliance with isolation orders for all returning citizens, who were quarantined in otherwise unoccupied hotels.[66] Progressives who, on that day, condemned excessive use of the government's punitive hand, took comfort when Morrison approved a welfare supplement package that would nearly double some aid packages, as many Australians became unemployed or went on welfare for the first time in their lives.[67] By the end of the month, Australia had registered roughly 4,400 cases and nineteen confirmed COVID-19 deaths, but the numbers that captivated the world's attention concerned the rate of new infections. In Australia, the rate was already in decline, while the United States and the United Kingdom were enduring a terrifying spike in death and illness.[68]

Australia, an island apart, had flattened the curve. As in China, however, its success in the early stage of the pandemic proved more uneven than it appeared, and more politically controversial, too. At first, public criticism focused on concerns over excessive restrictions on mobility and civil liberties, particularly in the state of Victoria, where residents were subjected to extended and recurrent lockdowns. In August 2022, journalists uncovered an abuse of political power that caused a major scandal. During a period that began in 2020 and lasted more than a year, Prime Minister Morrison had quietly made himself the nation's second health minister, finance minister, resources minister, and home affairs minister, as well as its co-treasurer. It was, Morrison later explained, an effort to centralize authority and ensure that the government could act quickly and forcefully during the health emergency; it was also, critics charged, an unprecedented power grab that compromised Australia's democracy. Citizens were not the only ones infuriated by this violation of political norms; senior Australian officials, including several of the ministers who wound up sharing power with Morrison, had never been informed of the new arrangement.[69] The prime minister had contained COVID, but only, as his successor, Anthony Albanese, put it, by "trashing democracy," and his own coalition government's status as well. In May 2022, Australians voted his coalition out of power, and Morrison stepped down as leader.

UNITED KINGDOM

Being an island nation did nothing to protect the country that, on paper at least, looked so well prepared for the crisis: Great Britain. The British media paid little attention to the coronavirus during January 2020. The national government, led by Prime Minister Boris Johnson, was rushing to make final arrangements for Brexit, its formal departure from the European Union. Until that happened, on the last day of the month, everything else was a secondary concern. But news about the dangerous new infectious disease emerging from China made it into the occasional television or tabloid story, igniting bursts of xenophobia, some quite public. On January 21, Piers Morgan, cohost of the popular ITV program *Good Morning Britain*, shocked viewers by mocking the Chinese language, saying "ching chang cho jo!" during a broadcast.[70] The next week, *The Guardian* published an essay about the threatening atmosphere for Asians in the U.K. The author, a student in Manchester, had witnessed a man scramble to avoid him when he sat next to him on a bus, and overheard people on a train saying, "I wouldn't go to Chinatown if I were you, they have that disease."[71] England would not report its first two confirmed cases of COVID-19 until January 31. They were both Chinese nationals.

On February 3, health secretary Matt Hancock told the House of Commons that, despite its limited spread in England, new cases worldwide were "doubling every five days" and "will be with us for at least some months to come." He announced that the government had begun evacuating British citizens in Wuhan and flying them back to the U.K., and urged residents to take "simple steps to minimize the risks to themselves and their families," like washing their hands and using tissues. England would soon make a major push to advance vaccine development, but it was wary about imposing what epidemiologists call "nonpharmaceutical interventions," such as lockdowns and border closures. As for face masks, "we are not recommending them for people generally," Hancock said. "But, of course, it's a free country."[72]

Preserving freedom in the face of the surging virus was a clear priority for England, and it defined the nation's initial response. Cases ticked up slowly, to twenty-three on February 29, and British officials, led by Johnson, expressed confidence that the National Health Service, along with their pandemic preparedness plans, would allow the country to fend off the threat. In March, as cases spiked in Europe and nations on the Continent began shutting down schools, sporting events, restaurants, and bars, Johnson touted the virtues of keeping Britain open. "As things stand, I'm afraid it bears repeating that the best thing we can all do is wash our hands for 20 seconds with soap and water," he announced at a March 9 press conference, before subtly criticizing the European governments from which he had recently severed ties. "We must not do things which have no or limited medical benefit, nor things which could turn out to be counterproductive."[73]

Expressing skepticism about the effectiveness of restricting public gatherings, his government decided, instead, to "go it alone" with an experiment that involved urging vulnerable people to remain at home while exposing the general population to the virus. While nearly every other nation aimed to reduce the spread of the coronavirus, England's top health officials refused to make its decision-making process open or transparent. Instead, relying on advice from the Behavioural Insights Team (colloquially known as the "Nudge Unit"), a consulting firm that originated in the U.K.'s Cabinet Office and advocates the "wider use of experiments in government,"[74] it concocted a plan to achieve herd immunity by letting the country's business proceed as usual. The strategy was not exactly anti-science, insofar as it was guided by economists who believed they could tweak behavior with the right "choice architecture," thereby leading people to make healthier decisions about, for instance, when to stay home or how frequently to wash hands. But it was predicated on the rejection of policies advocated by public health scholars with expertise in infectious disease prevention. As *The New York Times* reported, it reflected "the hyper-rationalist self-image of a prime minister who has not always hewed so closely to scientists in the past, as when he occasionally trafficked in discredited theories about climate change." [75]

To epidemiologists, former health leaders, and members of the opposition Labour Party, it also reflected an arrogance of power and disdain for the public, who were not only left out of deliberations about how to handle the outbreak, but also not fully informed about the reasons why Johnson and his cabinet decided to "go it alone" with an unproven and risky tactic. Civic groups and political officials demanded that the government offer evidence that its unusual plan would protect British people, as did more than five hundred British behavioral scientists, in their "Open Letter to the UK Government Regarding COVID-19."[76] Instead, they got only a theory, and in practice it failed to work.

On March 16, Imperial College London released a study predicting that, if England continued with Johnson's herd immunity plan, as many as 510,000 Brits could die of COVID-19.[77] The report put pressure on the government to change its public health strategy, and soon the government began shifting its position, discouraging visits to pubs, restaurants, and theaters, and postponing nonurgent medical procedures. Despite a lack of official guidelines or mandates on physical distancing, nursing homes discouraged or banned visitors, some colleges shuttered, and countless private citizens self-isolated. Older people, who faced the greatest risk of death from COVID-19, complained that the government's advice was opaque and confusing. National news outlets reported rumors "that the government will soon tell people over 70 to isolate themselves for four months, either at home or in care facilities, 'under a wartime-style mobilization effort.'"[78] Some said British football matches would remain open to the public, others that they would soon stop playing altogether. The national government delayed and equivocated. Not until March 23 did Johnson reverse his policy, issuing a nationwide stay-at-home order except for trips for food or medicine, closing all nonessential shops, and prohibiting meetings of three or more.[79] The fantasy of remaining open and free while the rest of Europe shut down was officially dead.

In late March, as the number of new British cases and deaths were doubling every three days and the country became a global coronavirus hot spot, Johnson himself contracted the virus, as did Hancock, the health secretary, and Chris Whitty, England's chief medical officer.[80] Johnson's symptoms grew increasingly severe. He was hospitalized on April 5, and transferred to the intensive care unit the next day.[81] British residents, now skeptical that the government had been candid about the crisis, openly speculated that the prime minister was on his deathbed, that the situation was worse than officials acknowledged. Johnson recovered, but while he was in the hospital, the Office of National Statistics publicly released data showing that the government's "Coronavirus Dashboard" was likely underreporting COVID deaths "by a significant margin."[82] Distrust had become a political problem, and it was contributing to the public health disaster as well.

By the end of April, the cumulative death toll from COVID-19 in the United Kingdom was at least 26,700, making it the second-deadliest place in Europe, behind only Italy, where the surge came earlier and left the government less time to respond.[83] The British public health system's performance was so poor that the House of Commons asked the Health and Social Care and the Science and Technology Committees to conduct an extensive study of what went wrong. "The veil of ignorance through which the UK viewed the initial weeks of the pandemic was partly self-inflicted," their report, "Coronavirus: Lessons Learned to Date," concluded. "This slow and gradualist approach was not inadvertent, nor did it reflect bureaucratic delay or disagreement between ministers and their advisers." It was, instead, a "deliberate policy. . . . It is now clear that this was the wrong policy, and that it led to a higher initial death toll than would have resulted from a more emphatic early policy. In a pandemic spreading rapidly and exponentially, every week counted."[84] Boris Johnson's government had gambled with the lives of its citizens, and lost. Before long, Johnson would lose his office, too.

UNITED STATES

If loss was on the minds of President Donald Trump and his cabinet members in the beginning of 2020, it had nothing to do with the new coronavirus or America's public health. On December 18, 2019, the House of Representatives had voted to impeach Trump for abuse of power and obstruction of Congress, making him the fourth president in U.S. history to face the prospect of losing office. That would be decided by the U.S. Senate, where members of the House would present their case to remove him in a trial beginning January 16, 2020. In the meantime, Democrats warned that the White House had placed the entire country in jeopardy, and that the damage could be severe. "The president and his men plot on," said Adam Schiff, the U.S. representative from California who led the impeachment inquiry. "The danger persists. The risk is real. Our democracy is at peril."[85]

"SUCH ATROCIOUS LIES BY THE RADICAL LEFT, DO NOTHING DEMOCRATS," Trump tweeted, while the House was voting to impeach him. "THIS IS AN ASSAULT ON AMERICA."[86] His administration, feeling reasonably confident that the Republican-controlled Senate would acquit the president, prepared for battle in the court of public opinion, unaware—or at least unconcerned—about the threat that would soon arrive on another front.

On January 21, a man in his thirties who had recently returned from a visit to Wuhan tested positive for the novel coronavirus in Snohomish County, Washington, becoming the first confirmed case in the U.S. The next day, at the World Economic Forum, in Davos, Switzerland, Trump declared he had no fears about the public health risks to Americans. "We have it totally under control," he told an interviewer from the business television channel CNBC. "It's just one person coming in from China. . . . It's going to be just fine." He was equally certain about the reliability of information he was getting from China, dismissing a question about whether he believed Beijing "will tell the world everything we need to know." "I do, I do," Trump replied. "I have a great relationship with President Xi. We just signed what's probably the biggest deal ever made." CNBC dedicated just one minute of the long conversation to the coronavirus, but that was enough for it to discern that "Trump believes that President Xi Jinping and health officials there are going to continue to tell authorities around the world everything they need to know about the virus."[87] The American leader conveyed remarkable confidence, projecting an image of an invincible nation, a superpower with nothing to fear from a bug.

There was no shortage of public health expertise in the U.S. government. Dr. Anthony Fauci, who had served as director of the National Institute of Allergy and Infectious Diseases (NIAID) since 1984, had access to the administration—contingent on whether they liked his message; the same was true for Dr. Deborah Birx, who would later become the coordinator of the White House COVID-19 Response Team, and was more willing than Fauci to bend in the president's direction. On January 28, National Security Advisor Robert O'Brien told the president that the U.S. was more vulnerable than he was acknowledging. "This will be the biggest national security threat you face in your presidency," O'Brien said. "This is going to be the roughest thing you face."[88] Trump showed no signs of anxiety, and on February 5, he confirmed that there was nothing to fear from the U.S. Congress, either. That day, the Senate formally acquitted him, and the president emerged emboldened. Nothing could take him down. Days earlier, he had closed the border to most, but not all, foreigners traveling from China to the U.S., and the military was in the process of evacuating and quarantining hundreds of Americans who had been in China. The CDC released its own test kits for the coronavirus, and Trump believed that they would soon be available to any American who needed them—not that there would be more than a handful of cases anyway. "We have 12 cases—11 cases, and many of them are in good shape now," he said on February 10.[89]

At that time, Trump and key members of his administration were publicly insisting that the coronavirus was no more dangerous than the seasonal flu, and the crisis would soon disappear. According to the reporting by Bob Woodward, however, on February 7 the president privately told him that the very opposite was true. "You just breathe the air and that's how it's passed," he told the journalist, on a recorded phone call. "And so that's a very tricky one. That's a very delicate one. It's also more deadly than even your strenuous flus." Why, Woodward asked, was the White House hiding this vital information? "I wanted to always play it down," the president said. "I still like playing it down, because I don't want to create a panic."[90] In late February, Trump grew irate after Nancy Messonnier, the director of the National Center for Immunization and Respiratory Diseases at the CDC, told the press that "we expect we will see community spread in the United States. It's not a question of if this will happen, but when this will happen, and how many people in this country will have severe illnesses." The president repeatedly asked his aides to have her fired for refusing to spread misinformation; eventually, she would resign on her own.[91]

A cocktail of deception and magical thinking shaped America's public health strategy. Trump promoted the idea that warm weather would kill the coronavirus altogether: "By April, you know, in theory, when it gets a little warmer, it miraculously goes away."[92] The United States was in desperate need of a comprehensive, scientifically driven infectious disease plan. Instead, it got shepherded to fantasyland. It didn't help that, when the president organized a task force to lead the nation's emergency response, he refused to cede control to a public health expert or independent figure who could speak with autonomy and credibility. Instead, Trump appointed the person who, besides himself, was most invested in the success of his administration: the vice president, Mike Pence.

In his book about climate politics, *Down to Earth*, the late French sociologist Bruno Latour characterized the message that the United States sent to the world when Trump pulled it out of the Paris Climate Accord. "We Americans do not belong to the same earth as you. Yours may be threatened; ours won't be!"[93] It's a variation on the theme of American exceptionalism, although instead of advancing the myth that the U.S. is uniquely virtuous and blessed with democratic values, it portrays America as deluded, if not doomed, by its refusal to recognize just how deeply it's tethered to the world. In the looming ecological crisis, Latour argued, the U.S. has two options. It can either "acknowledge the extent" of the problem, "finally become realistic and lead the 'free world' away from the abyss, or it can plunge further into denial." On climate, it was clear, Trump and his supporters "have decided to keep America floating in dreamland a few years longer, so as to postpone coming down to earth."[94] They did the same in the coronavirus pandemic, and—quite unlike in climate change—the consequences were immediately apparent.

The numbers, as the world now knows, did not stay where Trump wanted. On the contrary, the American dreamland quickly turned into the pandemic's epicenter. It's impossible to know how many Americans developed COVID during the first weeks of the outbreak, largely because the test that the CDC developed proved faulty and unreliable, and the federal government refused to authorize the use of alternative tests in local laboratories. The problem was apparent by February 20, 2020, when an article in *Science* explained: "The World Health Organization (WHO) has shipped testing kits to 57 countries. China had five commercial tests on the market 1 month ago and can now do up to 1.6 million tests a week; South Korea has tested 65,000 people so far. The U.S. Centers for Disease Control and Prevention (CDC), in contrast, has done only 459 tests since the epidemic began."[95] The *Science* article was prescient. Within weeks of the first American COVID-19 cases, it was already clear that the country experts had just ranked first for "pandemic preparedness" was, in fact, unable to achieve the most basic public health challenge: diagnosing the disease. The story contained only one significant error, the headline: "The United States Badly Bungled Coronavirus Testing— But Things May Soon Improve." They most certainly did not.

By mid-March, the U.S. did not need widely available COVID tests to know that the coronavirus was spreading exponentially. The country was barreling into a full-blown catastrophe, and the health system in its greatest metropolis, New York City, was on the verge of collapse. There, the most urgent problem was the lack of PPE for medical workers and lifesaving equipment, such as ventilators, for patients. The shortages were confounding. The U.S., after all, is an economic giant, with unmatched purchasing power and strong industrial capacity as well. One of the federal government's most important powers is the ability to command resources in a national emergency, and when the outbreak began, governors and health leaders throughout the country called on the administration to take over procurement and distribution. Trump rejected the request.

At a White House briefing on March 19, Trump said: "The federal government's not supposed to be out there buying vast amounts of items and then shipping. You know, we're not a shipping clerk."[96] He refused to invoke the Defense Production Act to ramp up production, on grounds that "we hope we're not going to need it."[97] But hospitals in the most hard-hit parts of the country did, urgently. Medical workers lacked face masks, surgical gowns, and gloves, and American medical institutions, which had long relied on Chinese producers for PPE, had no way to procure them. Images of nurses wearing garbage bags in a Manhattan hospital circulated widely on social media, prompting commentators to note that the world's most powerful nation looked more like a Banana Republic.[98] The White House had not merely left governors and local health officials to fend for themselves; it effectively turned them into competitors in a high-stakes auction for basic medical resources. When plague-ridden states hit the open market to purchase PPE, sellers reacted just as the cruel logic of supply and demand dictated, by driving up the price.[99]

From his first days in office, Trump had used the price of another essential American commodity—equities in the financial market—as a barometer of his performance. There are, of course, good reasons for a government leader to focus on the economy during an unstable time; a sustained market crash can do major damage to a nation's health and welfare, leading to hunger, unemployment, and insecurity on many levels. But Wall Street is not the economy, and the administration's fixation on stock prices during the first stage of the coronavirus outbreak struck policy analysts as odd and worrisome, since it signaled that the White House was more concerned about keeping the S&P 500 numbers up than about keeping the number of COVID cases down. On February 24, after the market dropped 3.5 percent, the president blamed Democrats for scaring the public, tweeting, "Stock Market starting to look very good to me!" The next day, his chief economic adviser, Larry Kudlow, made the rounds on cable news programs to amplify this message. "The virus story is not going to last forever," he declared, weeks before the first surge had begun. "To me, if you are an investor out there and you have a long-term point of view, I would suggest very seriously taking a look at the market; the stock market, that is a lot cheaper than it was a week or two ago."[100]

Such boosterism did little to lift the markets, and it didn't improve Americans' confidence or security, either. Case numbers continued rising; the markets grew more jittery. On March 9, the Dow Jones Industrial Average (DJIA) dropped some 2,000 points, or 8 percent of its value, and analysts immediately named it Black Monday. From there, the market became a roller coaster, surging and crashing at an unnerving rate. March 12, or Black Thursday, delivered a 2,300-point drop in the DJIA, losing 10 percent of its value.[101] On March 13, Trump declared a national state of emergency, which triggered the release of some $50 billion in funds for public health efforts and relief.[102] Two days later, the CDC advised against gatherings of more than fifty people, and the day after that it recommended limited gatherings to no more than ten. Trump began to refer to himself as a "wartime president." On March 16, the White House issued guidelines for Americans to follow—working remotely, avoiding unnecessary travel and social gatherings, practicing good hygiene, and staying home if you're sick or frail—during a fifteen-day campaign to "Slow the Spread."[103] The DJIA average fell 2,997 points, its steepest single-day drop in history (and greatest, in percentage terms, since the crash of 1987), amid fears that more extensive shutdowns were inevitable, and might last far longer than fifteen days.[104] On March 25, with the economy tanking, Congress approved a $2 trillion coronavirus stimulus package, including small business loans, direct deposits of just over $1,000 to almost all taxpayers with incomes below $100,000, and a $500 billion corporate bailout fund.[105] The president signed the bill into law on March 27.

March was also the time when states began to issue their own stay-at-home and shutdown orders: California on March 19 and New York on March 22, with the "New York on Pause" policy requiring all schools to close, all "non-essential workers" to stay home, and all public events and gatherings to be canceled. By March 23, nine states were under full stay-at-home orders.[106] In America's federal system, the president lacks authority to prevent these measures, but that didn't stop Trump from tweeting his disappointment about the wave of public health measures: "WE CANNOT LET THE CURE BE WORSE THAN

THE PROBLEM ITSELF."[107] Several conservative governors amplified this message, and some adamantly refused to mandate restrictions on economic or social activities in their own states. In Florida, beaches, hotels, bars, and restaurants were booming with Spring Break festivities.[108] In South Dakota, Governor Kristi Noem mocked leaders of other states for their "herd mentality" and denied calls to close businesses, schools, or churches. Individuals, she insisted, should "exercise their right to work, to worship and to play. Or to even stay at home."[109]

On March 26, the U.S. became the country with the highest confirmed number of coronavirus infections, despite the fact that tests remained hard to procure, and New York, the epicenter of COVID mortality, recorded one hundred Covid deaths that day. On March 27, facing a shortage of hospital beds, New York converted the massive Jacob K. Javits Convention Center in Manhattan into an emergency medical center. Three days later, the USNS *Comfort*, a navy medical ship, docked on the Hudson River after being deployed to Manhattan for the first time since September 11, 2001. The federal government sent refrigerated trucks to hospitals throughout New York City, because the morgues were filled to capacity, and in some cases, beyond. Researchers at Johns Hopkins University reported that at least 4,476 Americans had died already. With more than 200,000 positive cases, and the virus spreading exponentially, the U.S. was on track to lead the world in COVID-19 cases and deaths.[110]

The White House conveyed its deep displeasure about this situation. But its public statements expressed more concern about the impact of strict public health measures than about the nation's unmatched death toll. On March 24, at a Fox News town hall, Trump announced that he wanted the U.S. "opened up and just raring to go by Easter," April 12. As he saw it, it was to be a day of celebration, a resurrection of America's dreams. "You'll have packed churches all over our country. I think it would be a beautiful time."[111]

The week after Easter, the president denounced state governments that insisted on maintaining pandemic restrictions. On April 17, he called for political leaders to do the very opposite of what public health leaders advised. "LIBERATE MINNE-

SOTA." "LIBERATE MICHIGAN." "LIBERATE VIRGINIA," he tweeted.[112] Soon, Republican governors in Arizona, Florida, and Texas reopened businesses and loosened stay-at-home guidelines. Some states lifted mask mandates, and prohibited municipal governments from imposing them on their own. The Trump administration insisted that the pandemic was ending, even as new cases surged in states that followed its recommendations. In June, Mike Pence used his position as chair of the President's Coronavirus Task Force to assure Americans that the White House had defeated the invisible enemy and restored the nation's security. "There Isn't a Coronavirus 'Second Wave,'" he wrote, on the opinion pages of *The Wall Street Journal*. "We are winning the fight."[113]

CHAPTER 3

"Twenty-Four Hours a Day"

SOPHIA ZAYAS

She can still hear the sirens.

The ambulances are no longer a constant presence, as they were in March and April. But she hears them, even when it's silent, when she closes her eyes and tries to forget everything that happened, when she gets in her car and drives home from Manhattan at the end of the day, when her grandmother is in the living room of the apartment they share, blasting the TV volume, which is pretty much whenever she is home.

Sophia Zayas was thirty-five when the pandemic started, in the best job she'd ever had. A former beauty queen, with long black hair, caramel skin, and kind brown eyes, she was two years into a position as the Bronx regional representative for Governor Andrew Cuomo. The role suited her perfectly. Zayas, who's Puerto Rican and bilingual, grew up in the Bronx and still lives in her childhood home in West Farms Village, a housing complex near the Cross Bronx Expressway, with 526 units packed into a set of hulking six-story brick buildings and two twenty-one-floor towers. She's an extrovert, generous with her laughter, always searching for points of agreement, making connections even in divisive times. She's a believer, not shy about quoting scripture, and convinced she can help. She's spent her life surrounded by opportunities to do so.

Her neighborhood, West Farms, is highly segregated, with a population that's 91 percent Black and Hispanic (with a large group of Puerto Ricans who identify as both), concentrated poverty, crowded housing, heavy air pollution, high rates of obesity and diabetes, low life expectancy, and crime levels that rank among the worst in New York City. But walk through the neighborhood with Zayas, feel the warmth of the old-timers, the energy on the playground, the camaraderie in the parks and bodegas, and you can see why Zayas is a local booster. "I'm proud to be from the Bronx," she told me. "It's got its ups and downs just like every other area."

One of the downs, Zayas complained, is that people in the Bronx don't seem to matter as much as those in other parts of the city. It's like their humanity doesn't fully register, their problems don't count. At the beginning of 2020, Zayas was focused on that very problem, trying to get everyone in the borough to fill out the decennial census, the one that determines whether the district would get the public resources and political representation it deserved. The work was more challenging than she had anticipated. "A lot of people here, they just don't trust the government," she explained. "They're like: 'They never do anything good for us. Why should we even bother?'" The 2020 Census would be particularly difficult. Under President Donald Trump, the White House was acting like it wanted people in places like the Bronx to go uncounted. The Trump administration had tried to insert a question about citizenship status on the census, which would surely keep undocumented immigrants from completing the form. The Supreme Court blocked the question, but not the fears about what could happen once the government found you. When Zayas canvassed the toughest parts of the borough, she kept meeting people who felt damned no matter what.

Zayas has more faith in the world, and even in the system, but not because she came from privilege. Her mother died of massive heart failure at age twenty, just eight months after giving birth to Zayas. Her father, who had a son with her mother and two daughters with another woman, also had a penchant for getting in trouble. "When my mom died, he didn't man up. He just wasn't there. He went to a maximum-security penitentiary. Robbery.

Drugs. I don't even know. He was just always locked up, and he died before I was twenty." Zayas's grandparents, whom she sometimes refers to as her mom and dad, raised her father in West Farms during some of the neighborhood's roughest years, and the period when she and her brother were growing up wasn't much better. The public schools were poor, with high dropout rates and occasional outbursts of violence that put families on edge. Her aunt and uncle helped her get a scholarship at a local Catholic school, St. Thomas Aquinas, which had often been generous to kids in the neighborhood. As Zayas saw things, sometimes you just need to know who to talk to; doors open if you push them the right way.

Zayas graduated from a local public school, and surprised everyone by signing up for the Marines. "I was just like, I can do this," she told me. Zayas had always been thin and delicate, but she was strong in ways few people recognized, and now she could prove it. "I was so ready. You could give me a barbell and I would pull myself up. But then my father died and I got worried about my grandmother. So instead of enlisting I wound up going to Hostos Community College, in the Bronx. I studied photography and I loved it. But my grandmother said I had to do something else because there were no jobs in it." She transferred to Hunter College, where she got involved in politics as well as pageantry, one of which proved more brutish. "I did Miss Puerto Rico, New York. National level! But those women were catty. They'll do whatever it takes to win. One poured baby oil on my dress!" It was too much for Zayas. She put away her evening gowns and pursued politics instead.

"My first job was with the New York City Council. I was working for Joel Rivera, the majority leader from the Bronx. I really liked the public affairs part of it. Engaging the community. Helping people out. Elected officials are so busy, they have to ignore people. But I like to do things for people." She recalled a time when an administrator at St. Barnabas Hospital, a nonprofit institution that serves a primarily low-income population, kept calling the office. "Her name was Arlene, and she was like, 'I need a meeting with Joel! We're in a crisis. We need funding or we are in trouble!'" But it was the Bronx, and Zayas's older colleagues told her to get used to it. Everyone's in a crisis, everyone needs funds. "One day Joel came into the office. I'm at my desk, and she calls again. I said, 'Hold on, we're going to end this right here.' I put her on hold and transferred the call to his office. I walked in there and I answered the phone myself! I handed it to him. He was like, 'Fine, I will take five minutes with her.' And they ended up getting like, millions of dollars. They kept the hospital going, kept it open." Zayas doesn't take credit for it, but she'll never forget how good it felt.

Her next job was at a big Bronx hospital, Montefiore, the academic medical center for the Albert Einstein College of Medicine. She worked there for five years, moving up the ranks from executive assistant to supervisor of a house call program, and earning enough money to get a place of her own. But the job ended suddenly and acrimoniously, after a conflict with a director whom she accused of being abusive. "It was a horrible time," she remembered. "No one would hire me. They kept saying I was overqualified. I lost my apartment. My car got repossessed. I was on unemployment, and then that got cut off because you only get it for six months." She moved back in with her grandparents, feeling defeated. "I was in trouble," she told me. "I was trying to hold on, but I was in such bad shape."

Jobless, living at home, and ashamed of her situation, Zayas spent days wandering aimlessly, steeping in distress. "One day when I was walking, I remembered Arlene from St. Barnabas. After I helped her, she had said that I should call if I ever need anything, and I did. She picked up and I started crying, just cried and cried. And she said, 'I want you to come here and go to Human Resources. We're going to get you a temporary job and I will help from there. I'll get you something more, too.' That was a Tuesday. I swear, I went in for my first day on Friday. I worked at St. Barnabas for two years."

The money was okay, but Zayas decided not to get her own place again. Her grandfather had moved into a building for seniors, just across the street, and she didn't want her grandmother to be alone. She left the hospital because she wanted to get back into public service, and a friend tipped her off about a job running the New York City office for the Democratic Assembly Campaign Committee. Not long after she took it, a friend who had modeled with her called and asked if she was looking for a new job. "I said no, and she said, 'Are you looking for a better job? The governor needs a community representative in the Bronx. They're looking for a Latina, someone bilingual. You'd be perfect. You speak Spanish. You know everyone.'" She did. She was. Days later, Zayas had the job.

Community representatives are the faces of state government, the people who attend local meetings, who listen to constituents, who nod, shake hands, promise to tell the governor what you need. "We're lobbying for our regions," is how Zayas put it. "We meet with elected officials, with community stakeholders, business leaders, principals, hospital directors." If Zayas knew everyone in her neighborhood before she took the job, within a few months she knew all of the Bronx. "Everyone has my phone number. My work number, my personal number, I just gave them out," she reported. "That's basically the way you do this job. You're just always available. You show up."

"The job was tough before COVID," Zayas told me. "The Bronx is always the forgotten borough, on so many levels. Sanitation. When a snowstorm hits. Health disparities. So here we have to work double." When the virus arrived, she would work even more.

"Early on, no one knew what was going on," she recalled. "It was scary." On March 1, 2020, the city registered its first positive COVID case, a thirty-nine-year-old health care worker who had just traveled home to New York from Iran. The next day, Governor Cuomo and Mayor de Blasio appeared together for a press briefing at the governor's Manhattan office. Zayas, who helped prepare the room for the meeting, said that she and her colleagues were overwhelmed by the number of people who showed up. "We had to move chairs so everyone could fit." Cuomo spoke first, and he insisted that the threat was minimal. "Once you know the facts, once you know the reality, it is reassuring and we should relax because that's what is dictated by the reality of the situation. I get the emotion, I understand it, I understand the anxiety. I'm a native-born New Yorker, we live with anxiety. But the facts don't back it up here." He was especially confident about New York's capacity to contain the virus. "We have the best healthcare system in the world here. And excuse our arrogance as New Yorkers, I speak for the mayor also on this one, we think we have the best healthcare system on the planet right here in New York. So, when you're saying what happened in other countries vs. what happened here, we don't even think it's going to be as bad as it was in other countries. We are fully coordinated, we are fully mobilized, this is all about mobilization of a public health system."[1]

Zayas had always admired and respected the governor, but she couldn't help but worry. Fully coordinated? The governor and the mayor had long been rivals, sometimes even adversaries. American mayors may look powerful, but governors can override their decisions on almost every major policy issue, including health, transit, and schools. Since de Blasio took office, in 2014, Cuomo seemed intent on undermining his authority, blocking his attempts to curb the growth of car services like Uber and impose a tax on millionaires, shutting down the subway in a blizzard without notifying the city of his plan.[2] It was great to see their show of unity in the press room, but Zayas and her colleagues wondered how far beneath the surface it went.

As for the best health care system on the planet, well, Zayas couldn't say that about the Bronx. The borough had great hospitals—some, like Montefiore, large; others, like St. Barnabas, relatively small—and she had seen them save the lives of family members and friends. But most caregivers struggled to meet local needs during ordinary times, let alone crises. Zayas wasn't the only one concerned that they might not have enough resources for the trouble ahead.

No one was more alarmed than the people responsible for managing the Bronx's medical system. In March, as the number of new COVID cases rose steadily, hospital presidents began calling Zayas regularly, begging for help. "At first they needed the most basic things, like PPE"—face masks, gloves, and surgical gowns. Then the requests got more complicated. COVID tests were hard to come by. Ventilators, which could keep people alive, were even more scarce. Hospital beds filled up so quickly that no one knew where to put new patients. "Montefiore Hospital is the biggest institution in the Bronx," Zayas said. "It was a war zone. The ER was full. There was no capacity on the admitting floors. The isolation units were filled up. They started opening up parts of the hospital where they were doing construction." Soon after, the president of a smaller hospital called her, on the verge of tears. "His chief of surgery had died. His morgue was at capacity. They had bodies everywhere. They didn't know what to do."

"I felt helpless," Zayas told me. "It was painful to feel like I couldn't do anything. There were times when I would break down and cry." By mid-March, both her personal and work phones were ringing every few minutes. Her voicemail box filled to capacity, leaving her core constituents as well as old friends feeling ignored. Her office went remote a few days after the joint press conference with the governor and the mayor. Zayas was relieved not to be taking the subway to and from Manhattan, but working from home created new challenges. One problem was that her apartment is situated in the crossroads of the major Bronx hospitals. "There were ambulances going by my window every two minutes," she reported. "Depending on the direction, I knew which hospital they were going to. I could tell from the way the sound carried. And every time I heard the sirens, I could feel this wave of nerves go through my body. I knew it was another death. It was the most traumatizing thing that I've ever been through. I ordered earplugs on Amazon because I didn't want to hear it again."

Earplugs couldn't protect her family or neighbors from the virus, however. Zayas's sister had a job as a health aide in a local public school, but when cases began to spike she got reassigned to a hospital. "They didn't have a mask for her. They didn't have PPE." Within days, she had developed a dangerously high fever, then her husband and two children, ages five and nine, got sick, too. "She tested positive on March 15," Zayas remembered. "They all tested positive, each and every one of them. My sister felt awful. She could hardly breathe. And she was FaceTiming me saying, 'Sophia, I don't want to die!'"

By then, both Zayas and her sister were afraid of the hospital. It seemed like everyone who got admitted for COVID wound up dying there. As they saw it, the best survival strategy was to stay at home. Zayas got on the internet and looked up holistic remedies. "Vitamins. Steam baths. Eucalyptus. Lung exercises. I got her doing all those things," she recounted. "And I was just praying, praying. I was like, is this really happening? Like, when is this nightmare over?"

Zayas's sister began to recover. Next door, though, things were even more frightening. Luis, fifty-nine years old with asthma and hypertension, had lived in the apartment since he moved there from Puerto Rico in 1995, along with his wife, Miriam, and their daughter, Mylischka. Luis had been close to Zayas's father, and the two families spent so much time together that they considered themselves relatives. Luis had served in the military, but he had been on disability for decades. "My dad knew a lot of people in the neighborhood," Mylischka told me. "But he didn't hang out or anything, it was just a hi-and-bye thing. He was more at home with us, reading the Bible, watching action movies, the Food Network, cooking. His favorite thing was making lasagna, fully loaded, with meat and cheese." There was always enough for Zayas and her grandmother, too.

Zayas worried about almost everyone when the pandemic started, but Luis and Miriam seemed like they were protected, because they rarely went out. One day in late March, Luis went to the grocery store, and when he came home, he said someone sneezed on him—the guy hadn't even covered his mouth. A few days later, Luis started coughing. Naturally, Miriam and Mylischka were nervous, but they figured it was asthma or bronchitis. Nothing serious. Then he developed a fever, and the doctor told them to get a COVID test, just to be safe. "Three days later, the doctor called and told us he had COVID," Mylischka explained. At that point, Miriam was also feverish and coughing. She got tested, and it came back positive, too. The couple quarantined together in their bedroom, with Mylischka taking care of them, until the morning when Luis woke up feeling disoriented and struggling to breathe. She called an ambulance, and within minutes they were carting him away.

Miriam tried to get in the ambulance with her husband, but the paramedics said she couldn't go into the hospital, so she and Mylischka put Luis's mobile phone in his pocket and went back inside. The separation was torturous, the silence was worse. On television, they had seen video footage of the crowded hospital wards, heard stories about people lying on gurneys in corridors, waiting for attention from nurses and doctors. It was a dark, terrifying universe, and now Luis had been carried into it. There was no way to visit or track his situation. All they could do was hope he'd call again or pick up the phone.

Luis called when he got there and once again a few hours later, to report that he would soon be intubated and unable to speak. That didn't sound good, but in March 2020, no one really knew what worked and what didn't. At that point, Mylischka said, "We just kept calling the hospital, speaking to the doctors. I would call like three or four times a day. In the morning and at night, and sometimes even like three in the morning, if I was still up." For two days, the doctors reported that Luis was steady. They were monitoring his oxygen levels, experimenting with different medications, hoping something broke in his favor. "Then one night I called around twelve and they told me he was stable," Mylischka remembered. A few hours later, the hospital informed them that Luis was dead.

Zayas recalled hearing her friends crying and screaming in the apartment next door, their grief compounded by isolation. "You couldn't even console them," she told me. "You couldn't hug them. It was, like, trauma on so many levels."

Luis's death pierced through the professional armor that had protected Zayas during the first days of the pandemic; it filled her with anxiety and pain. "That's when it really hit me, that's when I crashed. I cried for nights. I felt like everything was closing in on me. I'd look outside and everything was dark. I didn't want to do anything. I didn't want to get on a phone call. I didn't want to deal with anybody." Her grandmother's insistence on watching TV news all day didn't help things. Nor did her "old-school" approach to stress. "She's eighty-four and she's tough," Zayas said. "She doesn't believe in anxiety. To her, mental health doesn't exist."

It was hard to deny the despair of Mylischka and Miriam. They were not merely barred from the hospital; they were quarantined at home because of Miriam's COVID, which was getting worse by the day. She had a cough, a fever, headaches, body aches, fatigue like she had never experienced. Her lips burned. She couldn't taste food. And neither she nor her daughter could keep from wondering what had really happened to Luis when he was in the hospital. Could someone have saved him? Was he completely alone when he died? "Thousands of families in New York State were asking those questions," Zayas explained. "There will always be a question mark."

Zayas, who spent the entire month of March working like a soldier on the front lines, was desperate for a break in the action, if not an escape. Instead, the cases surged higher, the demands from her constituents grew more frequent and dire. "I was getting thirty calls a minute," she remembered, and not for typical emergency requests, like PPE and food pantries. Health care providers needed COVID tests. They still couldn't tell who had the disease. But everyone could see how precarious people were. Funeral homes in the Bronx were so far beyond capacity that they could not take more bodies. At hospitals, the situation was worse. So many people were dying that their morgues filled, and some had to pile bodies on top of each other until they could set up mobile facilities. "They needed ice trucks," Zayas explained. The city helped procure a fleet of large trucks, only to discover that they didn't come equipped with adequate storage equipment. At one institution, the president and CEO organized a team of staff members who volunteered to build a shelving system, which they had to expand after filling a second truck with COVID decedents. "It was like the Twilight Zone," Zayas said. "Except this shit was real."

There's always a blur in time and space when you're a community representative for the governor. You travel often. You're always in public. Everyone's got your number, and there's always something to do. Before the pandemic, there were few hard stops in Zayas's workday, little separation between office and home. But

COVID hit her like a cyclone, upending any sense of order or balance and constantly sending new threats her way.

During April, Zayas said, the virus spread "like wildfire" in the Bronx, ripping through her building, where four people died of COVID, and reaching the seniors' building where her grandfather lived, just across the street. He had moved there twenty years ago, after retiring from his job as a forklift operator, separating from Zayas's grandmother, and renting a room a few blocks away while waiting for a unit to open up. The senior building had always been a safe place for him, still in the neighborhood but a world of his own. Although he lived alone, her grandpa was hardly independent. He'd survived a major heart attack four years earlier, but he suffered from congestive disease and required a home aide to support him, six days a week. He still socialized in the building, albeit not as energetically as he once had, and rarely in the common areas near the lobby, where the more garrulous men played cards and dominoes and reminisced about the way things used to be. He preferred to go outside and chat with the building staff. Leroy, the superintendent, had become a friend and confidant, as had Robert, the porter. "He's a social butterfly," Zayas reported. The kind of guy who makes everyone smile.

"My grandpa was kind of dismissive of COVID when it first started," Zayas remembered. "He was like, 'Oh, it's just another virus. It's going to pass, you'll see.' He almost sounded like Trump!" She worried about his situation, and particularly about his dependence on the health aide. "She's Dominican. She lives with a lot of other people, and she gets to him by taking the bus," Zayas explained. "I told her I didn't want her coming, but she said, 'Who's going to take care of him? How am I going to get paid?'" Conflicts like that were bubbling up all over the Bronx, however, because the borough is full of domestic workers who live paycheck to paycheck, and also of people who, like Zayas's grandfather, need assistance at home. "I didn't want to be insensitive, but I had to protect him," she said. "In the end I just said, 'Keep your mask on and keep a distance. And if something happens to him, that's your fault!'"

In truth, there were dangers everywhere at the time, a fact that soon proved undeniable in the building. Robert, who was fifty, got so sick from COVID that they thought he wouldn't make it. His illness scared everyone, Zayas said, because he had socialized with so many people in the building. Sure enough, soon there was an outbreak among the men who spent their days together in the common areas. "They were always in the hangout room, playing dominoes," Zayas told me. "Eight people. They all died from COVID." Her grandfather was shaken up, but not as much as she expected. "This is why I don't hang out down there!" he remarked. Soon after, Zayas, too anxious to sleep, found herself logging onto Facebook at four in the morning, where she discovered that Leroy, who was fifty-seven and healthy, had died as well. "I was devastated," she remembered. "And when I called my grandfather, he stood quiet on the phone. That's when it got dark for him, when he just didn't want to leave his home. He said, 'I'm not going to leave here.' He got really depressed."

The feeling was everywhere. At the outset of the pandemic, when governments everywhere ordered lockdowns and social distancing measures, scholars and officials warned about an "epidemic of loneliness," a "social depression" that would sunder the bonds people needed to survive.[3] There were, to be sure, deep emotional effects of the sudden isolation imposed by states and communities. But research showed that, for most of the population, levels of loneliness rose modestly, perhaps because people found new ways to engage each other, or rediscovered old ones, like conversations on the phone. Depression rates, however, spiked dramatically—to more than three times pre-pandemic levels, as a study in *The Journal of the American Medical Association* showed.[4] *Nature* reported that stress and anxiety among Americans soared even higher, from 11 percent of the population before the virus hit to a staggering 42 percent.[5]

For Zayas, the daily traumas proved overwhelming, inducing stress and anxiety so crippling that, by early summer, she asked for a medical leave. Although she had managed to avoid catching COVID, the symptoms of her condition were no less debilitating. Her doctor diagnosed her with malabsorption, because her body wasn't absorbing vitamins and nutrients. "Usually I weigh like 120," she told me. "And I lost, like, ten pounds. I felt like I was deteriorating." She had pounding headaches. She was sleepless, with constant fatigue. "COVID fatigue," is how she described it. Her chest was so tight and painful that it was hard to breathe. "I've become paranoid to the point where my doctor wants to put me on medication. I asked for X-rays of my chest and he told me it was just pent-up anxiety. He said, 'Unless you control it, you're going to lose your mind.'"

In early December 2020, during New York City's second surge of COVID, Zayas, Miriam, Mylischka, and I checked in by telephone. The three of them were all in Miriam and Mylischka's apartment, preparing for the holidays, their first without Luis. They had spent Thanksgiving together, and Zayas had told me that Miriam and Mylischka were suffering from their lack of a ritualized grieving. "In Hispanic culture, we have these customs where if somebody dies and even if you don't view the person, you congregate at home. You do a prayer service, you serve hot chocolate, you serve coffee, desserts. You take a break. You pray for like another hour. And it's like, you just can't do any of that. Miriam and Mylischka don't have that closure and they never will." The night we spoke, they were discussing what to make for Christmas dinner. "I want to make my dad's lasagna," Mylischka said. "Maybe not *so* fully loaded!" Zayas joked, lightening what had been a heavy conversation about sickness and loss. There were other sources of brightness. A new year was dawning, the skies were opening, too. Miriam told me that they would soon return to Puerto Rico, where they planned to scatter Luis's ashes in the ocean. Perhaps that would help.

In Zayas's world, the promise of help came not from release but from deliverance. The following week, New York would begin to administer the first doses of the Pfizer-BioNTech COVID-19 vaccine. A miracle, no doubt, but one that much of the population was reluctant to accept.

Health workers were the first priority, and government employees who participated in the mass vaccination campaign that would follow would soon be eligible. Zayas, who was back in the office, had already been told that she would play a big role in the effort. The Bronx had more than its share of essential workers and vulnerable populations, and the governor would need her to help get them inoculated, whatever it took. There were enormous logistical challenges, but Zayas was convinced that the cultural hurdles would be even greater. "We're a vulnerable population," she told me. "But people in Black and brown communities—we have trust issues. A lot of folks are like, 'Nope, this is a setup, they want Black and brown folks dead.' The community leaders here, the elected officials, the locals—they distrust it."

As it happened, so did Zayas.

On December 14, 2020, a nurse became the first American to be vaccinated outside of a medical trial, at a press event with Governor Cuomo in Queens. "I believe this is the weapon that will end the war," Cuomo declared, at a moment when researchers estimated that between ten and thirty thousand New Yorkers were getting infected by the coronavirus each day. "We have planes, trains and automobiles moving this all over the state right now. We want to get it deployed, and we want to get it deployed quickly."[6]

"I fear it's too fast," Zayas told me when we spoke that day. "We have a vaccine five months after this new disease. *Really?*" She paused for a beat, aware that not everyone shared her skepticism, but also that many of her neighbors in the Bronx did. "I personally don't trust it."

There was another moment of silence, before Zayas clarified her position. "I'm not antivaccine, I just want to give it more time."

The reality, Zayas knew, was that the state's political officials and health care leaders felt nothing but urgency, and that the vaccination campaign was about to take over her life. New York was in the midst of its second major surge in cases; in January, the number of people testing positive for the virus would reach its apex, surpassing even the scariest moments of the first wave. That month, the government, along with hospitals and pharmacies, would begin inoculating the most vulnerable people, including the elderly, those with underlying health problems, and designated essential workers. Zayas's job was to help everyone in the Bronx understand that the vaccine was safe and effective. The fact that she didn't quite believe it was a new source of stress.

Zayas decided that she would not get vaccinated, at least not right away. Despite the death of her neighbor, the despair in her community, the unrelenting anxiety that ravaged her mind and her body, she felt more fear of getting sick from an inoculation than from getting the virus itself. "I'm part of a vulnerable population," she told me, referring to her malabsorption as well as her ethnicity and race. "I'll be damned if I go and get vaccinated, and COVID didn't kill me but a vaccine did." Her colleagues in the governor's office had trouble understanding her decision. They tried to persuade her that she would be better off with the protection, but somehow hearing about the benefits of vaccination only added pressure to the vise that entrapped her. There were no good options, no ways out.

When the campaign started, Zayas found herself traveling everywhere in the borough. A mass vaccination event for Bronx residents at Yankee Stadium. A health care clinic. Churches. Public housing complexes. Although she stuck with her decision not to get inoculated, she could tell how much relief the shots gave to those who wanted them, and she gained appreciation for the project. She admired the way Governor Cuomo was talking about the health disparities that made COVID so much more widespread and deadly in her district. "It's abundantly clear that Black, Latino and poor communities have been hit the hardest by COVID," he told the press at Yankee Stadium, "and the Bronx is no exception."[7] Under his leadership, the state was targeting vaccination efforts in the places that had the highest rates of infection and the most severe vulnerability. "He's fighting for immigrants and minority communities," Zayas told me. "And a lot of these groups are really happy. They're ready for the vaccine."

It was a different story in Black and Puerto Rican communities, including her own. The conversations she had with her neighbors couldn't have been more different from the ones in her office. They noticed that Governor Cuomo was prioritizing vaccinations in their neighborhood, and in others like it. But they didn't buy his explanation, that the state, which had done so little to promote racial justice earlier in the pandemic, was suddenly committed to health equity. How did they know that they weren't just being used as guinea pigs? "What if," as Zayas put it, "the vaccines cause a whole new pandemic?" One even worse than COVID-19? She could tell, even before the city's official data confirmed it, that the Bronx, which was among the state's most deadly COVID hot spots, was about to become a hot spot of vaccine resistance as well.[8]

Once the vaccination campaign was up and running, Zayas was assigned to a distribution center in public housing complexes for the elderly and people with disabilities. The job required going into different buildings and posting flyers to promote inoculation. It meant leading meetings with New York City Housing Authority staffers, with tenant associations and community groups. It meant being there, in person, when the vaccinations started, fielding questions, handling problems, managing the crowd. "When I got the assignment, I fought it," she recounted. "I told them I wasn't comfortable going out there. I told my boss I didn't want to be that person who was not a team player, but I live with my grandmother [who was high risk], and they knew it." They needed her, though. Who else could communicate so well with people in the Bronx who needed to get vaccinated? Who else would they trust as much?

Zayas and I spoke a few days into her work in Co-op City, a massive housing complex with thirty-five high-rise buildings, seven townhouse clusters, 15,372 residential units, and roughly fifty thousand residents packed into a corner of Northeast Bronx. She didn't hide her distress. "It's just not safe there," she complained. "I mean, there's no ventilation. There are people with dementia, people walking around without masks. I just . . . I don't want to get COVID. You know? But I just know I'm going to. I'm scared."

Meanwhile, the coronavirus was relentless. On February 8, just a few weeks into the vaccination campaign, her grandmother woke up feeling tired. "She didn't have an appetite," Zayas said. "She had no energy. Some stomach problems. Her body ached. She just felt off." Zayas could feel her own heart racing. "I'm already a hypochondriac. Everything, I'm like, that must be COVID!" But this time it felt different. She didn't have much doubt.

She rushed to a health center and got herself a rapid test. Positive.

She got her grandmother to do one. Positive, too.

"My whole world went dark when we got those tests back," Zayas told me. "I started crying. I was just like, what now? You are told to go home and quarantine, but you don't know what it's going to be like when you wake up. You don't know what your symptoms are going to be."

When we spoke on February 9, Zayas was trying to calm her nerves and keep her grandmother stable. "I'm not symptomatic," she reported. "I feel fine. I feel the same." But she was taking precautions, doing home remedies that she had read about on the internet. "We're steaming our faces every hour for five minutes, with water and Himalayan sea salt. We're using Vicks VapoRub tablets in the shower, drinking a lot of teas. I'm doing vitamin D, vitamin C, and an antioxidant drip is coming tomorrow with a nurse." She was convinced that she had been infected a week earlier. That was good news, because it meant that in a few more days she would likely be rid of the virus, but also bad news, because it meant she had exposed the friends she had been hanging out with the previous weekend. She told them they needed to get tested. But she had been wearing a mask the whole time, and she wasn't surprised that they refused.

She wasn't proud of it, but Zayas acknowledged that she took some pleasure in telling her boss that she'd contracted COVID. "He was so nervous," she recounted. "He was silent, like he knew he had been wrong" to send her there for work. But Zayas didn't blame him entirely. "I always knew I was going to get it," she confessed. "At least now I don't have to worry about when it's going to happen." She told her boss that she would return when she was healthy, but that she was no longer going to the vaccine centers. "God has a way of intervening," she said. "He's like stop. You need to come home."

Zayas's grandmother never got dangerously ill from COVID. Zayas was less fortunate. Two days after we spoke, she started feeling tired. "At first, I was winded," she explained. "I was really dragging. I was sleeping more and more, and it was hard to get out of bed. And then I noticed, like, every time I woke up from a nap, I felt worse. My legs started to hurt really bad. I got afraid that, you know, maybe I had a blood clot. I got this excruciat-

ing, unbearable back pain, pain like I've never felt before. And
I started having these night sweats. I'd have to wake up in the
middle of the night and change." For a day or two, she thought
that bathing in Epsom salt and taking hot showers with vapor
would get her through the sickness. "I figured it was just a part
of COVID and I would have to live through it." But one morning she woke up and realized that "just inhaling and exhaling was
hurting me, and I couldn't even inhale all the way." She called
her doctor, and within a few minutes she was on her way to the
emergency room. The doctors ran tests and a CAT scan. She was
negative for blood clots, but positive for pneumonia. They gave
her medication, and sent her home.

> That week was rough. My lungs were hurting, and the
> cold sweats got worse. Now I was changing at least six
> or seven times a night. I haven't done my laundry, right?
> Because I'm sick. I have nobody to help me. And, oh my
> God, I'm running out of clothes. I don't have any more
> blankets because now they're all wet. My sheets are dirty,
> I'm trying to find clean sheets. And, you know, it was a
> horror.
>   So for a whole week I was freaking out. I was really,
> really cold, I mean, freezing cold. And it was almost like
> if you took an ice bucket and you just dumped it over
> me. Oh my God. My doctor told me that's part of the
> pneumonia, that it was normal to break a sweat. And I
> didn't shower for a few days because every time I got in
> the shower, I felt worse. But then at some point I was in
> the shower and I felt like I was gonna faint, like I was just
> gonna drop. There's a bar inside of the shower. I grabbed
> on to it, and I just closed my eyes. Please get me to the
> bed. And I rinsed off the little bit of soap I had on, shut
> off the water. I went to the bed and I sat on the corner.
> I said, "I'm gonna die." That's how bad I felt. I thought,
> "It's gonna kill me."
>   I just laid out on the bed. And I said a prayer: "God, if
> this is my calling and you pick me, then please, no pain. I

don't want to suffer. I don't want to gasp for air. I just want to go in peace."

God didn't pick Zayas that day, but the doctors wanted to see her immediately. They changed her medication regimen, told her to stay home and keep resting. The pneumonia would eventually clear up. Miriam and Mylischka cooked homemade soups to help her recover. She drank orange juice. Ate cereal. "I was like a preg-

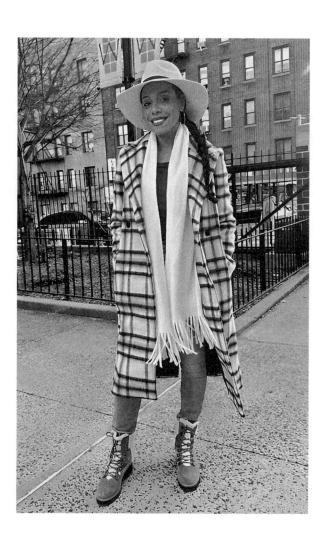

nant woman," she told me. "The only thing I craved was Lucky Charms!" She still felt crummy, still worried about her grandmother, but she could feel her strength returning, her energy picking up. "I started walking around a bit, doing some jumping jacks, getting my blood flowing, my oxygen levels up again." She waited a month from her positive diagnosis to get a reliable COVID test—partly because she wanted to make sure she had recovered, partly because she knew how much work there would be when she did.

For the time being, Zayas had other things on her mind. "I was thinking of going back home to Puerto Rico to see my family," she explained. "Santa Isabel. My father's sister is there. My cousins. My father's buried there, too.

"But you know what I really want to do right now?" she asked. "I can't wait until they open up those cruises. I want to go to the beach. I love cruises. They're amazing. I've done two of them. The first one left from Puerto Rico. It went to a different Caribbean island every day. The ships are beautiful, spacious. It feels like you're in a gigantic building. And the food is so good you'll gain like five, ten pounds! I mean, they take care of you. They take care of everything. Twenty-four hours a day."

CHAPTER 4

Trust

Uncertainty poses deep problems for modern states and societies. In ordinary times, governments predict outcomes and make plans based on historical experiences, with empirically grounded calculations of risk and vulnerability driving policy choices. Of course, data analysis does not always lead to the best decisions, but it sets the framework for expert judgments based on reasoned and informed debate. Governing under conditions of deep uncertainty requires interpreting partial or incomplete data and making leaps of faith. Scientific knowledge and personal experiences in previous or analogous events can be useful in these situations, but by no means do they guarantee success. This puts both political officials and professional experts in a treacherous position: in a high-stakes emergency, they have no choice but to do something, but doing the wrong thing will mean coming in for criticism, maybe even being condemned. It matters how they set rules, issue advice, and communicate the knowns and unknowns to the public. The things they say and do will inevitably affect how much people trust the government, medical scientists, and fellow citizens, when lives are on the line.

If living with uncertainty is challenging, managing a public health crisis amid widespread distrust—of political leaders, of scientists and experts, and of fellow citizens—is a nearly impossible task. In a pandemic, authoritarian states can achieve social control through aggressive surveillance, intensive policing, and strict punishments for people who violate rules around masking, distancing, and remaining locked down at home. Democratic governments can use these tools as well, but doing so without popular support invites backlash from citizens and competing political parties. In open societies, political leaders need to persuade the public that they are trustworthy, and that the experts they rely on for national security are reliable as well. This has never been easy to accomplish, and it's especially hard in a world where misinformation flows freely, scientific findings are routinely questioned by skeptics, and everyone feels entitled to their own facts. In this context, the sociologist Gil Eyal argues, "mistrust is not the puzzle. Trust, 'the leap of faith,' is."[1]

During the first year of the pandemic, journalists exposed a number of powerful political leaders whose refusal to follow their own rules made millions of others reluctant to take that leap. On March 13, 2020, Australia's chief medical officer, along with top medical officers from every state and territory, agreed that the nation should cancel all nonessential mass gatherings to prevent spreading the coronavirus. Later that day, the Council of Australian Governments convened in Parramatta, where they adopted the decision. Prime Minister Scott Morrison endorsed it immediately. "By Monday we will be advising against organized, non-essential gatherings of persons of 500 people or greater," he announced, calling the measure a "commonsense precaution to ensure we can manage the transmission of this virus in the most effective way possible."[2] It was unusual for leaders from opposing political parties to unite around such a dramatic policy, but political officials insisted that they trusted the medical experts who were leading the nation's emergency public health initiative. Australian citizens were prepared to comply with the restrictions, because they trusted the government's medical leadership, too.[3]

Many were puzzled, though, by something else that Morrison said at the press conference where he voiced support for the "commonsense precaution" of canceling large gatherings. Morrison explained that the next day, before the policy went into effect, he planned to attend a rugby (or, as the Aussies call it, footy) match to see his favorite team, the Cronulla Sharks, in person. When a journalist questioned this decision, the prime minister defended himself, insisting that the threat was not yet dire, and also that, well, he just did not want to miss the game. "The fact that I would still be going on Saturday speaks not just to my passion for my beloved Sharks; it might be the last game I get to go to for a long time," Morrison declared.[4] The policy would not be in effect over the weekend, so technically, the prime minister would not be breaking his own law. But for millions of Australians, Morrison's statement violated the spirit of the government's pact with its people. On Twitter and talk radio, they began asking a simple but essential question: Shouldn't rulers be required to follow the rules?

The media condemned Morrison's decision. "PM Can't Seem to Read the Room," ran a headline in *The Australian*. Fox Sports agreed: "'I'm Still Going to the Footy!' ScoMo's Weird Take After Announcing Crowd Ban Plan," its story said.[5] The Australian Broadcasting Corporation pushed the matter further. Morrison's behavior led the leading national news company to ask "The big question." Namely: "What trust can we place in the crucial decisions being made and the advice being offered to a deeply nervous public?"[6] Under pressure, Morrison made a last-minute decision to skip the match—which was just as well, because the Sharks lost, 22–18. But ABC continued to raise questions about the judgment and expertise of other Australian leaders. The treasurer, for instance, had pushed through a $17 billion economic stimulus package, and the chief medical officer had deemed it acceptably safe to continue public gatherings through the weekend, rather than canceling them right away. "This is all very accommodating," the ABC journalist David Speers wrote, "but what if it's the wrong call? What if allowing big crowds to assemble this weekend only accelerates the spread of the virus, causing far more suffering, not to mention far more economic pain?"[7]

"What if" questions were everywhere in March 2020, and not without reason. It was a moment of true uncertainty, in which there were no data from past events that could reliably guide present risk assessments or decision-making. The novel coronavirus, and the potentially lethal disease it caused, remained a mystery to medical scientists, public health experts, and policymakers. Virologists didn't know if the virus spread through droplets or aerosols, how far it could travel, how close to another person one could be without risk. There was no established science on why some people experienced severe symptoms from COVID-19 while others were hardly affected. Physicians could only guess which interventions would work best for serious illness, whether antivirals were useful or if ventilators helped. No one knew whether children were in danger, or how likely they were to spread the disease. It was impossible to predict how long the outbreak would last, or whether the virus would mutate into something more dangerous still.

Australia was one of many nations where critics were raising concerns about the trustworthiness of political leaders and the decisions of public health agencies during the first weeks of the outbreak. Nearly everything came under scrutiny. How did anyone know what was right? The United States did not ban large public events as they did in Australia, but on March 15, the U.S. Centers for Disease Control and Prevention recommended canceling or postponing public gatherings with more than fifty people, noting that the advice did not apply to businesses, universities, or schools.[8] In the absence of strong federal policies, state governors took on the primary responsibility for imposing restrictions. Their decisions about what could stay open and what had to close varied dramatically, and largely followed party lines. Inevitably, that variation helped animate and intensify ideological conflicts over how to treat the crisis, with Republicans promoting personal choice and individual responsibility, and Democrats favoring rules and regulations that emphasized mutual obligations, and protected those most susceptible to severe disease.

Initially, however, it was not clear exactly which rules and regulations would protect people and which would cause undue harm. Consider, for instance, the question of face masks. During the first months of the outbreak, the World Health Organization claimed that face masks were unnecessary for civilians, and, despite pushback from experts who suspected that the corona-virus was being transmitted through aerosols, the WHO insisted that governments should not recommend them for daily use. This recommendation had a major influence, particularly in Western nations that had been spared the worst of the SARS epidemic during 2003, and had little experience masking up to prevent infectious diseases. In the U.S., both the White House and the leading federal health agencies echoed the WHO's message, with massive consequences for the public's confidence in what counted for scientific knowledge about the pandemic disease. On March 8, 2020, Anthony Fauci went on the popular American news program *60 Minutes* to discuss the outbreak with the medical reporter, Dr. Jon LaPook.

"People should not be walking around with masks," Dr. Fauci explained.

"You're sure of it?" LaPook asked. "Because people are listening really closely to this."

"Right now, there's no reason to be walking around with a mask. When you're in the middle of an outbreak, wearing a mask might make people feel a little bit better, and it might even block a droplet, but it's not providing the perfect protection that people think that it is."[9]

Fauci stuck to this position until April 3, when the CDC changed its recommendations in light of research showing that the coronavirus was, in fact, transmitted through aerosols, and by asymptomatic as well as symptomatic carriers. From then on, he and other American public health leaders would emphasize that their initial advice was based on the best information they had in the early days of the crisis, and insist that critics remember the "right now" phrase in their language as well as their reminders that official health guidelines would likely evolve as new knowledge emerged. This, studies show, is the kind of rhetoric that usually helps officials establish and maintain public trust during periods of uncertainty, when facts are difficult to discern and scientific findings are tentative, at best.[10] In early March, neither Fauci nor his colleagues anticipated how their statements would play into the looming ideological battles over pandemic policies and politics. Soon, however, their words would become weapons, circulated widely online and in partisan news coverage, and wielded regularly in campaigns against mainstream medical expertise.

There's little question that the internet and the news media helped spread skepticism about the competence and intentions of public health experts and the effectiveness of government policies during the pandemic; after all, the internet and the media help spread everything, true and false, malicious and good. Millions of Americans joined Facebook groups to find communities of like-minded people who shared their political affiliation as well as their interpretation of medical facts. For Democrats, the COVID crisis represented a failure of President Trump's leadership, from gutting the CDC's disease surveillance operations in China to forcing state governments to find their own personal protective equipment and emergency medical supplies. As Republicans saw it, COVID was a "Trojan horse" that liberals were using to advance new forms of social control and economic regulation, and a political tool for undermining the president in November's election. Social media and partisan news outlets played key roles in fostering solidarity among people who shared a worldview and a political agenda; in so doing, they also fostered distrust between people with divergent viewpoints, and helped tear the body politic apart.[11]

But social media and partisan journalists were by no means the main drivers of public distrust in government during the pandemic. More fundamental was the blatant violation of official rules, regulations, and recommendations by high-ranking political leaders, from presidents and prime ministers to governors, mayors, and cabinet members, in nations around the world. In a host of nations, top officials acted as if the emergency restrictions they advocated did not apply to members of their own inner circle, and especially not to themselves. It's impossible to know exactly how much their behavior, once exposed, engendered distrust among those who already doubted the intentions of political officials and medical scientists, but there's no question that it undermined the spirit of mutual obligation or linked fate. At a moment when societies needed solidarity, political elites—left and right, and in countries around the world—used the privilege of their position to thwart it.

It's not unusual for states to ask citizens to make personal sacrifices in a crisis, reducing their consumption of certain foods and metals during an armed conflict or their use of water during a drought. In some cases, states ask for something greater. In February 2022, for instance, Ukraine responded to Russia's invasion by declaring martial law, prohibiting all adult males between the ages of eighteen and sixty from leaving the country, and ordering all conscripts and reservists for military service to report for active duty.[12] Although thousands of these men died in the fighting that followed, few questioned the rationale or the legitimacy of Ukraine's policy. But it was a very different story in states that imposed sweeping lockdown orders on all residents during the first wave of the coronavirus pandemic. Requiring civilians to maintain physical distance was bound to be difficult and controversial; demanding, under threat of fine or detention, that people in otherwise open societies confine themselves to their homes and avoid social gatherings with friends and family was an invitation to outrage and dissent. Political leaders who curbed individual freedoms in democratic states and nations faced extraordinary pressure to justify and legitimate their decisions. Complying with them in their own lives was the least they could do.

According to research by a group of behavioral health scholars who participated in the University College London's COVID-19 Social Study, this simple fact helps explain the dramatic drop in public trust of the British government in spring 2020. After initially rejecting advice from public health experts who recommended aggressive restrictions on social and economic activities, Johnson's government implemented a full national lockdown on March 26. Under the order, all nonessential businesses were ordered closed. All residents were required to stay home unless they were buying food, getting medical care, or exercising outdoors. Social gatherings were strictly prohibited. Johnson took to the media to promote his restrictions. "Follow the rules," he implored—so often, in fact, that a popular activist Twitter feed, Led By Donkeys, tweeted a montage of the prime minister repeating those words. "The police will have the powers to enforce them. . . . Breaking these rules now could undermine and reverse all the progress that we've made together."[13]

Between April and June 2020, researchers conducting the COVID-19 Social Study surveyed 40,597 individuals in England, Scotland, and Wales, measuring their confidence in government (on a scale of 1 to 7) as the pandemic evolved. When the study began, participants in each country reported that they mainly trusted government, with the average Scottish response around 5, the average Welsh response around 4.6, and the average English response around 4.5. There's minor fluctuation in the levels of reported confidence during late April and May, as all three governments struggle to deal with health and economic threats, but in late May, something dramatic happens. In England, and only in England, confidence in government plummets, falling to 3.7 and then, days later, 3.5.[14] There is a clear, demonstrable, crisis in national confidence—and there was little mystery about why.

The British press called it the Cummings Affair. On May 22, newspapers reported that Dominic Cummings, senior aide to Boris Johnson, had violated the government's lockdown rules by traveling more than four hundred kilometers to a family estate with his wife, who was rumored to have COVID-19, and their child. "Although some other officials and senior figures had also broken the lockdown rules," write the behavioral scientists Daisy Fancourt, Andrew Steptoe, and Liam Wright in *The Lancet*, "this transgression was the first to not immediately be followed by an apology and resignation."[15] Instead, Johnson defended his government's performance and brushed off demands for an investigation into the aide's behavior during a "fiery evidence session" at the House of Commons on May 27, where he insisted that the Cummings Affair was not a serious problem. Members of Parliament, including many from his own Conservative Party, saw things differently. Simon Hoare, a Conservative MP from North Dorset, declared, "My inbox tells me that as a result of the last few days, the response of the British people is going to be far less energetic than it was first time round, and that is as a direct result of the activities of your senior adviser. What do we say to our constituents who are likely to say you can keep your lockdown if it has to come back; if other people don't abide by it, why on earth should we?"[16]

The *Lancet* article by Fancourt, Steptoe, and Wright shows that this is precisely how the British public reacted, and other research indicates that the "Cummings effect" on trust in government grew stronger during summer, as political leaders refused to acknowledge the double standard, and citizens in England— though not in Wales or Scotland, which are part of the U.K. but have their own national ministers and parliaments—felt betrayed. In "Public Trust and COVID-19," a team of scholars from the University of Southampton report that the government's loss of moral authority in the aftermath of the scandal "has come up unprompted in every group when people were asked what issues the current government was most and least trustworthy on." They quote participants in their focus groups who lost confidence in the state after the Cummings Affair, turning the national response into a "free for all."[17]

At the time of the Cummings Affair, neither members of Parliament nor British civilians could understand why Johnson refused to condemn or apologize for his aide's violation of official policies. Why not make the prime minister's office a symbol of responsibility and a force for solidarity? Why not demand that everyone, including elites as well as ordinary citizens, commit to respecting the emergency rules? For months, it was a puzzling failure of political leadership, perhaps due to Johnson's quirky, belligerent personality, perhaps to his loyalty toward staff, though before long the relationship between Johnson and Cummings would grow cold. Eventually, a series of photographs leaked to the press revealed that Johnson may have had another motivation altogether. He, too, had been flouting his own restrictions during May 2020—even more recklessly and egregiously than his aide had, and with less salutary motivations. The example Johnson set would surely have given Cummings reason to believe that 10 Downing would excuse political elites who discreetly exempted themselves from COVID regulations.

Inevitably, the British media called it "Partygate." The illicit behavior began on May 15, nearly two weeks before Cummings fled London, when Johnson attended a garden party outside his offices on Downing Street. Images from the occasion show the prime minister drinking socially with his romantic partner and a small group of colleagues while other small groups of partygoers are assembled nearby. They must have enjoyed the occasion, because days later, on May 20, his office emailed invitations to share "socially distanced drinks in the No 10 garden this evening" to somewhere between one hundred and two hundred people. Johnson's communications director initially expressed concerns about the event, emailing the planners that "a 200-odd person invitation for drinks in the garden of No. 10 is somewhat of a comms risk in the current environment." But this cautionary note did not deter Johnson. The prime minister was one of about thirty people who attended the celebration, and when it ended, without any immediate complaints or public notices, his private secretary expressed relief that "we seem to have got away with" it.[18]

After the initial party photographs emerged in late 2021, the Metropolitan Police initiated an investigation into potentially illicit behavior on Downing Street, and Sue Gray, the second permanent secretary of the British government, compiled a separate Cabinet Office report. Both inquiries listed a series of apparently illegal gatherings held on government property, both indoors and in the gardens, during the first year of the pandemic. The police fined Johnson for violations, making him the first sitting prime minister in British history to be found guilty of breaking the law, and named eighty-two others who defied the rules as well.[19] The so-called Sue Gray report offered detailed descriptions of drunken parties with loud music and offensive behavior held during periods of the lockdown when all government employees were aware that social gatherings were forbidden. Neither of the official documents said much about how the conduct of Britain's political leaders affected the public's confidence in its pandemic policies, but for critics, this was Johnson's most unforgivable crime.

"While we were sacrificing and mourning . . . they were drinking until they were sick, laughing at security guards, laughing at cleaners . . . Laughing at us all," the *Mirror* reported on the cover of its tabloid. The *Metro* sounded a similar note. "We got away with it," its lead story reads. "Brazen Downing St staff knew they were all breaking the rules." The *i* newspaper put it more plainly: "Failure of leadership," it said. By the time the Sue Gray report was released, however, the Conservative Party was closing ranks around Johnson, fighting to preserve his government and political career. The right-wing media, which had once criticized the prime minister for his illegal behavior, now dismissed the seriousness of the charges. "Is that it?" wrote the *Daily Mail;* the more reputable conservative papers, the *Telegraph* and the *Times,* chose another topic for their lead story, encouraging their readers to move on.[20]

Few people could, however, and in 2022, when more scandals about violations of COVID restrictions at 10 Downing dominated the news, Boris Johnson was forced to resign.

The most powerful man in England was not the only political leader who urged voters to move on from their hard feelings and support their government despite the betrayals of trust. In May 2020, Austrian police found President Alexander Van der Bellen and his wife eating in a restaurant after a curfew that he had imposed on the rest of the nation. In May, Ludovic Orban, prime minister of Romania, was fined after photographers caught him drinking and smoking with cabinet members at the very kind of social gathering that he had outlawed.[21] In July, Sakaja Johnson, a Kenyan who chaired the Senate Ad Hoc Committee on COVID-19, was arrested for flouting pandemic restrictions. Although Sakaja Johnson resigned, both Orban and Van der Bellen remained in office after their violations, and their governments lost credibility at the moment they needed it most.

Among the political leaders whose violations of public trust did damage, few faced as much backlash as Gavin Newsom, the Democratic governor of California. During the initial outbreak, Newsom had been unusually successful in managing the pandemic, with sweeping closures, mask requirements, and distancing guidelines that kept residents far healthier than those in comparably large and populous states. Although California was one of the first states to report confirmed cases of COVID-19 and likely cases of community transmissions, as of April 13, 2020, its COVID mortality was roughly fourteen times lower than New York's. Public health experts praised Newsom for his proactive mentality and aggressive emergency measures. California "acted more quickly than New York once it became clear that coronavirus was starting to spread in the US," *Vox* reported. "The San Francisco Bay Area issued America's first regional shelter-in-place order on March 16, and California Gov. Gavin Newsom issued a statewide stay-at-home order three days later."[22] But in June, soon after the government relaxed its pandemic restrictions, the virus rushed into the Golden State, causing a dramatic spike in cases and deaths.[23]

By summer and fall, public health policies such as mask mandates and restaurant closures had become ideologically charged and controversial. Newsom's government had tried to find a compromise that allowed businesses to operate and social life to continue without unduly endangering residents, but it was hard to find the right balance. On September 12, the state issued a ban on all gatherings "to protect public health and slow the rate of transmission of COVID-19."[24] California permitted outdoor dining in restaurants, but only under strict conditions. An October 3 tweet by the governor's office stated, "Going out to eat with members of your household this weekend? Don't forget to keep your mask on in between bites. Do your part to keep those around you healthy."

On October 9, the state updated the order, loosening but by no means lifting the restrictions. "Gatherings that include more than 3 households are prohibited," the California Department of Public Health declared, in a section on private events. "All gatherings must be held outside. Attendees may go inside to use restrooms as long as the restrooms are frequently sanitized. . . . Gatherings should be two hours or less. . . . People at gatherings may remove their face coverings briefly to eat or drink as long as they stay at least 6 feet away from everyone outside their own household, and put their face covering back on as soon as they are done with the activity."[25] It was not an absolute lockdown, but the California government was asking residents to sacrifice quite a lot of social life.

This context helps explain the public outrage after photographs showed Governor Newsom dining indoors in a group of twelve at the Michelin-starred restaurant French Laundry. The meal, on November 6, was a birthday party for an influential and well-connected lobbyist, and two high-level members of the California Medical Association were reportedly also in attendance.[26] Journalists reported that the price for private dining during the pandemic was somewhere between $350 and $850 per person, and that the wine bill from the party was $12,000 alone.[27] For a governor who had pleaded for people to sacrifice their personal privileges for the public good, the optics were terrible, and the news generated a fierce backlash. At a press conference, Newsom apologized for attending the dinner, saying that he believed it would be held outdoors and that the group would be smaller. "Instead of sitting down, I should have stood up and walked back, gotten in my car and drove back to my house. Instead, I chose to sit there with my wife and a number of other couples that were outside the household. . . . You can quibble about the guidelines but the spirit of what I'm preaching all the time was contradicted and I gotta own that, so I want to apologize to you. I need to preach and practice, not just preach and not practice. . . . But we're all human and we all fall short sometimes."[28]

Newsom's plea for understanding may have satisfied some of his supporters, but California Republicans were unforgiving. In the media, critics pounced. "As the pandemic spikes, the economy convulses and democracy fissures, the urgent need to restore faith in government cries out for leaders with authenticity," wrote Miriam Pawel, a contributing opinion writer for *The New York Times*. "Instead, in one costly dinner, Gov. Gavin Newsom dramatized the chasm that divides California—more severely than North versus South or inland versus the coast. Flouting his own guidelines and exhortations to Californians to avoid socializing, Governor Newsom and his wife joined a birthday celebration for a friend—and prominent lobbyist—at the luxurious French Laundry restaurant in the Napa Valley. It is hard to say which was more astounding, the hypocrisy or the hubris."[29] The conservative media were even more damning. "So if you're wondering why, if you live in California, you can't have Thanksgiving this year or visit your mother as she dies alone in the hospital, it is because of them [Newsom and the medical professionals] and people like them. And yet there they were, eating $300 truffle pasta and living like this pandemic thing never even happened," the Fox News host Tucker Carlson explained. "The picture of them doing it . . . is the year 2020 condensed to its essence. Here you have plutocrats dining with lobbyists, ignoring the very orders they're so self-righteously imposing on others, gorging themselves in seclusion as the people they're supposed to be helping wither and die. And then when they're caught, they lie about it."[30]

For Newsom, and for California taxpayers, the dinner would prove far more expensive than the initial bill. The governor, who was wealthy, handsome, and progressive, was a star in the Democratic Party, and his name was included on lists of potential candidates for national office. Naturally, he was also a target of conservative ire. Back in June, Republicans who disdained Newsom's tight pandemic restrictions had ramped up their campaign for a recall election, with little success. The French Laundry dinner changed everything. Soon, a petition to hold a special election gained momentum, with a website that listed the top reason for booting Newsom from office as "Rules for Thee, but Not for He = French Laundry Indoor Dining, No Mask, 22 guests."[31] The message worked. Some 1.5 million Californians signed the petition, and in 2021 the governor, whose approval ratings had dropped from 58 percent before the dinner to 46 percent two months later, was forced to defend his office from an insurgent right-wing campaign.[32]

Newsom won the recall election easily, but the effort required to run could not help but distract the governor's office from the state's more dire problems, including COVID, the housing crisis, economic insecurity, a spike in crime, a historic drought, and millions of children whose education had been disrupted. At a time when California needed every dollar available for services, the recall election cost some $276 million in public money, and analysts estimated the total price at nearly $450 million.[33] The larger problem, though, was that the entire ordeal tore at the state's social fabric, making the pandemic even more divisive. The French Laundry dinner party was a vivid reminder that Californians were not "in it together." Everyone, including advocates for collective public health programs and the governor's most ardent supporters, lost faith.

Public distrust in government and political leaders was only part of the equation; the government's distrust of ordinary people also helped produce negative results. From the initial outbreak of the coronavirus in China, political leaders in a number of states and societies kept vital information from people who could have used it, including scientists, medical doctors, journalists, and citizens, as well as other public officials. Health officers in Wuhan and Beijing chose to conceal news about the "pneumonia of unknown origin" because they feared causing public anxiety, political backlash, or a diplomatic crisis.[34] The Brazilian president, Jair Bolsonaro, described COVID as a "little flu" or a meager "cold," and accused the media of manufacturing "hysteria";[35] the Italian prime minister, Giuseppe Conte, insisted that the rising number of cases in his country was due to an increase in testing, rather than to rapid spread of the virus; New York governor Andrew Cuomo suppressed data about the catastrophic spike in nursing home deaths.[36]

According to a Cornell University study of 38 million English-language articles published in media outlets around the world, one man, Donald Trump, was by far "the largest driver of the COVID-19 misinformation 'infodemic,'" which the WHO defines as "an overabundance of information—some accurate and some not—that makes it hard for people to find trustworthy sources and reliable guidance when they need it."[37] The president acknowledged that some of his fabrications, such as the claim that the virus was not being transmitted through aerosols even after top government scientists told him otherwise, were designed to advance a style of leadership and a set of policies he favored. In the early weeks of the outbreak, Trump believed that downplaying the threat of a lethal pandemic would help Americans retain their confidence in the country and the economy, and in subsequent months he spun fabulous tales of his administration's success with COVID as a campaign strategy for the November election.[38]

That month, the *Atlantic* magazine compiled a list, "All the President's Lies about the Coronavirus," that documents the scope of the president's falsehoods during 2020. In February, Trump repeated the lie that the coronavirus would weaken "when we get into April, in the warmer weather—that has a very negative effect on that, and that type of a virus," and pledged, with no evidence, that "it's going to disappear. One day, it's like a miracle—it will disappear." On multiple occasions, he claimed that national case numbers were going down even when they were rising. On Independence Day he proclaimed that 99 percent of COVID cases are "totally harmless," discounting the severe and sometimes long-term illness it causes. On July 6, he boasted, falsely, that "We now have the lowest Fatality (Mortality) Rate in the World."[39] In August, he said that America had "developed, from scratch, the largest and most advanced testing system in the world." He often said that children were "totally immune" to COVID-19, and that everyone who recovered from it would become immune, too.[40]

The president of the United States is always among the world's most powerful people. During 2020, Trump enjoyed not only the authority of the White House, but also nearly unmatched influence on social media, where he spread lies about the pandemic with impunity and apparent delight to tens of millions of followers. His public statements, status updates, and tweets circulated widely and made a discernible impact in debates about the crisis. The researchers who analyzed the 38 million pieces of content about the virus found that "Trump mentions comprised 37.9 percent of the overall 'infodemic.'" He drove "major spikes in the 'miracle cures' misinformation topic" after speculating, in a press conference, that injecting disinfectants could cure COVID, and advocating the use of the antimalarial drug hydroxychloroquine for protection from disease.[41] He inspired people to form new groups dedicated to alternative science on the pandemic, and, on the other side, groups intent on defending mainstream medicine and epidemiological research. Above all, Trump encouraged people who trusted him to distrust Democrats and established experts. Republicans had spent decades whipping up a culture war against "government scientists," "mainstream media," "egg-heads" in academia, and "global elites," all of whom, the right insisted, aimed to weaken America. The president harnessed the energy of this campaign and used it to charge up his core sup-porters, placing the blame on their ideological adversaries. "The Democrats are politicizing the coronavirus," Trump declared. "This is their new hoax."[42] Instead of promoting unity, he turned the Oval Office into a wedge.

Inevitably, the mistrust multiplied, and spread. When the president condemned or dismissed the advice coming from the government's epidemiological or medical science agencies, other Republican officials followed, and voters did as well. Prominent conservative doctors also attacked the government's policies. Joseph Mercola, an osteopathic physician and author in Flor-ida with more than 2.7 million Facebook followers and another 700,000 on Twitter and YouTube, claimed that masks did not pre-vent transmission of the virus and promoted a blend of vitamin supplements as a more effective alternative.[43] Dan Erickson and Artin Massihi, doctors who own urgent care centers in California, told the media that the results of some five thousand COVID-19 tests they had conducted proved that the disease was no more dangerous than influenza. Elon Musk, who had been pushing to reopen his factories in the region, tweeted out the story of the Trump-supporting doctors who refused to wear masks or accept the CDC's recommendations, and Fox News invited them on national television.[44] A host of other doctors took to cable news and social media to push similar views, accusing "medical elites" of abusing their power to curtail Americans' freedom. President Trump led the charge, repeatedly attacking the credibility of Anthony Fauci. He was "a disaster," the president said, responsi-ble for hundreds of thousands of deaths.[45] Fauci, who had served both Republicans and Democrats and considered himself non-partisan, quickly became the right's symbol of repressive, wrong-headed, establishment science. By April 2020, the doctor would need stepped-up security to protect him from death threats.[46]

During 2020, distrust for public health experts and medical doctors, if not outright disdain, became an increasingly common conservative position. According to polling by Gallup, until recently, people who leaned Republican reported having higher levels of confidence in the advice of their own physicians than people who leaned Democratic. In 2002, for instance, 70 percent of Republicans and 62 percent of Democrats said they trusted their medical doctor, and in 2010 the numbers were 73 and 68 percent. The two sides flipped around 2012, and the trends accelerated in opposite directions during the pandemic. In May 2020, surveys by Pew Research showed that people who leaned Democrat were gaining faith in medical scientists at a rapid clip, whereas people who leaned Republican were not; in October 2021, a Grinnell College poll found that 71 percent of Democrats, and just 48 percent of Republicans, expressed "high" levels of trust in doctors. By the end of 2021, a new Gallup poll revealed the extent of the partisan gap: Republicans' confidence in their own doctors had plummeted to 60 percent, while Democrats' confidence had gone up to 71 percent.[47] Prescription drugs and medical treatments for COVID were now either conservative or liberal. Each side had its own facts, and each scoffed at the other for its ignorance.

In this context, distrust of other people—particularly those who have other political preferences or values—runs rampant. For decades, the fault lines dividing American political constituencies had been growing deeper and more dangerous, threatening not only the nation's capacity to manage a pandemic, but its ability to govern democratically as well. "In the early 1970s half of Americans said that most people can be trusted," wrote the philosopher Kevin Vallier in December 2020. "[T]oday that figure is less than one-third." What's more, he explained, "the U.S. is the only established democracy to see a major decline in social trust. In other nations the trend was in the opposite direction. From 1998 to 2014, social trust increased in Sweden from 56.5% to 67%, in Australia from 40% to 54%, and in Germany from 32% to 42%. Meanwhile, the U.S. is becoming more like Brazil, where trust is around 5%. What makes America unique?"[48]

In his book *Trust in a Polarized Age*, Vallier argues that conventional accounts of rising social distrust focus on three key drivers: corruption, ethnic segregation, and economic inequality. Although levels of perceived corruption in the U.S. rose steadily from 2015 to 2020, the country is not an outlier among affluent democratic nations, ranking 25th among the 180 nations in Transparency International's Corruption Perceptions Index.[49] Ethnic segregation and economic inequality are long-standing problems in the U.S., but they are not increasing at the rate that distrust is going up. On the contrary, Vallier claims, in recent decades both ethnic segregation and economic inequality have been relatively stable, and by some measures they have gone down.[50]

Vallier is among a number of scholars who suspect that political polarization, and the cultural conflicts that come with it, is a likely driver of rising interpersonal distrust. If, for instance, liberal Americans do not trust the doctors who tell them masks are useless and suggest they take hydroxychloroquine, they are also unlikely to trust people who eagerly accept and even celebrate that wisdom. It reflects a different worldview, a different understanding of knowledge, belief, even, in a different set of facts. Well before the pandemic, American citizens were expressing strong concerns about the character and motivation of people who supported the opposing political party. "In 2017," Vallier writes, "around 70% of Democrats said that Donald Trump voters couldn't be trusted, and around 70% of Republicans said the same of Hillary Clinton voters."[51] In 2019, Pew Research reports, "55% of Republicans say Democrats are 'more immoral' when compared with other Americans; 47% of Democrats say the same about Republicans," a sharp spike from 2016, when the numbers were 47 and 35 percent, respectively. Pew also finds that the differences extend into personal matters. "Majorities in both parties say those in the opposing party do not share their nonpolitical values and goals," they report.[52] This gulf helps explain another striking fact about how polarization and distrust affect American social bonds: marriages across party lines have fallen dramatically, and people in "politically mixed" marriages seem to be less happy than those who share the same party identification.[53]

Sharing the same political ideology also helps create bonds in the place where people spent an outsized proportion of their social time during 2020: the internet. Among social scientists, there is a long-standing debate over whether using social media and online news is a cause of political polarization. Some, such as the Harvard law professor and political scientist Cass Sunstein, argue that people online tend to spend time in "echo chambers" that solidify their convictions and sometimes make them more extreme.[54] Others, including the Stanford economists Levi Boxell and Matthew Gentzkow, as well as the Harvard economist Jesse Shapiro, point out that the growth in American polarization is most pronounced among the demographic groups who are least likely to be on social media.[55] The internet, they claimed in a 2017 paper, is unlikely to be the cause of that. But in recent years, new platforms that are specifically designed for building or strengthening communities have changed the social landscape. They make it far easier for people to make connections and organize projects with others who share their values, beliefs, and ambitions, and also far easier to identify and oppose those who don't.

Facebook Groups are, by far, the most popular of these digital spaces. The company now known as Meta launched Facebook Groups in 2010, but it was not until after 2017, when founder and CEO Mark Zuckerberg declared that its core mission was to help people build "meaningful communities," that it fully promoted the platform and added a "Groups" tab to its mobile display. In 2020, the company claimed that more than 70 million people had registered as Facebook Groups moderators, and that some 1.8 billion people were using Groups on a monthly basis.[56] By April, Facebook reported that more than 4.5 million Americans had joined support groups related to COVID-19, as had more than three million Italians and two million in the U.K.[57] Some of these were hyper-local mutual aid organizations that used the technology to build sophisticated social support systems—for food donations, home deliveries, cleaning supplies, burial assistance, and the like—that would have been difficult to organize without social media. Others were ideologically driven interest groups sowing seeds of distrust or scammers peddling unproven medications. Disinformation was everywhere, and although Facebook insisted it would ban content that caused harm, it lacked the capacity to keep it off the platform.

In February 2020, the WHO issued its first warning about
the emerging infodemic, and by early March, it was apparent
that the internet would be a breeding ground for propaganda,
profiteering, and patently false news. Conspiracy theories that
China—or perhaps the U.S.!—had engineered the coronavirus
as a biological weapon, and that Bill Gates had created the virus
to promote vaccines. Rumors that there were far more—or far
fewer!—cases and deaths than countries were reporting. Promises
that a secret medication or rare herb—for sale here!—could prevent or cure COVID. In the *American Journal of Tropical Medicine
and Hygiene*, an international team of medical researchers reported
that misinformation about the efficacy of drinking highly concentrated alcohol to cure COVID had resulted in some 800 deaths,
5,876 hospitalizations, and 60 cases of complete blindness among
people who consumed methanol as medication during the first
four months of 2020. "Trust between healthcare workers and the
affected community is essential to deal with the pandemic crisis.
However, medical conspiracy theories can lead to mistrust with
governments and health professionals that can impact people's
healthcare-seeking behavior," the scholars concluded. "National
and international agencies, including the fact-checking agencies, should not only identify rumors and conspiracy theories and
debunk them but should also engage social media companies to
spread correct information."[58] In the U.S., and in all other open
societies, no agency was up for that task.

As a sociologist, I understood the value of observing how
rumors, conspiracy theories, and outright fabrications were circulating on social media during the pandemic, and—given its
unmatched popularity—I was especially interested in the action
on Facebook Groups. A postdoctoral researcher, Melina Sherman, and I identified public Facebook Groups in the U.S. with
more than ten thousand members that explicitly identified as
being conservative, on the one hand, and Democrat or progressive, on the other. We selected four self-identified conservative or
Republican groups, two self-identified Democratic groups, and
two self-identified progressive groups to observe. In total, the
eight groups had more than 374,200 members. We used Crowd-

Tangle, a platform that helps researchers analyze social media posts, to track status updates, photos, links, livestreams, and videos shared from Facebook, YouTube, and other platforms, with any of the following keywords: COVID, COVID-19, coronavirus. We contained our search within a specific date range, starting on January 1, 2020, and ending on April 1, 2021. We also limited our search to posts written in English. Cumulatively, we analyzed over 17,800 posts, which on average received 207 interactions.

What we discovered, after spending far more time reading social media posts than any doctor would recommend for psychological wellbeing, is that active members of politically partisan Facebook Groups experienced dramatically different pandemics, and worried about utterly different threats. In the confines of their interest group, members developed narratives that were rooted in a specific diagnosis of the underlying condition that most threatened America: an inept and authoritarian president, an unjust social and economic system, an insurgent party of radicals hell-bent on political transformation. Each diagnosis called for a different remedy, and a different vision of what the nation should do next.

For groups aligned with the Democratic Party, the COVID-19 crisis in America was fundamentally driven by the corruption and incompetence of Donald Trump and his Republican followers. On November 15, 2020, for instance, a member of the group "Riden with Biden 2021!" shared a long status, written as a letter to Republicans, which read: "We are no longer going to allow you to kill more Americans. We are asking for each one of you to either act now and save our United States. Tell Trump you will no longer endorse his delusions and that he has lost: He will no longer be the President of the United States. . . . We are tired of you Republicans being more concerned with your stock portfolios, then [sic] with the lives and wellbeing of the rank and file American." This post, which received 1,276 interactions—nearly twenty times the average number of interactions for posts in the Riden with Biden group—calls on Republicans to take responsibility for a tragic loss of life, making it clear that it is not a virus per se, but rather a political party that is responsible for the COVID-19 death toll. The post also shows what social in-grouping can look like on the internet. It calls not for unity or understanding in a time of crisis, but for accountability.

The use of Facebook groups to establish social distance from outsiders is even more apparent in posts from Democrats that gleefully reported cases where conservative leaders contracted the virus after downplaying the threat of COVID or dismissing the need for distancing and masks. On October 2, 2020, several Riden with Biden members posted about the news that President Trump had contracted the virus. They were overwhelmingly celebratory, with one member exclaiming that the president and first lady "deserve this outcome" because of "their arrogance and complete disregard for the American people." Members of the group took particular delight in posts that found humor in the situation. "Well I think the hoax just got real!" said a post that received 6,960 interactions, more engagement than any other of the 6,563 posts we analyzed in the Riden with Biden group.

For progressive groups, the American COVID-19 catastrophe was the inevitable result of broken social and political systems, one that tolerated extreme inequality, lacked universal health care coverage, and devalued the lives of poor and working-class people. On February 29, for instance, a member of "America for Bernie Sanders 2020" shared a story from *The Guardian* where a journalist cites America's "greed-driven, grotesquely unequal and cruel 'healthcare system' as being uniquely vulnerable among industrialized nations to the threat of the global pandemic." The poster commented on the headline, writing that "This is a critical reason why we need Medicare for All. This is a critical reason why we need Bernie! #PublicHealth #CorporateGreedKills #Pharma-GreedKills #MedicareForAll #BernieBeatsTrump #Bernie2020." Similarly, on March 21, 2020, in the group "Alexandria Ocasio-Cortez Progressives," a member shared an article with the headline: "The coronavirus crisis shows we need an entirely new economic system." Posts such as these typically received several hundred or thousands of interactions, significantly outperforming other content in the group.

It's notable, too, that members of progressive Facebook Groups were particularly attentive to people that were disproportionately affected by COVID-19, and were demonstrably less concerned with individual political leaders or the actions they took—or failed to take—to combat the disease. In the AOC Progressives group, members posted updates pointing out that the pandemic was hitting the poor especially hard and advocating for universal health care as a way to prevent future crises. In several posts, members in both the America for Bernie Sanders 2020 and AOC Progressives groups call attention to the fact that Blacks, Native Americans, Latinos, and immigrants were more likely to contract and die of the virus. There was nothing natural about this disaster, they insisted. It was a social and political breakdown, and it was important to name it as such.

For conservative groups, the COVID-19 crisis was a social drama that liberals were manipulating, if not manufacturing, to advance a socialist agenda and undermine President Trump's reelection campaign. At first, though, Republican groups emphasized that the virus had been engineered and unleashed by the communist regime in China as a way of gaining power over the capitalist, Western world. Within weeks, conservatives shifted to the threat of socialists within the U.S. who, they claimed, were exploiting the pandemic to seize political control. On March 8, 2020, a member of the MAGA Institute group posted, "This isn't about COVID-19. The media weaponize fear to control behavior. The vector is irrelevant. Snow. Hurricane. Virus. All the same." On July 2, another conservative member quoted from a *Breitbart* article, "Democrats want a second American revolution: a socialist one," which argued, "Democratic leftist totalitarians [are attempting] to capitalize on tumult caused by the COVID-19 pandemic to seize power." Posts like this triggered a relentless series of messages about "globalists"—a code word for Jews—who were trying to "reorder" the world. Such devious behavior, members of right-wing Facebook Groups repeatedly explain, is impossible not to see.

Like liberals, conservatives used Facebook Groups to establish their own moral standing, and to distinguish themselves from their malevolent political adversaries. A member of the "Conservative Causes Connection" Facebook Group posted a link to an article about Debra Messing, a celebrity who allegedly suggested that MAGA supporters will die of COVID-19 due to Trump's lies. "Democrats want mass deaths just so they can blame Trump. This is how sick these people are." In the group "Making America Greater Together!" a participant claimed that liberals were more calculating and determined than his conservative allies appreciated. "IT APPEARS THAT COVID-19 WAS PLANNED STRATEGY FROM THE BEGINNING . . . TO MAKE THE US HAVE THE MOST PEOPLE WITH THE VIRUS! YES, IT WAS RELEASED IN CHINA, THE FINAL DESTINATION IS AMERICA! IT CAME FROM A LAB RUN BY A LIBERAL HARVARD PROFESSOR IN CHINA!😩." Another member pushed things further, calling on "all patriots" to "BE AWARE. THIS IS THE FIRST STAGE OF THE REVOLUTION TO INSTALL THE NEW WORLD ORDER. WE HAVE TO MAKE A STAND-PATRIOTS NATION WIDE. THE GREAT AWAKENING IS HAPPENING ALL OVER THE WORLD." These messages would likely alienate those who did not already accept them, but they engaged members of groups like Making America Greater Together!, helping them find the "meaningful community" that Facebook promised to engineer. For people who shared their perspective, the platform was working. They had identified an enemy, uncovered a plot, drawn the battle lines. Now they were connected and getting organized. Eventually, they would fight back.

There were no comparable conflicts in Australia during 2020. The federal government endorsed the chief medical officer's pandemic response plan, which involved closing national borders, pubs and clubs, gyms, theaters, and entertainment venues, and limiting restaurants to takeout or delivery. It also supported each state's right to set its own local policies, even those where restrictions were particularly stringent. In late March, for instance, premier of Victoria Dan Andrews prohibited all indoor socializing of more than two people who lived in different homes, including couples in romantic relationships (though that was reversed within days), and any outdoor gathering of more than two people who did not share a household. Residents of Victoria were allowed only four reasons to leave their homes: for exercise, for food and supplies, for work or education, and for medical care or caregiving.[59] No American governor issued lockdown orders that were this severe, but President Trump denounced those, such as Andrew Cuomo, whose restrictions he deemed excessive, and governors returned the attacks in kind. Morrison, a conservative who favored more libertarian policies, refrained from such public denunciations. Although they occasionally disagreed with the prime minister, neither the leaders of Australian states and territories nor the nation's top medical officers had good reason to fight.

The country remained politically divided, with strong ideological disagreements creating contentious debates over issues such as climate change, education, labor, and immigration. Like Americans, Australians used social media to complain about their adversaries, organize mutual aid networks, rally support for their favored political party, and build community ties amid stringent lockdown and distancing measures. In Victoria, where the lockdown orders were especially restrictive, groups of libertarians used sites like Facebook and Telegram to protest against public health policies that they considered repressive. Although a journalist investigating one group discovered that its organizer had ties to the extreme right, the content of the group's messages was less incendiary than those that circulated in American far right communities, and the network was significantly less active.[60]

It helped, of course, that Australia's response to the outbreak was so effective, and that the country was one of the healthiest places to be in 2020 and beyond. (In 2022, its COVID mortality rate was one tenth the rate in the U.S.) This was not a preordained outcome. Yes, it's a large island, but so is the U.K. Australia's median age, thirty-eight, is the same as America's. It has similar levels of urbanization. It's a popular destination for tourists and business travelers from China, and it gets nearly 10 million international visitors in a typical year. But its public health policies for managing the pandemic were stronger and better executed than those in most other nations, and Australians, as surveys show, trusted that their government would get it right. "When the pandemic began, 76 percent of Australians said they trusted the health care system," *The New York Times* reported, "compared with around 34 percent of Americans."[61] Over the course of 2020, Australians' trust in the system would only grow higher; in the U.S., however, it collapsed.

Perhaps more importantly, the success they achieved, collectively, by complying with public health restrictions encouraged Australians to grow even more trustful of their fellow citizens. Some "93 percent of Australians reported being able to get support in times of crisis from people living outside their household," *The New York Times* explained, and Australians were more likely than people in other countries, including Americans, to believe that "most people can be trusted."[62] During 2020, most Australians were willing to look out for each other and respect public health orders, from mask mandates to distancing requirements and stay-at-home orders. Their pro–social behavior helped generate a virtuous circle, as opposed to the American death loop.

Compliance with the rules was by no means perfect or universal, however, and Australian states deployed police officers to reprimand, fine, and ticket those who violated restrictions. At times during 2020, and more frequently in 2021, Australians pushed back against a culture of confinement and a level of government control that so clearly broke with national norms. Had they known about Prime Minister Morrison's move to seize additional political authority during the early stage of the pandemic, they surely would have pushed back harder. They knew that people in other countries enjoyed more freedom to socialize, travel, eat out, attend sports events, and dance in clubs. It's impossible to enjoy any of these things unless you're living, however, and Australians were far more likely to be doing that at the end of 2020 than people in comparable nations. ("If the United States had the same Covid death rate as Australia, about 900,000 lives would have been saved," *The New York Times* reported, some two years into the pandemic.[63]) No one loved the sacrifices that the effort required, but nearly every family experienced the benefit. Less illness. Less death. More faith in neighbors and fellow citizens. The belief, as things got better, that they could handle the next challenge, that they were ready to move on.

CHAPTER 5

"Nothing Left to Lose"

DANIEL PRESTI

At last, 2020.

Daniel Presti, thirty-three years old, 120 pounds, with a bald head, a neat goatee, and the temperament of a bucking bronco, could hardly wait to change the calendar. The year 2019 was supposed to be a breakthrough; instead, it had been an exercise in frustration, with backbreaking work followed by endless waiting and bursts of bad news. It was hard to imagine things getting worse.

At the start of 2019, Presti and a close friend, Keith McAlarney, were planning to open a new pub, Mac's Public House, in Grant City, a quiet residential neighborhood in Staten Island, just a few miles from where Presti grew up. Presti and McAlarney had been managing a restaurant there for the previous two years, and they'd had their eyes on a dive bar nearby with a reputation for fights, prostitution, and indifferent proprietors. Presti always avoided the place, for fear of getting caught up in trouble, and he advised his staff to do the same. But he also saw potential in the site. "We always wanted to have our own little spot," Presti told me. "A neighborhood spot." The space was well located. The neighbors wanted a change and were demanding that the city shut it down. When it happened, the two friends pounced on the opportunity. All they had to do was sign a lease, fix up the bar, and line up some local support.

Presti knew how hard it could be to build his own business. In 2013, he and a college pal started Downtube, a brewery in Johnstown, New York. They had been home brewing, successfully, and they discovered how enjoyable it is to share craft work with friends. Scaling up production didn't seem like it would be too difficult. Why not try to make a living doing something they love? Leasing a building in the small town was surprisingly affordable. They did some basic math and figured that they could make decent money, maybe even more. "You hear horror stories," Presti recounted, but "we were like, 'What could go wrong?'" A lot, it turned out. It was hard to find loyal customers. The town didn't get much traffic. The bar got even less. "My buddy and I, we just started fighting every day, butting heads." Within a few years, the company's name proved prophetic, but it wasn't beer going down the tubes, it was the entire business. Presti filed for bankruptcy, and returned to Staten Island.

Back home, in 2019, Presti was convinced that things were set up for success. He and McAlarney had plenty of experience working together, and they fed off each other's energy. What's more, McAlarney had money to invest in the project. Presti would put in sweat equity, restoring the old bar, shopping for new fixtures, changing the vibe. He'd be the general manager, overseeing operations and running it like he was an owner. It was exactly what Presti wanted.

Presti lived a few miles from the new bar, with his wife, a teacher, and their three children, all under the age of four, so he could help out around the house after he woke up and work at night. He knew the people who would be his customers: the bowling league members, the local parents, the firemen and police officers and government workers who lived on the island because it was in the city, but not quite of it. "We said, 'Let's be there for the community,'" he told me. "We like them, they like us."

The relationship with the police proved important, because more than a few residents were determined not to let another bar operate in the neighborhood. Police play a big role in Staten

Island, not just in law enforcement, but in local culture and politics, because so many officers live in the borough. Presti and McAlarney needed strong advocates. They called the precinct and pitched their idea. Mac's would be an ideal tavern: A home away from home for residents and workers. A sponsor for Little League teams and softball leagues. "When we met with them, the main guy said: 'I hated the place before, but I really love you guys. We'll tell the community board that we're okay with you guys there and you have our support.'" The precinct's endorsement was exactly what they needed. Presti and McAlarney got their permit, and quickly got to work restoring the bar.

The initial plan was to open the bar in June of 2019, just as soon as the state of New York approved their proposal for a liquor license. Presti told me that they expected the process to take three months, maybe four. "Not really that long." But all they got was silence, and every time they called to ask for an update, the state gave them the same response: "We'll get to you when we get to you." Presti found the process infuriating. Here he was, a neighborhood guy, trying to open a small business, doing it responsibly, and right, and some bureaucrats in state government treat him with callous indifference, as if his livelihood didn't matter, as if he didn't, either.

The license finally arrived in November. Mac's opened late that month. It's "kind of the worst time," Presti said. The summer sports leagues were over, so there were no more postgame gatherings. On Staten Island, people hunkered down at home for Thanksgiving and spent December preparing for Christmas. Instead of a roaring start, business was quiet and slow. Still, they began to get customers, some regular, and they started to build that neighborhood tone they'd always wanted. Obviously, there would be no more illicit behavior or fighting. They didn't want ideological conflict either. "Keith and I are the furthest from political you can find," Presti told me. "We never had the news on. We don't talk politics, ever. We threw people out of the bar just for speaking politics, because of what it does to people. Yeah, do not say anything. We're not getting into it."

Some news you can't keep quiet. In December 2019, the Democrats in Congress launched impeachment proceedings against Donald Trump, a popular figure in politically conservative Staten Island, where 57 percent of voters cast ballots for him in 2016 and even more were ready to support him in 2020. Cable news on TV or not, there's no way to muzzle that conversation in a bar. There was also a story about a new coronavirus in China. It was killing people and circulating at an alarming rate. Was it coming this way, too?

The stress of the previous year had also taken a toll on Presti's personal life. He and his wife separated, and though it was amicable, divorce was expensive and painful. He'd put his own money into the redesign of the bar. He had given up the income from his previous job managing a restaurant. He needed Mac's to work.

That's when COVID arrived in New York. At first it was just a few cases. First New Rochelle, a suburb north of the city. Next, Manhattan. Close, but Staten Island is another universe. It wasn't their problem. Not yet. At first, it seemed like New York's political officials believed they could contain the virus. New York City mayor Bill de Blasio advised residents: "If you're not sick, you should be going about your life." Despite warnings from top officials in the local health department, the mayor urged healthy people to go out to bars, restaurants, and theaters. "I'm encouraging New Yorkers to go on with your lives + get out on the town despite Coronavirus," he tweeted on March 2, the day after New York City reported its first COVID case. He even issued a movie recommendation. "Thru Thurs 3/5 go see 'The Traitor' @FilmLinc. If 'The Wire' was a true story + set in Italy, it would be this film."[1]

And then the message changed. On Saturday, March 14, de Blasio declared that all bars and restaurants must close by Tuesday. "This is not a decision I make lightly," he said. "These places are part of the heart and soul of our city. They are part of what it means to be a New Yorker. But our city is facing an unprecedented threat, and we must respond with a wartime mentality."[2] Public schools, which enroll 1.1 million children, would shut down, too. On Monday, New York governor Andrew Cuomo expedited the timeline, using Twitter to announce that all in-person service in bars and restaurants had to stop by 8 p.m. that night.

For Presti, the declaration was ominous. The bar would have to close, but he came up with a new strategy. "I revamped

Mac's into a takeout, delivery spot," he told me. "We started to be known for having the best cheesesteaks on Staten Island. We kind of make it like a chopped sandwich. I don't know if it's the flat top we use, the way we put the cheese on top. All of the sudden, online, everybody said this is the spot to go to. And community was there for us. Orders started to come in, probably more than we wanted." Presti was spending his days watching the kids, his nights cooking meat in a hot kitchen, and the early morning hours making sure Mac's was clean and COVID safe. "I'm so tired," he recalled. "I'm exhausted." But what choice did he have? Presti had never worked harder, and he loved the camaraderie with McAlarney and their small staff. But now he had no liquor sales, full rent, utilities payments, and unusually high food costs. The websites that people used to order online took a hefty bite out of each sale, as much as 30 percent. "We're almost losing money every time we make something," Presti reported. "It's literally a broken system."

Initially, Presti accepted the measures. He knew COVID was serious. He didn't want to see anyone else get sick. But what began as a temporary effort to flatten the curve, a few weeks of closures, maybe a month, soon turned into something long and indefinite. "They just kept on pushing it back, pushing it. On the slower nights it would be just two of us at Mac's, and I'd be, like, 'I think they're going to do martial law.' How long can we get shut down for, without getting anything?"

They weren't the only ones asking those questions. Throughout the city, thousands of bar and restaurant owners, and even more of their employees, were growing anxious. When could they reopen? How would they make ends meet? Who would protect their interests? Did anyone in government care? Presti knew that everyone was struggling, but for bars, whose main purpose is to provide a gathering place for socializing, the threat was existential. "If you don't want the social gatherings, fine. Shut the bars down completely? Fine. But you have to do something for us. You have to give us assistance, but to do nothing? We'll all go out of business."

Eventually, Mac's did get something: According to Presti, about $4,000 in federal aid. He can't explain the number. They'd asked for more, but the bar was so new when COVID hit that they had no record of proven losses, and they had no idea how their claim would be received. The cash showed up in their account one day, without justification. "That was the only money we received in the entire pandemic," Presti said. "They gave hundreds of millions of dollars to these big corporations that didn't even need it and neglected the mom-and-pop places. And they were like, 'Whoops, we made a mistake!'"

With frustration mounting, a group of bar and restaurant proprietors in Staten Island and South Brooklyn set up the Independent Restaurant Owners Association Rescue, or IROAR, and Presti and McAlarney jumped into the campaign. "At first it was just a group to vent and ask if somebody has a cook or can't get one, and it was good," Presti recalled. "But then we had lawyers getting in touch with us."

The association began to lobby the government for help. Some members threatened lawsuits. Did the governor really have the right to keep their businesses shuttered? Didn't they deserve compensation for complying? What would happen if they refused? Presti was dubious. "It's a joke," he told me. "A joke where the punch line is 'The Restaurants Act still hasn't passed.' New York kept saying, 'We're gonna do this. We promise you there's gonna be money from us and the federal government is coming. It's just gonna be another two weeks.' But you know, they're not helping us. How are we supposed to survive?"

In June, Mayor de Blasio announced that restaurants could begin serving people in person again, but only outdoors, and Mac's didn't have any space. Governor Cuomo released a reopening plan for early July, but he postponed it, indefinitely, after seeing other states experience surges when they allowed indoor dining. As the summer went on, hundreds of city restaurants began to shutter, permanently, and the crisis for bars was even worse. Some owners served patrons on the sidewalk, only to have the State Liquor Authority crack down on them for violating social distancing rules, issuing fines, and, in some cases, suspending their license to operate. Presti couldn't get over the irony. The same state agency that needed eleven months to approve his liquor license, the officials who couldn't be bothered to explain why he couldn't open his new business and provide for his family . . . here they were, "hiring an army of people" and searching for establishments to punish and harass. "It's almost extortion," Presti said. "It got so serious, where if you came into my place at noon, just like saying hi, we would tell you, like, you got to keep moving, keep moving. If the Liquor Authority comes in, and you're just here speaking to me inside, they're gonna fine me $10,000. And this was actually happening."

Although bars and restaurants in other parts of the state were allowed to open for indoor service, in the city, Presti told me, the shutdown felt endless.[3] They were finally allowed to serve food or drinks inside on September 30, but only at 25 percent capacity. That, too, would prove short-lived. On October 6, Governor Cuomo initiated a zoned shutdown in response to spikes in various New York City neighborhoods.[4] By early November, as cases surged, de Blasio was insisting that the city reevaluate indoor dining altogether. He imposed a 10 p.m. curfew and warned that indoor service would likely be banned soon after the Thanksgiving holiday, around the one-year anniversary of Mac's opening night. Then Staten Island, which the city and state had shut down earlier in the pandemic, when COVID rates in the borough were low, turned into a hot spot. The city placed Grant City into the "Orange Zone," which meant the bar could not operate. Presti was apoplectic. This was more than he could take.

Presti felt desperate. He couldn't support his family. He didn't know how he'd pay for his car, his mortgage, his insurance, his food. He couldn't see a future, didn't know what to do. "Something had to happen," Presti told me. "And I was someone very dangerous, because I had nothing left to lose."

He and McAlarney met and decided to do something radical. They were going to reopen. Indoors. Regardless of the prohibition. Regardless of the fees and sanctions. Regardless of what would happen to their liquor license. Come what may. They told members of IROAR about the plan and tried to recruit them to do it with their places. No one was interested. Too much risk of losing their hard-won liquor licenses. Presti saw it differently. For Mac's, it was either comply with the state and go out of business, losing everything they had built, or stand up to the government and keep things open. He knew the fines would keep coming. Thousands of dollars. Tens of thousands. What did it matter? Presti had gone bankrupt before and if it happened again, so be it. He had tried to get an audience with the governor and the mayor. Neither responded. "So we said, we have to take it to an extreme now. We'll be the ones."

Presti and McAlarney understood that there was no sense taking a stand if they were going to be silent and invisible. "If we just open, the sheriff or somebody from the NYPD will come right over and shut us down before anyone notices." There was no point in that. Presti didn't know many people with strong ties to the media or experience with publicity. But he had started following Scott LoBaido, a Staten Island flag artist and self-proclaimed "patriot activist" who had been advocating for the rights of small business owners during the pandemic. Maybe he could help promote the story of Mac's on social media and around the community? "I'd met him once or twice," Presti said. "He's very controversial. He knows how to get a lot of attention. He's caught up in the political thing."

LoBaido listened to Presti's story and took in his idea about reopening despite the state prohibition. "If you're serious, I'll come there and meet you tomorrow," is what Presti remembers LoBaido saying. "One thousand percent serious," Presti replied. And he was.

The next day, November 20, LoBaido arrived at Mac's and told Presti that he had a plan. "We're going to make this an Autonomous Zone," he said. LoBaido had designed a poster that looked like a warning sign, with bold letters declaring "!ATTEN-TION!" "AUTONOMOUS ZONE" amidst blocks of white, orange, and yellow, and text declaring "We refuse to abide by any rules and regulations put forth by the Mayor of NYC and the Governor of NY State." He sent Presti to print them out at Staples, and then used thick orange tape to write AUTONOMOUS ZONE and mark the perimeter around the sidewalk in front of the bar. When Presti returned, he and Keith put the posters on the windows. "Scott went on Facebook Live with them, and basically said, 'I'm at Mac's Public House. These guys are standing up for what's right and what they believe and they don't want to get trampled on any longer.' It was about a minute. I'd never been in front of a camera before. And then he's like, 'I helped you with my part, hope the best for you, and I hope you know what you're getting into. You guys are on your own from this point on!'"

"So, that's when Keith and I got caught up in a political mess," Presti told me. Political movement would be more accurate. "Scott is a very heavy, conservative Republican," he explained. He came with a strong take on what was really threatening America in 2020. It wasn't the pandemic, but an assault on individual freedoms and a plot to turn the country into a socialist haven, with the government as a nanny state. LoBaido offered more than an interpretation of the crisis; he also brought an affect, marked by outrage and a deep sense of victimhood, that resonated with millions of disaffected Americans who felt betrayed by the government and the highly educated professional class. Most of all, he came with followers, thousands of them, in search of a cause. People who wanted to push back, open up, not wear masks, and fight. Soon, Presti said, "We've got Trump flags getting waved out front and people are like, this guy Keith and this guy Danny, they're just a bunch of Trumpers, far-right-wing guys, and they support the Proud Boys and all this. We're like, no, we're just two guys that wanted to bring attention and awareness to how bad it is for small businesses." The activists embraced them, and Presti and McAlarney embraced them right back. That, Presti said, is when "it just blew up."

In much of America, things were already out of control that November. President Trump had just lost the election to Joe Biden, but instead of conceding and helping coordinate a smooth transition of power, Trump challenged the results and tried to get other powerful Republicans to invalidate votes and keep him in power. Across America, including Staten Island and parts of New York and New Jersey, conservatives stewed in anger and, following the president, insisted that the election had been stolen or rigged. They were agitated, and primed to protest.

The Autonomous Zone got everyone to pay attention. The Sheriff's Office, which is run separately from the local police precinct, took interest, and the State Liquor Authority got more involved. Mac's started getting heavy fines on a daily basis, including one for $15,000 that, Presti said, got voided soon after it was delivered, and several others for $1,000 or more. On Friday, November 27, the Liquor Authority voted to suspend Mac's license to serve. That night, Presti opened Mac's and went on camera in the loud, crowded bar to announce that they would not pay a dime of the fines. "The Health Department has given us a closed business order. The Liquor Authority has now revoked our liquor license. . . . We're still doing things in a safe way. We're still open! . . . It doesn't seem like we can do business. So here's what we're going to do: We're going to give everything away for free! You can drink for free. You can eat for free. We just ask that you make a donation towards us."[5] Naturally, the donations poured in.

On November 30, McAlarney went on *Fox & Friends* to explain the situation. Two days later, he was invited to go on air with Tucker Carlson. With millions of Fox News viewers watching, Presti complained that the mayor and the governor had set policies unilaterally, without consulting proprietors about how they could stay open safely. "I was put against the wall. Either I took a stance and continued to open up my establishment, hoping that people spend money, so I can pay bills, and end up providing for my family. I'm so behind on bills that I really felt that I had no other choice."

"I feel for you," Carlson replied. "Turns out your white privilege isn't paying the bills automatically." He then asks McAlarney if he worries that the city and the state will come after him for taking a stand. "They're coming after me already," McAlarney said. He detailed how the Sheriff's Office had been coming to the bar to fine him for staying open despite city orders, and accused them of targeting him because he had upset the mayor. "You're a brave man, and I wish you godspeed," Carlson says. "I hope you'll come back and tell us how it goes."

It went . . . predictably. McAlarney's appearance on Fox News was fodder for social media and promotion for their cause. Advocates for "opening up New York City," including members of the extremist Proud Boys organization, flocked to Mac's, creating a spectacle of right-wing protesters shouting "I am a proud Western Chauvinist," singing "We Will Rock You!," and carrying signs saying "Don't Give Up" (a reference to Trump's attempt to overturn the election) and "DickTator Cuomo" in the largely liberal, pandemic-scarred city.

Mac's, meanwhile, remained open, and they had never had so much support. Right-wing activists throughout the region arrived at Mac's to protest. The rallies continued nightly, and the bar filled up with new patrons who were there to support the cause. Presti and McAlarney created a Facebook page, and used it, along with YouTube, to post video status updates to their growing list of followers from across the U.S. and, as their story circulated through right-wing news outlets and social media platforms, around the world. "We got overrun with people," Presti recalled. "One hundred people would show up. Everybody coming was kind of like, far-right-wing. They're like, 'No masks!'" At this point, no one was in control.

Of course, the mayor's office noticed. The police officers in Staten Island had been sympathetic to Presti and McAlarney for most of the pandemic. Before the Autonomous Zone opened, they would issue warnings for rule violations, but they rarely gave tickets or fines. After the orange tape and posters went up, officers they knew came by and implored them to take it all down. "'You can operate under the radar,'" Presti remembers them saying. "'Take all this down and we'll just drive by tomorrow. Keep driving. You can even have people inside. We don't care as long as this isn't here.' And I told them, 'You're missing the point. This is something that I have to do because no one's paying attention to us. This industry is dying right before our eyes. I can't survive. I'm not saying that this is right.' I was like, 'This is the best course of action.'"

On Tuesday, December 1, the Sheriff's Department closed down the pub and arrested Presti for multiple city and state violations. "I started the Facebook Live feed when the sheriffs came," Presti recalled. "They weren't going to arrest me that day, but I refused to leave. They looked at me and said, 'You leaving with or without cuffs?' I said 'With cuffs,' and they hung their heads. They said, 'You're really gonna make us do this?' I was like, 'Yes, you understand why.'" A crowd had assembled, and Presti used the moment to declare his refusal to comply with the forced closure. LoBaido was there with his camera, broadcasting on Facebook Live. "He's like, 'This is crazy! I want thousands of people on Staten Island. We're holding a rally!'" On Wednesday, hundreds, and by some counts more than one thousand people assembled for a rowdy demonstration that attracted local and national media. Armed sheriffs blocked the doorway to Mac's, and protesters in the police-friendly borough duly insulted them. "Where is your backbone?" one exclaimed, through a megaphone. "Where is your morality?"

Presti, who was released after spending forty-five minutes in a holding cell, returned to the pub the next day, and again each day after. By then, Mac's felt like something more than a neighborhood pub. As Presti saw things, it was a fortress, a last bastion of liberty in a state that had become hostile to everything he thought it valued. On Friday, he heard from staff members who told him that people wearing black, maybe members of antifa, they speculated, were throwing bottles at the windows and threatening violence. "For the last four years, my whole focus has been my kids and getting this bar operating," Presti told me. "I was like [antifa], I don't know who they are!"

Now Presti was getting a crash course in conflict. The pressure was crushing, the stress unbearable. He was too anxious to sleep and too agitated to eat. "I almost looked like a druggie," he told me. "I dropped almost fifteen pounds. I only weigh 120, so I usually can't afford to lose two pounds. I've been the same size since high school. People around were like, 'Danny's gotta eat something,' like 'We're getting worried about you.' I'm like, 'I can't. If I eat something, I'm literally gonna throw it up.'"

It was in this state that, early on Sunday morning, December 6, after another Saturday night of illegally serving drinks to a room full of maskless, defiant conservatives, Presti had his most explosive encounter with the authorities. The pub closed early, around 10 p.m. He and the staff stayed past midnight to clean the place, as was their custom. The sheriffs had come by earlier to issue fines and tickets, but they left right after, and the bar had stayed open without incident. Presti dismissed the staff, locked up the bar, and began walking to his car, which he had parked down the street. "I get to the corner and I auto-start the car," he told me. "All of a sudden, someone yells out, 'Hey Presti!' So I glanced over my shoulder. It's like midnight, right? And there's two people charging me. Oh my God. And I'm like, nope. My stress levels, I can't even tell you what they were. I still can't eat anything. I'm in front of a news camera every night. Jesus, people were trying to break into the bar. I thought that they were coming to kill me. And the only thing I thought was I'm not dying in the middle of the street. I'm getting home to my kids."

Presti took off running. The men, dressed in black, followed in pursuit. He got to the car first, jumped in, and slammed the door shut. "I go to shift the car and the car won't shift," he recalled. "I'm addled. And I remember that you can't shift until you hit the button." He found it, hit it, and put the car in gear. When he looked up, though, one of the men was standing in front of the car and one was beside it. He didn't want to run over anyone. Then again, he didn't want to get killed. "So I hesitated. I go slower." One of the men went up on the hood briefly, then fell off. "I get to the end of the street and there's a car that comes out of nowhere, just tries to ram my car. So now, not only are people facing me down on foot. Now we have drivers trying to run me off the road." The motion sensor on Presti's car forced it to stop, and suddenly he was surrounded. "I'm like, 'I'm dead.' Now I hear sirens, and I think they're coming to save me."

Presti said it took a moment to realize what was actually happening. The officers weren't coming to save him; they were the ones chasing him. The guy who had fallen off his hood—he was from the Sheriff's Office. A deputy. So was the guy who opened Presti's car door after they had trapped him, ripped him out, and arrested him. So were all the guys driving all the cars that were now surrounding him, too.

Although the officers later swore under oath that they had identified themselves, Presti insisted they could not have, because he never heard it. "Two people yell out my name in the middle of the night and then start charging at me. They didn't say like,

'Stop! Police!' No one announced themselves. Ever. Nobody identified themselves. Not a single person." He drove off, even with an officer in front of his car, because he thought they were about to attack him. He gave the same reason for refusing to stop when the sheriff's car tried to corner him. "It's a tan car. No lights. No sirens. Not a sheriff's car. And it tries to ram me off the road."

The officers put him in handcuffs, read him his rights, and took him to the station for booking. This time, the accusation went beyond serving liquor without a license and violating the shutdown order. The sheriffs, who told Presti that the officer he hit had broken both his legs and been placed in a hospital intensive care unit, were charging him with felony second degree assault for causing physical injury to an officer; menacing; reckless driving and endangerment; fleeing an officer; and resisting arrest.

They released Presti on bail, a controversial decision that raised the ire of advocates for racial equity in the criminal justice system. "While Mr. Presti, a white man who stands accused of assaulting a police officer with his motor vehicle, is at home with his family, able to continue operating his business and has unfettered access to his defense lawyers, thousands of equally presumed innocent Staten Islanders are sent to Rikers per year on far less serious charges," said Marie Ndiaye, an attorney with the Decarceration Project at the Legal Aid Society. His release, the organization said, was proof of a "disparate legal system that benefits white New Yorkers with means over Black and brown New Yorkers."[6]

Presti may well have gone home, but he was anything but comfortable. Nor was he presumed innocent, at least not by the national and international audiences that learned his story the next day, when television and major newspapers and social media were buzzing with accounts of the Proud Boys sympathizer on Staten Island who drove his car into an officer while resisting arrest for illegally operating a bar. The news would have been sensational under any circumstances, but the media got hold of surveillance video of the incident, beginning with Presti running away from the officers and driving his car into one of them, and ending with his arrest. Everyone with an internet connection could see that

Presti's crime looked egregious, and his guilt certain. Both the governor and the mayor condemned Presti for the act of violence. "It's repugnant to the values of any real New Yorker," Cuomo said. "You never assault a police officer. Tough guy drives his car into a police officer, nah, it's disgusting. And a coward." De Blasio was even more threatening. "Our sheriff's deputy's life was in danger because of what this guy did and it's absolutely unacceptable. He should pay very serious consequences."[7]

Presti's lawyers instructed him to maintain his silence until they could defend him in court. Privately, Presti was fuming. "They slandered me," he said. "Resisted arrest! Mowed down a deputy! Broke his legs!" The whole story was ludicrous, he told me. In the days leading up to the arrest, he had accepted the tickets, taken the fines, let the officers issue whatever charges they wanted. Why would they suddenly come after him when he's walking to his car in the middle of the night? He'd never committed a felony, never once resisted arrest. What he really couldn't understand is why they sent so many deputies and squad cars for the crackdown. "What was this Osama bin Laden, special Black Ops mission where they had to smash and grab and disappear me?" Presti asked. He only had one theory: they wanted him silenced.

In public, Presti was a pariah. It's one thing to fight for the rights of small business owners. Mowing down a cop? No one, especially not on Staten Island, is okay with that. But then Presti heard that Kenneth Matos, the deputy he hit with his car, had not broken his legs, after all. Nor had he been treated in the ICU. That story, Presti insisted, was fabricated to make him look like a monster. "Saying that he broke his legs is an outrageous, outright lie," Lou Gelormino, Presti's attorney, told the press. "If he ran over a sheriff's deputy, they would've asked for a half a million dollars in bail."[8] Something was fishy, and Presti became even more angry. His sense of persecution and contempt for the government grew.

In January 2021, Staten Island district attorney Michael McMahon brought Presti's case to a grand jury. Prosecutors charged Presti with multiple felonies, with some, like assaulting an officer, carrying heavy prison time. Ordinarily, Presti said, his attorneys would never let someone accused of a crime like that testify before a grand jury. In his case, however, they insisted that he take the stand and tell his story. They weren't worried, Presti explained, because they knew he was telling the truth. Presti gave a brief statement about what happened that night, from his perspective. "Then the prosecutor grilled me, and I was able to answer every question really clearly," he said. He went home that night and waited for the jury to deliberate. Presti's attorneys told him he'd done perfectly, but the stress was overwhelming. He hardly slept.

The next morning, the court announced that the grand jury had reached a decision. The jury dropped every charge except those related to licensing violations, but none of those worried Presti. He knew the business would go bankrupt, and he had no intention of paying the fines. What mattered was that he had been exonerated of resisting arrest and assaulting an officer. Now he could tell his story and change the way other people saw it. "I got my voice back," he told me. And he needed it. He was preparing for "a huge fight."

There were two fronts, at least, to the battle. First, Presti and McAlarney, emboldened by the jury, decided that they would fight back against the shutdown orders, challenging the city and state's legal rights to keep them closed in the pandemic, and pushing to get their liquor license restored. Second, Presti committed himself to the larger campaign against the government's public health restrictions, from shutdowns to mandates for masks and vaccines. He began speaking out more often, and more forcefully, on social media and at rallies. He got more active on Facebook, where Mac's Public House group page gained thousands of followers. In May, he set up a brand, Freedom Over Fear, that sold clothing marked with "76" or the message "Freedom Over Fear." Its website asks: "Are you tired of being pushed to the side while your Liberties are stripped away, one by one? Then welcome to the tribe. We hold our Freedoms and Liberties above all else, and realize that if we don't take a stand here, there will be nothing left to fight for. Unite with us using a unified voice and we can all stand behind. The time to be silent has passed and we will be afraid no longer." In June, he used Facebook to organize protests: "Any parents on here have their kids at JCC [the Jewish Community Center] on Manor Rd and want to join me in getting masks off kids? I need good people willing to fight alongside me. Also have no problem advocating at another school with you if you want to join the fight."

At this point, however, Presti was giving me the silent treatment. He stopped returning my phone calls and messages. I could not ask him to explain what led him to embrace the political ideology and activism that he had once rejected or what he now wanted to accomplish. A few months earlier, he had friended me on Facebook, and I suspected that he'd cut me off because he noticed we did not share the same views. I'd never learn the answer. From then on, I'd have to follow his story in other ways.

Presti had gotten active on Twitter, where he adapted his voice to suit the medium. "The Constitution tells us we can overthrow the Gov't for exactly what's going on," he wrote in April 2021. "NY Senate just passed a bill essentially making all mandates a LAW. For those who thought you would get your liberties and rights back after an 'emergency,' take a look. You never get them back. How does a mandate become a law? When there's no resistance." In August, when New York City announced a vaccine mandate for teachers, Presti tweeted: "It's just about time to nut up or shut up here in NYC. We're going to find out who really wants to fight for their freedom and what you're willing to sacrifice. This is where we make our stand. I'm all in." A few days later he directed his message to fellow parents: "School is about to start here in NY soon. If your child is healthy and you are complying with sending them in with masks, you are part of the problem. Don't tell me there are no options. We all have a choice . . . Fight back."[9]

Things had escalated all through the summer of 2021. In July, Presti and Gelormino, his attorney, announced that they were suing the sheriff and the city for "illegal conduct," including defamation and wrongful detention.[10] In August, *The New York Times* named Presti as a close friend and ally of John Matland, the medical technician who was leading a "full-blown public protest" against Staten Island University Hospital for requiring employees to get vaccinated or agree to regular COVID-19 testing. The medical workers had taken to calling themselves "the Resistance," after the rebels in *Star Wars*. They questioned the science showing that vaccines were safe and effective, complained that their civil rights were being violated, and threatened to quit or move to more permissive states, like Florida.[11] The *Times* cites Presti as the figure who established a local precedent for these tactics. Presti embraced the role.

Throughout this time, Presti maintained that he was nonpartisan. "I am neither left nor right," he tweeted in September 2021. But the positions he took were almost perfectly aligned with those of the right-wing protesters who flocked to Mac's in defense of his right to serve liquor indoors during the most dangerous stages of the pandemic. The hostility he expressed toward political officials was directed toward Democrats and progressives, beginning with de Blasio and Cuomo and going all the way up to President Biden. On Twitter, his rhetoric was indistinguishable from that of Donald Trump's most ardent supporters. "How many more rigged elections do we have to witness?" he asked. "It's all decided ahead of time. Until we all say No."[12]

In some ways, such positions are consistent with Presti's views on regulation during the pandemic. He insisted on his right, as the manager of a small business, to stay open and operate, regardless of the health risks, no matter what scientists or public health agencies prescribed. But Presti did not always take such a radical libertarian position, and certainly not when the pandemic started. In our conversations, he often asserted that a shutdown would have been acceptable had the government provided funds to keep small businesses solvent and their employees economically secure. When I asked him whether America's failure to do that in the first year of the pandemic was largely due to President Trump's policies, he quickly changed the subject.

In September, a criminal court on Staten Island dismissed seven summonses issued against Presti in December for violating the state's Alcoholic Beverage Control Law. Presti and his attorneys blasted the Sheriff's Office for prosecuting the case further. "This decision just adds more value in our quest for damages," said Mark Fonte, who is representing Presti in his lawsuit against the city. "If the sheriff wants to issue these summonses for a third time, we will amend our complaint and add a charge of malicious prosecution."[13]

On October 20, Mayor de Blasio announced that all city employees, including police, firefighters, and sanitation workers, had to be vaccinated by 5 p.m. on October 29. Those who got their first dose before then would be paid a $500 bonus, while those who did not would be placed on unpaid leave. Presti, who had let his beard run long and wild, helped lead the pack of protesters who refused to conform. "NYC is on the verge of collapse," he tweeted under a bio he'd changed to "Freedom Fighter." "We allow a tyrant to control us. 9 days until we have 100% compliant, obedient, subservient betas in every city position. I will be in the streets the next 9 days. I will be loud. I will fight for the freedoms of all. Last stand to save the city."[14]

On October 28, the day before the deadline, Presti carried trash bags to Gracie Mansion, the mayor's house on the Upper East Side of Manhattan, and stood before the cameras. "We're asking everyone to bring trash because, mainly, we're standing behind our sanitation workers and the rest of the city workers. They've been doing their part and not picking up the trash, so we're bringing it directly to the mayor's doorstep, in part, also, because he is a piece of trash."[15] For all that trouble, the mayor's day was decidedly better than that of Presti's other object of contempt. In the afternoon, Governor Cuomo was formally charged with groping a female employee's breast at the Executive Mansion, "for the purposes of degrading and gratifying his sexual desires."[16] Presti did not tweet about it.

The Twitter account @macspublichouse no longer exists, and Mac's is no longer in business. It's a free country, though, and Presti's legal team told the press that he and McAlarney are "looking for another location." They will need a new liquor license. They will also need the endorsement of the police precinct as well as the neighbors. At the moment, it may seem like a long shot. But on Staten Island, Presti is a man of the people. Some consider him a local hero, and he still has plenty of support.

"Too many people still think we worry about dying from covid," Presti tweeted in fall 2021. "Fact is we don't care, and our freedom and defending it are the most important things right now, and always. I'll gladly die before I let my kids grow up in a world where they aren't free. Battle ready. LIVE FREE OR DIE."[17]

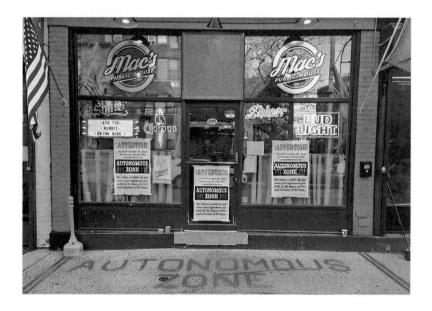

CHAPTER 6

The Meaning of Masks

On the surface, it seems so simple.

When a person suddenly confronts a dangerous new virus and there is no vaccine or medical treatment available, there is one easy way to protect oneself from infection in social spaces: wear a face mask. But the dynamics that shape social life are hardly superficial, and—as the first year of the pandemic made clear—the decision to wear a mask is anything but easy. In some parts of the world, mask mandates were adopted quickly and respected widely, without much public debate. In others, however, the question of whether, where, and when a government or business could require people to wear a mask proved contentious and divisive, inciting private objections, fiery protests, even homicidal violence. Masks, it turns out, are made of social fabric, and they are saturated with meaning. If, for some, they are fundamentally about promoting personal and collective health, for others they are about muzzling, controlling, and suppressing individual freedom, or submitting to state domination. The question is why.

Of course, culture matters. How could it not, since the concept of culture specifically refers to a group's beliefs, values, norms, and practices—the very things that determine how someone facing a risk or a rule will act. Social scientists have a long record of showing the influence of cultural factors on health behaviors. Psychologists, for instance, have published reams of research showing the differences in behavior between people whose cultural identity is marked by "collectivism," defined as "the tendency to be more concerned with the group's needs, goals, and interests than with individualistic-oriented interests," and those more influenced by "individualism," or "the tendency to be more concerned with one's own needs, goals, and interests than with group-oriented concerns."[1] These studies are analytic, not normative. They take no position on whether, as conservatives generally believe, individualism in a free market results in better conditions than does collectivism in a highly regulated economy and generous welfare state, or whether, as progressives generally believe, the reverse is true. But the studies leave little doubt that people in more collectivist groups would be more likely to wear masks during an infectious disease outbreak. In fact, we already have evidence that they did.

In 2021, a group of American and Chinese scholars led by the MIT social psychologist Jackson Lu conducted four large-scale studies of the relationship between cultural orientations and mask-wearing during the pandemic, controlling for all kinds of factors, from demographics and population density to government response stringency and time. They were interested not only in understanding cross-national differences, such as those between, say, South Korea, Germany, and Brazil, but also cross-state and cross-county differences within one particularly polarized country, the United States. The psychologists got access to three separate datasets: one based on information from 248,941 individuals representing all fifty U.S. states and 3,141 counties; one based on 16,737 individuals across fifty states; one based on 367,109 people in twenty-nine countries; and another based on 277,219 Facebook users in sixty-seven countries. The data on mask-wearing is based on self-reporting, so it's not entirely reliable. (People have a tendency to report behavior that comports with their own group's norms, even if they don't always follow them, and they also sometimes don't recall exactly how they have behaved.) But the evidence from every one of the studies established and confirmed the same core finding—and a not altogether surprising one at that: collectivism, whether at the county, state, or national level, predicts mask-wearing; individualism predicts that people are far more likely to thwart masking rules.[2]

Often, however, we label cultures with a level of generality that veers into stereotype, crudely characterizing entire populations as, say, "obedient" or "unruly," and blinding ourselves to important variations within and between them. On the question of why some groups adopt mask-wearing and others reject it, Jordan Sand, a historian of Japan at Georgetown University, argues: "The cultural explanations that newspapers have offered have relied on familiar clichés about Western and Asian attitudes towards authority and group norms." Sand condemns the way that Western pundits crudely lump together nations across the Pacific Rim, noting that "the pandemic has actually revealed profound differences among Asian societies." In Japan, for instance, surgical masks were used widely before and during the pandemic, yet "neither obedience to authority nor collective reasoning seems to have much to do with why people wear them."[3] Instead, historical experiences more distinct to Japan, from the association of masks with biomedical progress to the notion that facial covering is an easy and efficient way to preserve health, lie behind their widespread adoption.

History, more generally, plays a crucial role in shaping the cultural meanings of masks. Since the COVID-19 pandemic began, medical anthropologists have emphasized the importance of direct experience with infectious disease outbreaks in evincing the value of masks for personal and public health. The anthropologist Christos Lynteris reports that face masks for reducing the spread of infectious diseases were invented in 1910 and 1911, during the Manchurian plague, and adopted not only as "personal protective equipment" but also as symbolically powerful objects that produced "a categorical transformation of their wearers into 'reasoned' subjects of hygienic modernity." The use of masks, he explains, became "ritualized" into epidemic control efforts, at once "a supposedly foolproof way of halting airborne plague-related contagion" and visual and material "proof" of Chinese scientific achievement and of a supposedly unified Chinese population, committed to the cause of combating disease.[4] By the Great Influenza pandemic of 1918–19, the mask would distinguish Chinese society from those that lacked its cultural virtues. It was a mark of distinction, particularly against societies in the West. So, too, was China's resilience. Although the country was affected by influenza, the authors of a historical study published in the *International Journal of Infectious Diseases* report that "it was relatively mild and less lethal than elsewhere in the world, despite the generally poor levels of health at that time."[5]

In other nations, the commitment to combating infectious disease with facial coverings ebbed and flowed during the tumultuous twentieth century, rising during the Great Influenza pandemic and falling as world wars and other new threats emerged. Roughly 50 million people died of flu between 1918 and 1919, but even that was not enough to inspire universal support for mask-wearing. In the United States, where 675,000 people perished, mask mandates sparked anger and resistance. "By the fall of 1918, seven cities—San Francisco, Seattle, Oakland, Sacramento, Denver, Indianapolis and Pasadena, Calif.—had put in effect mandatory face mask laws," the medical historian Howard Markel told *The New York Times*. "As bars, saloons, restaurants, theaters and schools were closed, masks became a scapegoat, a symbol of government overreach, inspiring protests, petitions and defiant bare-face gatherings."[6] Although the protests were nowhere near as widespread as they were in 2020, they generated considerable press coverage and undermined efforts to mount a united public health campaign. Moreover, as the historian Brian Dolan recounts, the groups that organized to fight mask mandates established precedents for framing facial coverings as instruments for "muzzling" and depriving Americans of "freedom and liberty."[7] Their rhetoric became part of the American cultural repertoire, readily available when government attempted to require masks again.

The United States had no need to attempt a mask mandate during the outbreak of the coronavirus SARS-CoV-1 in 2003, because the nation recorded only eight confirmed cases. In other countries, however, the SARS experience proved transformative, generating new policy initiatives for controlling infectious diseases and teaching civilians that facial coverings could protect them. There were several reasons that SARS proved so alarming. Typically, coronaviruses produce only mild to moderate upper-respiratory-tract illnesses; but SARS-CoV-1 was terrifyingly lethal, with an overall case fatality rate around 10 percent and far higher fatality rates for the elderly.[8] It was also worrisomely contagious. Health officials learned this on February 21, 2003, when Liu Jianlun, a sixty-four-year-old doctor from Guangdong, China, where SARS-CoV-1 originated, spent the night in a Hong Kong hotel. Liu became ill that evening, and in the following days eight cases of SARS were linked to hotel guests who had stayed on the same hotel floor, some of whom would carry it on flights to Singapore, Toronto, and Hanoi. Soon after, Hong Kong had more cases than any nation except for China, where the virus originated.[9]

"SARS," the WHO reported, "travelled more widely, swiftly, and lethally than any other recent new disease so far." Whereas, HIV/AIDS "took two decades to cover the globe," and Ebola and the "new Asian diseases, caused by the Nipah and Hendra viruses have not travelled extensively," SARS infected at least 8,456 people across thirty countries, and resulted in 809 deaths between February and June 2003.[10] "SARS is the first new disease to show the damage possible in a globalized world," said the author of the WHO's health updates. "Symbolized by the image of masked faces, SARS struck fear into the public across the globe, triggering drastic measures: mass quarantine in hospital wards enforced by armed guards, infectious passengers hauled off planes, and closed businesses and schools."[11]

Fortunately, SARS-CoV-1 was not quite as contagious as scientists feared—and not nearly as communicable as SARS-CoV-2. Although asymptomatic and pre-symptomatic individuals could transmit the disease, people with clear symptoms of the SARS disease were far more likely to infect others, and hospitals, working in close collaboration with government health agencies, could identify and isolate them. By July 2003, the outbreak was effectively contained. "SARS changed the world," the WHO claims. But some places changed considerably more than others.[12]

Nations that were geographically close to China were deeply affected by the epidemic, as were those in more distant countries, such as Canada, where misfortune delivered an unexpectedly high number of cases. In East Asia, the Columbia University sociologist Gil Eyal writes, a set of "experts who enjoy more prominence and trust than others" came out of the crisis as "SARS Heroes," scientists and public health officials who "accumulated credibility"—not only by successfully combating the virus, but also by challenging China's false claim, in the early stages of the outbreak, that the virus was not especially dangerous.[13] The work of SARS Heroes was important because it transformed the epidemic experience into a set of specific historical lessons and shared memories that leaders could invoke in policy debates and in future events. When SARS-CoV-2 arrived in early 2020, several East Asian health officials warned that "SARS is back." Their expertise commanded respect.

When news about the novel coronavirus that caused COVID-19 trickled out in early 2020, leaders throughout East Asia advised civilians to wear face masks for protection, and the spike in consumer demand for masks in nations hit hard by SARS led to dire shortages. China is the world's largest manufacturer of N95 masks, and demand there was so great that importers feared that Beijing would block exports. Other nations, including some that had initially donated masks to China due to humanitarian considerations, quickly threatened to do the same.[14] In February and March, governments across East Asia pushed manufacturers to accelerate production of face masks, and implemented plans for mass distribution as well. Japan delivered reusable cloth masks to more than 50 million households, free of charge.[15] South Korea and Taiwan shipped masks to local pharmacies, which rationed them to families in the area while also offering advice about the importance of physical distancing and contact tracing.[16] The policy goal was to provide universal access to the basic tools of infectious disease prevention. Masks were not the only resources available, but in this region, at least, officials and civilians were convinced that they were essential.

The World Health Organization, a specialized agency of the United Nations founded in 1948 to manage global health challenges, could have helped to promote this message when the

COVID crisis was emerging, particularly in places where widespread use of face masks during virus outbreaks was less common. Surprisingly, however, it did the reverse. During the first months of the outbreak, WHO leaders—concerned that shortages in the global supply of masks would leave medical providers without them, confused about whether the disease could be spread through aerosols or droplets, and lacking empirical evidence that facial coverings were reducing the spread of COVID—consistently expressed doubt that mask-wearing would protect people from the virus during ordinary social interactions. Some even suggested that, when used improperly, facial coverings could do harm.[17]

Instead, the organization used its influence to emphasize that the situation appeared ordinary and manageable. On January 5, 2020, when WHO reported on "cases of pneumonia of unknown etiology" in Wuhan, it also noted that "pneumonia is common in the winter season." Although there were already cases of infected people who did not have direct exposure to the wet market in Wuhan, the WHO had no capacity to independently assess claims that the pneumonia might be caused by a novel coronavirus that would spread across the human population. "Based on the preliminary information from the Chinese investigation team, no evidence of significant human-to-human transmission and no health care worker infections have been reported," it explained. "WHO advises against the application of any travel or trade restrictions on China based on the current information available on this event."[18]

One week later, on January 12, WHO reported that China had identified the genetic sequence of a new, potentially lethal coronavirus. Again, however, it amplified Beijing's advice that visitors and residents take only routine cautions. "The government reports that there is no clear evidence that the virus passes easily from person to person," the organization explained. "No case . . . has been reported elsewhere other than Wuhan."[19] Days later, cities across China and countries throughout the world announced that they, too, had cases of COVID-19, and in the following weeks the numbers soared. On January 22, members of the WHO's Emergency Committee convened via teleconference to decide whether to declare the outbreak a Public Health Emergency of International Concern, or PHEIC. The stakes were enormous. WHO defines PHEIC as "an extraordinary event which is determined to constitute a public health risk to other States through the international spread of disease and to potentially require a coordinated international response," and it applies the term only when a situation is "serious, sudden, unusual or unexpected; carries implications for public health beyond the affected State's national border; and may require immediate international action."[20] That day, the WHO reported, "members of the Emergency Committee expressed divergent views on whether this event constitutes a PHEIC," and Tedros Adhanom Ghebreyesus, the Ethiopian doctor serving as director-general, decided not to sound the alarm. Instead, WHO advised governments to "be prepared for containment, including active surveillance, early detection, isolation and case management, contact tracing and prevention of onward spread."[21]

The WHO's decision not to declare a PHEIC drew criticism from international observers, who worried that the organization was involved in infectious disease diplomacy, uncritically accepting China's public relations efforts—perhaps in hope of gaining access to Chinese laboratories and medical data, perhaps in hope of staving off panic or xenophobia—rather than guiding a global public health response. The Council on Foreign Relations blog accused Director-General Tedros of being an "outspoken advocate for the Chinese government's COVID-19 response," because he had "commended China for 'setting a new standard for outbreak control' and praised the country's top leadership for its 'openness to sharing information' with the WHO and other countries."[22] Clearly Beijing had done neither. When the Emergency Committee reconvened on January 30, there were more than twelve thousand suspected cases of COVID-19 in China, and confirmed cases in eighteen other countries as well. This time, the director-general decided that "the outbreak now meets the criteria for a Public Health Emergency of International Concern." The WHO noted that the declaration "should be seen in the spirit of support and appreciation for China, its people, and the actions China has taken on the front lines of this outbreak, with transparency, and, it is to be hoped, with success."[23] The decision initiated the sweeping global response that many had been waiting for, but it still did not involve a recommendation on masks.

New COVID-19 cases and deaths rose ominously in February and March, especially in the U.S. and Europe, where public health agencies were reluctant to initiate extensive lockdowns, testing, and tracing efforts, and people were unaccustomed to wearing masks. In the U.S., members of the Trump administration ridiculed nonpharmaceutical interventions. Surgeon General Jerome Adams tweeted: "Seriously people—STOP BUYING MASKS! They are NOT effective in preventing general public from catching #Coronavirus."[24] During this fateful period, facial coverings were ubiquitous in East Asia but largely unavailable in Western nations, except in their various Chinese, Korean, and Vietnamese neighborhoods, where local suppliers who regularly purchased food and commercial products from Asia were now ordering masks as well. Health officials across East Asia were puzzled and concerned about the rejection of masks in other parts of the world. In an interview with *Science*, George Gao, director of the Chinese Center for Disease Control and Prevention, argued that "the big mistake in the U.S. and Europe, in my opinion, is that people aren't wearing masks. This virus is transmitted by droplets and close contact. Droplets play a very important role—you've got to wear a mask, because when you speak, there are always droplets coming out of your mouth. Many people have asymptomatic or presymptomatic infections. If they are wearing face masks, it can prevent droplets that carry the virus from escaping and infecting others."[25]

As late as March 30, however, WHO leaders maintained their skepticism. "There is no specific evidence to suggest that the wearing of masks by the mass population has any potential benefit," said Dr. Mike Ryan, executive director of the WHO Health Emergencies Programme, during a press event in Geneva, Switzerland. "In fact, there's some evidence to suggest the opposite in the misuse of wearing a mask properly or fitting it properly." The claim sparked widespread criticism, though, because it hinged on the notion that evidence about the protective value of masks in other viral outbreaks, including SARS, should not inform public health guidelines for COVID. WHO was rejecting the precautionary principle, and insisting that only established scientific research on what was, after all, a novel disease, could justify a policy push for masks.

At this point, officials in some parts of Europe and the U.S. had decided to ignore WHO and issue clear mask recommendations or requirements. In March, the Czech Republic and Slovakia became the first two European nations to impose mask mandates in public settings, despite the fact that masks themselves were in short supply.[26] In early April, Laredo, Texas, was the first U.S. city that threatened fines for anyone baring their face in public, and other cities, including New York and Los Angeles, urged residents to keep their faces covered in shared spaces as well.[27] It was not just logic that suggested masks would likely work about as well for the new coronavirus as they had for other airborne viruses; early research findings, as well as epidemiological trends on the relatively modest spread of COVID in East Asia, offered additional support for this view. So, too, did the precautionary principle, since, for any given individual or society, the potential benefits of wearing a mask far outweighed the potential harm.

From the WHO's perspective, though, the most significant risk of issuing a mask recommendation was that, in the early stage of the pandemic, the global supply was woefully inadequate. When Ryan explained the organization's opposition to mask mandates on March 30, for instance, he quickly jumped from concerns about efficacy and emphasized, instead, an anxiety that was far more difficult to dismiss: "We have a massive global shortage," he reported. "Right now, the people most at risk from this virus are frontline health workers who are exposed to the virus every second of every day. The thought of them not having masks is horrific."[28] This argument resonated among political officials and public health leaders in Western nations. "You don't want to take masks away from the health care providers who are in a real and present danger of getting infected," said Anthony Fauci, a member of the White House COVID-19 Response Team.[29] It was an indisputable point.

By April, however, another indisputable point about SARS-CoV-2 pushed the U.S. Centers for Disease Control and Prevention, along with health agencies in other parts of the world, to break from WHO guidelines and adopt strong mask recommendations. The virus, as a team of scientists reported in *The New England Journal of Medicine*, was not only being transmitted by droplets. It was also spreading through aerosols, which are comparably infinitesimal, and they can travel on air currents for hours without weakening.[30] What's more, new research established that asymptomatic people were spreading the virus, which made masking up even more essential for reducing transmission—particularly in places like the U.S., where testing capacity was limited and only sick people could get one.

On April 3, the CDC officially changed its guidelines. The agency was still concerned about the short supply of medical masks, but now it advised all Americans aged two and above to wear nonmedical fabric or cloth face coverings whenever they were in public.[31] That day, President Trump appeared before the press for a coronavirus briefing and delivered the news. "The CDC is announcing additional steps Americans can take to defend against the transmission of the virus," he said. "From recent studies we know that the transmission from individuals without symptoms is playing a more significant role in the spread of the virus than previously understood. So, you don't seem to have symptoms and it still gets transferred. In light of these studies, the CDC is advising the use of nonmedical cloth face covering as an additional voluntary public health measure." Immediately, however, Trump undermined the message. "So it's voluntary, you don't have to do it. They suggested for a period of time, but this is voluntary." He paused for a beat, then clarified his position: "I don't think I'm going to be doing it," he acknowledged, and then, minutes later, "I'm choosing not to do it."[32]

Trump's declaration marked a turning point in the U.S. debate about face masks. Before then, Americans, like so many people in the West, were largely confused about the benefits of masks for staving off COVID. Their attitudes were inconsistent, as were their behaviors, especially since masks were so hard to find. In March, for instance, the market data firm Statista had surveyed 1,986 adults about their views on masks, and found that 49 percent of Americans "believed that face masks were very or somewhat effective for preventing the spread of the coronavirus," 42 percent "believed that face masks were not very effective or not at all effective," and 8 percent had no opinion or did not know.[33] When Statista released the report, they provided no information about how political party identification affected people's beliefs about masks. At the time, it seemed irrelevant: Why would someone's political preference affect their perspective on the health benefits of a mask?

The president's public rejection of the CDC's mask recommendation changed everything. In the following days and weeks, Trump and his allies made a point of flouting the federal government's own guidelines. Soon, refusing to wear a mask became a litmus test of every Republican's fidelity to the administration, and the White House was monitoring the situation. Trump and his cabinet members proudly bared their faces in public settings, including a Honeywell factory that produced PPE and a Ford plant in Detroit. In late April, Vice President Mike Pence, who led the White House COVID-19 Response Team, took this symbolic display of defiance to another level, spurning hospital policy and refusing to wear a mask during a tour of the Mayo Clinic, where he spent time alongside medical staff and a patient.[34] Pence was the only person in the medical facility who visibly ignored its mask mandate. Television crews captured the moment and projected it onto screens across America. The message that the vice president conveyed was unmistakable: the administration did not care what the nation's leading medical doctors, scientists, and public health officials had to say about the benefits of face masks, nor would they respect local rules.

By late spring, American public opinion on masks grew politicized and divided. New Facebook Groups organized around the mask controversy quickly gained followers. An article in *PLOS* by scholars from the University of Oregon shows that, in April and May, debates about masks on social media became contentious and heated, with exponential growth in pro-mask and anti-mask hashtags on Twitter and "sharp rhetorical polarization" creating an adversarial climate online.[35] The conflicts were hardly limited to the internet. Americans with and without masks glared at each other in public settings, judging, trading insults, ratcheting up the hostility in what was already a tense election year. By summer, surveys from Pew Research show, Americans' views on a variety of public health issues that were widely accepted in the early stages of the pandemic—including distancing, school closures, restrictions on public gatherings, and face coverings—were hardening along partisan lines.[36] That's also when news media began reporting on an alarming trend, apparent in supermarkets, gas stations, and transit hubs across America: disagreements about masks were leading to violence.

The United States was not the only country where people disagreed about the benefits of facial coverings during the first year of the pandemic, but in no other nation were disputes over mask-wearing so frequent and ferocious, nor was political identity so salient. Consider England, where levels of self-reported mask use in July 2020 were startlingly low. That month, data from the market research company YouGov showed a mere 38 percent of British people said they wore masks in public, compared to 90 percent of Singaporeans, 88 percent of Spaniards, 83 percent of Italians, and 73 percent of Americans.[37] The numbers suggest that Britain was primed for ideological battles over facial covering, but ideology proved not to be a major source of tension. Research by the London School of Economics professors Chris Anderson and Sarah Hobolt showed that in Britain political partisanship was not driving public opinion about the value of masks. "The major parties have been far more aligned in their messaging on masks than they have in the US," they report. "It is therefore not surprising that we find near-identical levels of willingness to wear masks among partisans of different stripes in Britain."[38] Mask-wearing was far from universal, but the Britons who wore them were as likely to be Tory as Labour. Contrast that with the U.S., where a YouGov survey from the same month, July, indicated that 89 percent of Democrats would support a mask mandate, compared to just 51 percent of Republicans.[39]

In the summer of 2020, as Americans grew absorbed in fiercely contested national and state elections, political leaders seized upon the face mask as a totemic symbol of their core principles. "Totemism," the sociologists Émile Durkheim and Marcel Mauss explain, "is, in one aspect, the grouping of men into clans according to natural objects," and "it is also, inversely, a grouping of natural objects into accordance with social groups."[40] For Democrats, the mask became a mark of social solidarity, mutual obligations, shared responsibilities, human decency, linked fate. Democratic political candidates, including Joe Biden and Kamala Harris, donned masks in their public appearances and political advertisements (as did some Republican candidates who believed masks worked or were trying to win over swing voters in contested elections). On social media, liberals and progressives mounted a grassroots campaign to promote facial covering, changing their profile picture to display an image of their own masked face, or putting hashtags such as #WearAMask in their bios. For conservatives, it was hard to see this as anything but virtue signaling. Judging, shaming, and shunning those who refused to wear a mask became commonplace. Instagram accounts featuring photographs of Americans flouting mask mandates emerged. What mask advocates perceived as righteous concern about the public health risks of rule violations and the reckless behavior of selfish neighbors, mask skeptics experienced as condescension.

For Republicans, the mask was a mark of repression, submission, and social control by a corrupt regulatory state intent on muzzling individual freedoms, a sign of weakness and fear. Political candidates showed their solidarity with President Trump by refusing masks and mocking those who endorsed them. On social media, conservatives reappropriated the language of liberal adversaries, with hashtags saying #MyBodyMyChoice and, to slight the activists rallying for Black Lives Matter in the wake of George Floyd's murder, #ICantBreathe. A new batch of empirical studies offered powerful evidence that face masks were, as the authors of an influential article in the journal *Proceedings of the National Academy of Science* put it, "the most effective means to prevent interhuman transmission," and that "this inexpensive practice, in conjunction with simultaneous social distancing, quarantine, and contact tracing, represents the most likely fighting opportunity to stop the COVID-19 pandemic."[41] The accumulated evidence was enough to persuade WHO to finally change its position and recommend mask use in public.[42] But prominent conservatives ignored this advice, and right-wing media outlets repeatedly attacked mask mandates and mask advocates as anti-American, or worse.

Consider the words of Fox News talk show host Tucker Carlson, whose opening commentary on an edition of his nightly television program was the basis for an article he wrote on the Fox News website, titled "The Cult of Mask-Wearing Grows, with No Evidence That They Work," with the subhead "Our Leaders Think They Are Holy Amulets Protecting Us from Disease. Why?" Carlson began his case against masks by associating them with violent criminals and racists. "What kind of person covers his face in public? Armed robbers do that sort of thing. So do Klansmen and radical Wahhabis. The rest of us don't." He recalled the history of Americans who protested against masks during the Great Influenza pandemic, and claimed that "a study found that compulsory mask use likely had no effect on curbing the Spanish flu." Carlson cited studies that, in his telling, demonstrated the folly of mask-wearing for COVID protection, and quoted officials, including Anthony Fauci, who had advised Americans against wearing masks in the early stage of the pandemic, but then changed their story. All of this, he concluded, revealed the inherent deceitfulness and illegitimacy of government and government scientists. They were corrupt and power-hungry. They should not be trusted. "To pretend that you are speaking God's word and rearrange our society on the basis of that and never acknowledge that you were completely wrong, that your assumptions were false, that's the definition of dishonesty. It's also the hallmark of the people who lead us. They know nothing."[43]

In this political environment, public encounters between masked and unmasked Americans were loaded with potential for conflict, as if each face were a uniform, and everyone knew their side. The stakes of this division are apparent in one of the more peculiar artifacts of the pandemic, the vast record of viral videos documenting what the talk show host Howard Stern called "Face Mask Freak Outs" from public settings—including supermarkets, coffee shops, convenience stores, and airplanes—across the United States. "I've made it clear: I can't stand seeing people walking around without a mask," Stern said on his June 16, 2020, program. "This is what we're dealing with." He then played a compilation of video clips that had gone viral on social media during previous weeks, as businesses issued mandatory mask requirements. In one, from Florida, a maskless man in a tank top shouts and makes threatening gestures at a grocery store worker who denies him entry. "You are in violation of my fucking constitutional rights and my civil rights! I've already fucking warned you! I'm filing a fucking class action lawsuit! . . . You're terrorists!" Another clip shows a man being led out of a Giant Eagle store in Pennsylvania. "I have a doctor's note!" he yells. "I'll sue you!" Clips of angry white women follow. One complains: "There's so much research that says we are actually in danger of having this mask. I'm breathing my own CO_2. Do you understand?" In Trader Joe's, a woman taunts fellow shoppers: "A 99 percent survival rate and you're all wearing masks, like sheep!" A masked man pushing his cart turns and gives her the finger. "Just so you don't think I'm being an asshole," Stern says, "there were over 17,000 new coronavirus cases yesterday. I mean come on, what are we doing?"[44]

Occasionally, the conflicts turned violent. In Alabama, an off-duty officer at Walmart "body-slammed" a female customer for refusing to wear a mask. In New Jersey, a young woman threw an older woman to the ground, breaking her leg, after the older woman asked her to wear her mask correctly. Tens of millions of people watched, commented on, and shared these videos during 2020. At a time of lockdowns, shutdowns, quarantines, and distancing, watching clips of bitter conflicts over mask-wearing quickly became a common way of sharing the pandemic experience. Through face-off videos, Americans came together, one screen at a time, and collectively observed their society splintering apart.

What cultural values and political issues gave fuel to these fights over facial coverings? Melina Sherman and I analyzed hundreds of recorded conflicts over masks in public settings, and identified four deep sources of disagreement that intensified these disputes. First, and perhaps more fundamentally, is the tension between individual liberty and shared responsibility. Conservative and liberal Americans have sharply different views of where the balance lies. Second are the wildly divergent ideas about what the U.S. Constitution allows people to do. Conservatives make direct appeals to the document as a cultural and legal justification for the right to act as they wish, and often buttress their claims with threats to sue a business or worker; liberals deny their interpretation. Third, parties to mask disputes mobilize sharply different ideas about what "the science really shows" to justify their behavior, with pro-mask and anti-mask actors expressing genuine conviction that they understand what's true and what's false about stopping the virus. Fourth, when confronted with demands to cover their faces, a surprising number of white Americans explicitly assert that their racial and national identity gives them the privilege to act as they like. When the person asking them to mask up appears to be not white, these assertions are made more forcefully, escalating the conflict.

These tensions are on display in a video shot in early July 2020 when Teri Hill, a white woman, allegedly removed her mask to speak to a staff member at a Home Depot in Illinois. After doing so, she was quickly confronted by Sydney Waters, another white female shopper, who asked Hill to put her mask back on. According to Waters, her comment caused Hill to explode, ripping Waters's mask off and threatening to cough on Waters. Hill also allegedly hit Waters, causing her to fall to the floor. The video, which went viral almost immediately after its publication on Facebook (and had 1.6 million views on YouTube by November 2020), is filmed following this initial tussle, with both women in a phone-to-phone standoff, devices held defiantly in front of their faces as they film one another. In a shaky voice, Waters demands, "Tell me how you cough on people again . . ." Hill laughs and raises her middle finger.[45]

After a few more exchanges, Waters tells Hill that taking off her mask is "disrespectful to everyone else in the store" and that her "entitlement" to do so is "disgusting." Continuing to film her opponent, Hill agrees. "Yes," she explains, "I am entitled. I'm white. I'm a woman." Waters, clearly shocked, asks Hill, "What does you being white have to do with you being able to get your way?" Hill replies, "'Cause I'm a white woman. That's what happens." Waters balks, offended by Hill's response. "You're a disgusting, racist piece of trash, literally." Hill is unfazed. "I believe in white power," she states. Waters, now furious, advances toward Hill. "White power!? You believe in fucking white power?" As she nears Hill, the other woman strikes her. According to other sources, the confrontation ended with both women on the ground. Hill was charged with battery and disorderly conduct.

Another viral video, from a Starbucks in California, features a young white woman denouncing a Black barista who serves her but asks her to wear a mask. "I know you're discriminating against me because I'm a Trump supporter," she exclaims, before shouting, "It's a hoax. I don't have to wear a mask and I'm not going to wear a mask! This is America!" The barista remains polite, even friendly, but she insists that the customer leave. The woman does, but she immediately turns around, agitated, reenters the shop, and screams, "Fuck Black Lives Matter!"[46]

Race and whiteness are also brought to the fore in the mask confrontation videos made in smaller shared spaces, including the inside of private car services such as Uber and Lyft. In one widely circulated video, a white man enters a Lyft without a mask. The driver, who is Latino, politely asks him if he has a mask that he can put on. The man says he doesn't, and the driver asks him to pull the top of his shirt up to cover his mouth. The man refuses, but places his palm over his mouth instead. After a minute of driving, the passenger tells the driver that he has made a wrong turn, and that he should go left unless he wants "to drive around all night with me without a mask." He pauses, then shouts, "I don't like you!" at the driver. The driver, surprised, asks if he would like to exit. The man shrugs and says no, but the driver pulls over anyway, announcing that the trip has ended. "I'm not getting out right now!" the man exclaims. "I've got a contract with you." "Nope," the driver refutes. "Your contract ends now."[47]

The two men go back and forth for a while, with the passenger saying that he is entitled to both his contract and to free speech while the driver waits for him to leave the vehicle. "I could just fucking crush your fucking skull," the man says. The driver tells him that he is on video, and the man begins to mock his accent. "You got bee-dee-yo? You got bee-dee-yo? You ever

take English classes?" The driver responds, "Did you take mor-
als classes?" The passenger scoffs. "Where are you from, *boy*,"
he asks. When the driver responds, "The U.S.," the passenger
does not believe him. "No you're not. You're a fucking wetback."
The driver looks back. "And *you* are?" The man smiles. "I'm an
American, motherfucker."

It's remarkable, how often people who refused to respect mask
mandates in private business insisted that being American gives
them the right to bare their faces in public. "I'm an American!
This is fucking America! I don't have to do this shit!" a Walmart
shopper insists, after an employee asks him to use a facial covering. In a Costco, an unmasked shopper who insists on this same
right threatens to publicly shame the worker who's trying to
enforce the store's mask mandate, raising his camera and telling
the employee that his act will be witnessed by some "three thousand Instagram followers." The employee, in response, smiles
into the camera. "Hi everyone! I work for Costco, and I'm asking
this member to put on a mask because that is our company policy.
So either wear the mask or—" The shopper interrupts him and
turns the camera back on himself. "And I'm not doing it, 'cause
I woke up in a free country!" He declares his position to the
small crowd that has assembled for the spectacle. "I'm not a fucking sheep."[48] Another video involves a parade of anti-maskers,
marching through a mall during the holiday shopping season and
chanting, cacophonously, protests of all varieties. "USA! USA!"
"This is America!" "You don't have to wear it! It's not a law!" The
leader carries an American flag. One demonstrator hoists a plac-
ard saying, "This is not China!"

The clashes over masks played out along the social fault lines that
shape life in contemporary America, but the tremors that made
the nation's divisions so consequential were activated by political
leaders, sustained by influential voices in the media, and amplified by social media, which is so often a radicalizing force in public disputes. What distinguishes America's experience with mask
controversies is not that so many American people refused to use
facial coverings; for the first six months of the pandemic, Ameri-

cans were actually more likely to report that they wore masks in public settings than were Australians, Brits, and Germans.[49] Nor is it that people in the U.S. felt uniquely emboldened to protest mandates in the name of individual rights and liberties; Australians, Brits, Canadians, and Germans organized demonstrations against mask requirements and other public health restrictions, too.[50] But the U.S. was exceptional in the extent to which the mask became a symbolic weapon in the nation's raging culture war, a battle which, in 2020 at least, had enormous political stakes.

Politics, not mere cultural differences, made the mask such a potent source of disagreement in America's first plague year. Political leaders and the media outlets that lobbied for them invested masks with deep meaning, transforming them from flimsy medical devices into totemic markers of partisan identity and ideology. President Trump played the leading and decisive role in this project, from the initial press conference when he insisted that he would not follow the very same CDC mask guidelines that he was announcing to his routine practice of mocking everyone who wore a facial covering, including Joe Biden, and expressing doubt that masks worked.[51] Unlike England, where the Conservative Party never fully embraced Boris Johnson's initial mask skepticism, in the U.S., most influential voices on the right amplified Trump's anti-mask position. When liberals and progressives countered by publicly endorsing the use of facial coverings and respecting the CDC's guidelines, they effectively elevated the mask's symbolic significance.

By the time of the presidential election, the mask had become a cardinal feature of American politics and culture. No matter how light in substance, in the U.S., the mask carried considerable weight.

CHAPTER 7

"Something's Missing in My Soul"

ENUMA MENKITI

Enuma Menkiti hasn't sung in ages. "Something's missing in my soul," she said.

Before the pandemic, her choir, Peace of Heart, rehearsed weekly, sometimes more, and did regular performances at nursing homes, hospices, homeless shelters, community centers. "We did uplifting music," she told me. "Beatles songs. Stevie Wonder. Feel-good stuff. We'd go to places where there were either older people or sick people. It was a nice way to be part of the city, to help people feel some joy."

The joy of connection. The chorus that gets everyone singing, maybe even on their feet. That feeling that you're with your people, together, raising each other up. Those are the things that brought Menkiti to Brooklyn in 2005, when she was in her mid-twenties. She grew up biracial in Boston, with a white mother and a Black father who taught philosophy at Wellesley College. They owned a poetry bookstore and filled their home with music. "I learned to sing and play the viola," Menkiti told me. "The arts are in our blood." Her parents were not wealthy, but they helped her get a scholarship to a prestigious private school in Newton, and education became a springboard. A bachelor's degree from Williams College. They were prestigious, beautiful places, but their overwhelming wealth and whiteness make them feel a bit isolating. At Williams, Menkiti became vice president of the Black Student Union, joined the minority coalition and the Gospel Choir. She developed close relationships, but she told me that, as a Black student in a small elite college, "you feel like you're a little out of touch with your full self, kind of like, performing all the time."

In her last year at Williams, Menkiti was selected for Teach for America and assigned to a public school in Jersey City. She lived there for four years—three of them while teaching, and the fourth when she started graduate school in education at Columbia University. "I liked Jersey City, but it could be rough back then," she explained. "There were good blocks and bad blocks, and gangs that were a little too close." On the weekends, Menkiti and her friends would go to Brooklyn. "We'd go to music and poetry readings, museums and parks. One thing I loved is that there were just all kinds of Black people. Caribbeans. Africans. African Americans. Multiracial people. All these Black experiences, all this culture. I felt connected to the people. I ended up moving there. It felt like being home."

It didn't take long to settle into Brooklyn, but settling into adult life was a longer process. Menkiti spent her twenties and early thirties the way most New Yorkers do, searching for her people, the right neighborhood, the right job. One night, on a dating app, she began chatting with a man named Persol. "Normally you meet someone online and they ask you out for drinks or something," she told me. "But it seemed like he hadn't really done it much, because he'd just send me messages like, 'Hi!' or 'How you doing today?' Maybe he was just curious, but he wasn't trying to make anything out of it." Menkiti let the conversation keep going. One day, when Persol asked what she was up to, Menkiti told him that she was going to Prospect Park for a Femi Kuti concert. "He was like, 'I'm on my way there as well!' So we met at the bandshell. Over Afrobeats music! Very appropriate, and we ended up dating from there."

Music was at the heart of their connection. He played saxophone and loved jazz; she was still singing and playing viola whenever she could. They practiced, went to concerts, listened to the stereo. It didn't take long to find a common groove. Inevitably, though, there were discordant notes to process. Menkiti grew up in an artsy, middle-class family in Boston, and was working as a teacher. Persol spent much of his childhood in the projects, with a loving but strict mother who demanded that he and his siblings come home early and focus on school. He made it to the University of Buffalo, where he got a degree in social work, but his career plans took a turn when, at age twenty-four, he became a father of twins. He needed a stable job with good benefits, and the best one he could find was at Rikers Island, the notoriously difficult and dangerous jail in New York City. Persol became a corrections officer. He didn't love the work, but it allowed him to provide for his family, and it shaped the way he saw the world, too.

"It's a running joke with us," Menkiti told me. "We'll be talking at the end of the day, and I'll tell him about something that happened at school. My school will say something like, 'This student is in a tough environment. We're not gonna punish or suspend anyone. Let's have a restoration discussion!' And we'll wind up in a heated debate." Enuma is a nurturer, generous and forgiving. Persol is also caring, but he believes in tough love and discipline. "He doesn't excuse anyone who makes bad choices," she explains. "He always says, 'My family didn't have a good environment, so we had to take control of what we could.' He was home at five p.m. every day, doing homework. All his siblings made it to college. They learned to work hard."

Persol was always working. At Rikers, he had no choice in the matter, because corrections officers don't have full control of their schedule, and sometimes he would show up at work and find out he needed to work overtime, or even a second shift. "He's like, a prisoner at his job sometimes," Menkiti said. "Persol can't play in a band because he can't commit to rehearsal times. It's hard for us to plan things with family and friends." Being at Rikers was stressful and taxing, she continued. "It's a toxic environment. The corrections officers there, they have very high levels of depression, high blood pressure, high suicide, high divorce rates." Persol doesn't like to talk about the situation. He tries to keep work issues locked up on the island, away from home. "He's a man of few words, but he sends me articles about what's going on there. It's his way of saying, 'Look what I'm going through.'"

Rikers is infamously troubled, with crowded facilities and

a vast population of detained people with severe mental health problems. Corrections officers often feel overwhelmed by the situation, and sometimes they lash out in response. One year, an investigation by the city's Department of Health and Mental Hygiene turned up 129 cases in which detainees suffered "serious injuries" at the hands of security guards, all within eleven months.[1] The problems persisted, and the climate at Rikers grew so bad that in 2019 the New York City Council voted to close the entire complex by 2026. By all accounts, Persol was a straight shooter, tough but responsible and decent. Yet the brutality he witnessed so regularly got under his skin, too. "There's a lot of people in his situation," Menkiti said. "College-educated people who never thought they'd work in a jail or a prison. You get paid more, yeah, but it comes at a high price."

The toll felt steeper than ever after 2017, when they had their first child, a daughter they named Eden. They relied on Persol's paycheck and benefits, but Rikers claimed his time. Menkiti wasn't surprised by the situation, but that didn't make it easier for her at home. Things got better when Eden was old enough to go to day care. They found a good one, based in the provider's home, nearby. Menkiti loved being a mother, and she was flourishing at work. In spring 2019, she started a new job as director of college counseling at a charter school in Brooklyn. In August, they had their second daughter, Ella, and moved to a larger apartment where the girls could have more space. Everyone was busy, but in a good way, Menkiti told me. Persol had only a few more years of work to do before he could retire and get his pension. They could see a new chapter coming, with plenty of time to join a band.

Menkiti can't remember exactly when she first heard about the new coronavirus. It was probably on a TV news program, or maybe someone at school. Initially, the reports of people getting sick in China didn't worry her. There's always a new virus, always scary speculation; there's rarely anything that causes trouble at home. "I thought, you know, the media is hyping it up, trying to cause a frenzy," Menkiti told me. She had more urgent problems to manage. Ella, her baby, was getting old enough to join her big sister, Eden, at day care, and the change, while welcome, caused anxiety. Who knew how it would feel, or how Ella would react? At work, Menkiti was busy preparing for the year's major event, a college trip to Washington, D.C., and Maryland that, for many of her immigrant and low-income students, would be their first time visiting a university. In April, her seniors would find out where they had been accepted or rejected. She was already managing their emotions. So much was on the line.

Then, suddenly, nothing was more important than the virus. There were cases in New York City. More every day. Persol was sure that there would be an outbreak at Rikers. So many people came through the complex daily—the staff, of course, but also attorneys, family members, new detainees. How could they prevent it? At school, parents began asking if their children's schools would be shuttered. Teachers were worried, too. On March 11, the National Basketball Association announced that it was temporarily canceling all scheduled games because a player had tested positive for COVID. For Menkiti, that was the turning point. "First it was Tom Hanks getting it," she recalled. "And when the NBA shut down—like wow, okay." The crisis was real.

On March 16, a few days before New York City's system-wide shutdown, Menkiti's charter school closed. Like so many mothers, she felt a mixture of relief and anxiety. She would not be exposed to her students for a while—the administrators expected that they would be out for two, maybe three weeks. But she would have to keep working with families on college admissions, and she would be doing it from home, where it would be impossible to avoid the constant demands of domestic labor, too. She didn't know how she would manage.

Nor did anyone else. In March 2020, the social structures that shape daily life throughout the world were dissolving—slowly in some places, and in others, like Brooklyn, at the speed of sound. Work. School. Child care. Libraries. Playgrounds. Chorus. Rock-solid things that Menkiti and her family had counted on were there one day, gone the next. She was tumbling in space, grasping for something stable and doing everything she could to keep the people in her orbit from floating away.

Predictably, the home day care closed. They still employed a nanny for Ella, an older Caribbean woman who came to their apartment five days a week. Menkiti had been reading local parent blogs about how to avoid the virus and take care of everyone in the household, including domestic help. People were figuring out how to turn their social networks into small, protected pods, and there was fierce disagreement over whether it was safe to employ cleaners and nannies, as well as whether it was okay to have them take buses and subways. One day, she recalled: "I'm on Park Slope Parents, and there were a bunch of sanctimonious parents saying 'Oh, we put our nanny in an Uber every day' and 'We're paying her the full rate and she doesn't have to come in.' Everyone's trying to be one better than the other. Of course, I think, 'Okay, maybe I should drive my nanny home so she doesn't have to go on public transportation.'" That night, Menkiti offered her a ride. "It's not too far away," she said, "but it was cold and we had all the windows closed." The next day, the nanny called to tell Menkiti that she was feeling sick and could not come to work.

She never returned.

A few days later, Menkiti felt feverish, with chills and an upset stomach. "I remember texting my friends, 'I think I have COVID,'" she said. "It seemed surreal. I kept thinking, okay, percentage wise, I should be okay. But obviously there's no treatments at that time, and people don't understand the disease. It's just a very scary thing to have looming over you." She had more specific reasons to feel anxious. Although scientists were still learning about COVID, they already knew that people with underlying health problems were especially vulnerable. Menkiti, who was relatively young but was being treated for high blood pressure, knew this made her vulnerable. Her social media was filling up with reports about friends and relatives who were getting COVID. The husband of a colleague caught it. He would soon be dead. A friend's father was in the hospital, on a ventilator. "A ton" of the corrections officers who worked at Rikers were getting sick, Persol told her, including a man with whom he had just shared a shift driving a van around the facility, and a friend of his who worked the gate. It was hard to believe how fast the disease was spreading in their circle. And it was impossible to deny how many of the people getting sick were, as is so often the case, Black and brown.

Sick, confined, with no treatment available, Menkiti couldn't stop thinking about what might happen. One possibility got under her skin. "The news was filled with stories of people who go to sleep, and then the partner would be sitting out there outside of their room and they go to find them in the morning. They had stopped breathing. Horror stories." She tried to calm herself by avoiding news programs and focusing on her kids, but the nightmare of dying in her sleep would begin as soon as she put her head on the pillow. She couldn't keep her eyes closed. "I was just afraid that I would stop breathing," she recalled, and the only thing that worked was going to the living room and trying to sleep while sitting erect, propped up on pillows. "It just felt better, air-wise." But it wasn't helping her body recover.

Menkiti could feel the disease coursing through her, from her stomach to her head and muscles, and then, as she dreaded, into her lungs. "I felt like I was choking," she told me. Her chest felt compressed and heavy. It was hard to breathe. A few days after the symptoms started, Persol began feeling ill, too. His breathing was even more labored, his anxiety more severe. He went to a health clinic nearby, where he was diagnosed with pneumonia. He asked for a COVID test, but they denied him, saying that they had to save the few they had for people with severe underlying conditions. "He tried four or five places," Menkiti recalled. "Nobody would give him a test." She had more luck at an urgent care center in the neighborhood. "Based on my weight and my high blood pressure, they were able to test me," Menkiti said. They also gave her chest X-rays. The diagnosis was what she expected. She had COVID and pneumonia, and surely Persol did, too. There wasn't much anyone could do to help them, either. They stayed home and prayed.

Prayer didn't do much to cure the infection, however, and as Menkiti's chest kept tightening, her mind moved toward other options. "I was really struggling to breathe," she recounted. "And I heard that hospitals were giving people supplemental oxygen." But hospitals terrified her, especially the ones in her neighborhood. She and Persol had gone by them a few times when they went out to the clinic or to get groceries, and they couldn't help but notice the refrigerated trucks where the corpses of COVID victims were being stored, nor stop imagining the grim situation inside. "I would scroll through death rates and hospital reviews," Menkiti explained. "There were certain hospitals where you were much more likely to die. I was like, 'I'm not going to those. I don't want to wind up dead.'" She got on Facebook, where friends from high school, Williams, and Columbia were sharing information about how to deal with the virus. "I said that I was sick and asked if anyone had connections at hospitals." The headmistress from her high school was close to an infectious disease specialist at one of the city's finest hospitals, Weill Cornell Medical Center, on the Upper East Side of Manhattan. Although health care facilities in Brooklyn, Queens, and the Bronx were overwhelmed with patients, prestigious places like Weill Cornell had relatively few cases. The headmistress told Menkiti that her friend, the doctor, could advocate for her if she wound up on a ventilator. All Enuma had to do was leave her neighborhood, and go.

"So, basically, I was trying to estimate whether it was more dangerous to go to one of these local hospitals or drive alone into the city," Menkiti recalled. "I'd have to be in the car for thirty minutes, and I was worried I wouldn't be able to make it." But the prospect of one difficult car trip was infinitely more appealing than checking into a facility where, it seemed, no one checked out. She said goodbye to Persol and the children, and drove away. It was a trip Enuma had taken countless times in the decades she had lived in Brooklyn. Never had it been so daunting; but also, never had it been so fast. "I was really focused. I wanted to get to that emergency room," she explained. "And nobody, nobody was on the streets!"

She got to the hospital so quickly that she hadn't braced for the wave of anxiety that hit when she entered the emergency room, and immediately found herself in the heart of a system where people were dying every day. It occurred to her that she could soon be among them, and that she hadn't prepared for the possibility. "I went down the rabbit hole of what happens to COVID patients," she told me. "I was trying to remind myself that, you know, statistically I was unlikely to die. But I got worried about what would happen if I was on a ventilator and I couldn't talk. I was a new parent and I hadn't done any estate planning, hadn't done any of that stuff. So, I pulled my little notebook out of my bag and just started writing my will. It wasn't like, a whole will, but I was writing out what I would want to happen."

It was surprising how little she waited before the medical staff arrived to evaluate her. They took her temperature, measured her blood pressure, listened to her breathing, and used a pulse oximeter to assess how much oxygen was in her blood. Her blood oxygen level was 93, about one point higher than the standard for being admitted to the hospital. They told her to go home and rest, and to return only if things got much worse. "At first I was really upset," Menkiti explained. "I was struggling to breathe and I was worried that I could tank quickly." That had happened to her friend's husband. It had happened to people whose deaths got reported on the news. Enuma was hoping that the excellent doctors at Weill Cornell would monitor her for a few days and make sure she stayed stable. It was comforting to know that they thought she could recover without them, but as she drove back to Brooklyn she found herself worrying what would happen if they were wrong.

That night, home and, once again, doomscrolling through the internet in search of something comforting, Menkiti came across an article touting the benefits of hydroxychloroquine. "It was on the news and people were talking about it," she recalled. "And I would do research online about what people were saying." There was nothing like definitive evidence that hydroxychloroquine worked on COVID, but she was willing to take a chance if it meant reducing the risk of dying at home. There was nothing else available, after all. And even if it didn't help her breathing, there was a chance that it would calm her nerves. "One of my friends is married to an orthopedist," she explained, "and he put in a prescription for me at a small pharmacy. I go there, and this pharmacist says that he will give it to me if I pay $250. I'm cheap enough that I was like, no, I don't want to pay $250. And then I was like, well if I die, I'm going to be really mad that I had a chance to live for $250. So, I took it."

While Enuma experimented with an unproved medication, Persol's breathing became strained and shallow, his chest pains more severe. At that point, he was inundated with stories about COVID spreading through Rikers Island. Officers. Staff. Detainees. Everyone was catching it, and some were getting seriously ill. They bought an oximeter and Persol's numbers didn't look scary. "I kept telling him, 'Babe, I think you're having anxiety.'" But now his mind was spinning through worst-case scenarios. He wanted assurance, and he didn't care which hospital treated him. Persol called 911 and a few minutes later an ambulance arrived, sirens blaring, lights flashing. The girls got excited by the stimulation, but it was confusing to see the men in masks take their father away. Like Enuma, Persol was sent home within a few hours. The doctors said it was a healthier place for him to be.

It didn't take long for Menkiti to discover that hydroxychloroquine wasn't calming her nerves any more than it was curing her COVID. Before she took the drug, she was fixated on all the ways it could help her; after, she got focused on the potential for harm. She called another doctor, a cousin, and he said hydroxychloroquine could damage her heart. Later that week, she went to another emergency room and asked them to check her. "They took a scan of electrical activity and they said there had been a change in my heart rate," she told me. "They couldn't say it was for sure because of the hydroxychloroquine, but they said that alone should be enough for me not to take the thing. So I threw it out."

A few weeks later, Enuma and Persol recovered. The timing was fortunate. Rikers needed as many corrections officers as it could get back into the facility. Enuma, however, didn't want Persol to return. "His coworkers were dying, and I told him, 'We can make things work without your salary. It's not worth the risk.' There was no vaccine then. We didn't know if the girls had gotten sick. COVID was running rampant and I just wanted him to be safe." But the job kept Persol in bronze handcuffs. Quitting meant relinquishing his pension and benefits, which meant decades of hard labor that, with just a few more years at Rikers, he could otherwise avoid. Enuma couldn't argue with his decision; she respected his dedication, too. She couldn't stand the fact that

New York City put so many people in jails and prisons, but as long as they were in there, they were better off having people like Persol looking after things.

Enuma was on call, too. Work—remote work, now—picked up again at school, because Enuma's students received their college admissions and financial aid offers in April, and everyone needed her help. So, too, did Ella and Eden. The family still had no nanny, no home day care, no neighbors or friends or family members who felt comfortable visiting during the raging pandemic and offering a hand. Menkiti did her best to take care of the kids when Persol returned to work, but it's impossible to juggle an infant, a three-year-old, and a classful of high school seniors (not to mention their parents), when all of them want your attention, urgently. Instead of fighting off COVID, she was spending her days putting out small conflagrations. Change a diaper. Explain the difference between a public and private university campus to a first-generation college family. Clean a spill on the carpet. Debate whether a "dream school" is worth the extra debt. Make lunch. Clean another diaper. And then a message from Persol: They're short-staffed at Rikers Island, again. He's working overtime, maybe even a second shift. "We asked the home day care when they were opening back up," Menkiti explained, "if the kids could go back." The provider kept telling them that she wasn't ready. "I presumed it was because her daughter had health issues, or because she was fearful of kids coming into her house. I mean, people were really dying, people were scared. I had a lot of empathy for her."

In mid-April, when the weather improved and COVID cases in New York City finally began to plummet, Enuma and Persol started taking the girls outdoors more often. They were still leery of benches and door handles. "Remember," Enuma said, "back then we thought that the virus spread through contaminated surfaces. We were wiping down our groceries with Lysol!" But they live near some of New York City's greatest public spaces, including Prospect Park and Sunset Park, and they joined the throngs of people who began using them daily, enjoying the reprieve from a month of lockdowns and isolation at home. One day, Menkiti recalled, they bumped into another family from the day care and began catching up. She asked the father how they were dealing with child care. "Oh, my son has been back at day care for a while now," he replied. "It's open."

Menkiti's heart sank. Open a while now? Why aren't we back, too?

Obviously, they had been excluded. "Basically," Menkiti explained, "they kicked us out." She sent a note to the day care provider, asking what was happening. "A week later, she called to say, 'I hate to do this. It's so hard to make decisions during a pandemic . . . but you know, the other families . . . they're not comfortable with your daughter coming here due to the exposure that Rikers presents.'" They were trying to create a bubble, a protected environment where every family could feel safe from the virus. "Everybody could go back," Menkiti told me. "But not us. All the other parents were working remotely. I guess they saw us as disease vectors. And I wanted to say to her, 'We're probably the safest people to send to your day care because we already had COVID!' But, you know, if someone says they don't want you there, you're not gonna argue to be there. It just hurt."

It was also infuriating—"hypocritical bullshit," is what Menkiti called it. The home day care was not just a service center; it was a community, the first that they had embraced as a family, the one they had expected to grow into as Ella joined her big sister that year. "The provider is also biracial," she explained, "and I always felt like I identified with her." Menkiti understood why she and other families felt anxious about COVID. But their refusal to let her child return, and their failure to communicate the reason until after she discovered what happened, felt like a betrayal. "It was classist, in the sense that people who are essential workers, who don't have an option about having to go out there and taking care of all the needs that the city has, you're getting discriminated against. It seemed like the day care was progressive, multiracial, an idyllic Brooklyn community," she said. "I had hoped we'd be a part of it. But to suddenly be cast out because you're an essential worker? The loss, you know, it was bigger than just losing child care."

Persol and Enuma didn't get many breaks in 2020, but they got a big one soon after this experience. Colleagues at Rikers told Persol that New York City was offering child care for essential workers. "We started calling and we found this place in Red Hook [another Brooklyn neighborhood not far from their apartment], a corporate day care center that I guess the city was sponsoring," Enuma explained. "And I guess not many people knew about it, because there were only four kids there. Our kids got so much attention—and it was free!" The program lasted through the summer, long enough for Persol and Enuma to decompress from the months of trauma and stress. When it ended, they were able to find a new nanny. Just in time for Enuma to return to her job at school.

"We were lucky," Enuma told me. And the sentiment was heartfelt, even though, when she compared her family to those that had made up their community at the start of 2020, they clearly were not.

Menkiti spent much of the first plague year thinking about the disparities between different families in her city, and not just because of her own experience. The ways that money, race, and resources mattered were even more apparent when school reopened, and everyone who worked there was struck by how social class shaped students' development during the crisis. The institution, which calls itself "intentionally diverse," aims to fill half of its spots with low-income students, many of whom are from immigrant families, or have parents who did not attend college. "Building a diverse and inclusive community is our most important goal, our hardest challenge, and the driving force behind everything we do," the school's website declares. Bridging the gaps between different students was even more difficult in the fall of 2020, Menkiti told me. One reason, she said, is that privileged families kept their kids engaged in formal education when the school was shuttered and classes were remote, while poor and working-class families had less capacity to focus on their children's learning. "We have families whose parents don't speak English. They work in grocery stores, or they're drivers. They're not on email, and our administration sends everything on email, sends out Zoom links for classes and meetings, sends grades on a portal where parents have to log in. A lot of our parents miss out on all that, they're iced out of education. And if their kid is struggling with motivation, the family has no way to understand what's going on."

Kids from wealthier and more educated families got more than adult oversight; the sheer fact of living with college-educated, professional parents meant that they enjoyed constant exposure to the world of higher education, just by being at home. "Our first-generation and low-income kids, they get that from the school, they get that from us," Menkiti said. "So not being here, having our college trip canceled, our local trips canceled, not having college fairs or visits from college representatives— all these things that build the mindset for college, they missed out on it. We got back to work with them on school applications, and there's a big disconnect for them." In fall 2020, few of the low-income students who walked into Menkiti's office were prepared for the college application process, some didn't know if they would still be able to go. The situation made her work feel more urgent, more necessary. It was so easy to see how the pandemic had derailed hardworking young people; kids whose futures seemed so promising before the crisis were on a precipice, and who, if not Menkiti, would get them back on track?

The problem was that throwing herself back into the charter school meant pulling away from her own children, whose own development had been altered in ways she could not yet decipher. Things worked well enough when Eden could go to pre-K and the sitter watched Ella, but the pandemic came in surges, and each new wave knocked their family off-balance. During one spike in cases, for instance, Eden's entire class (of kids who were too young to be vaccinated) went remote because a student tested positive for COVID. Remote school isn't easy for anyone, and it's especially challenging for three-year-olds, for whom sitting still in front of a screen while doing educational activities is, as Menkiti put it, "basically impossible." In their case, it was even more challenging, because both Enuma and Persol had to be at work, they had only one laptop, which Enuma needed, and the nanny, whose main job was to engage one-year-old Ella, did not know how to use Zoom.

"The teacher expected all the kids to be on Zoom at 8:30," Menkiti told me. "And it's like the whole public education system thinks that everyone is working from home, with time to be with their kids. I was thinking, okay, maybe I should email the teacher and tell her that we don't have the ability to do Zoom. But then I was like, I don't want to be a bad parent! So, today, I was actually late to work because I wanted to make sure my daughter could log on. And when we did, every single one of those kids was there, with their parents holding them on their laps!" Menkiti paused for a beat, choking up a little, before catching her breath. She exhaled, laughing at the absurdity of her family's predicament, the parents' work so essential that they could not fulfill their parental responsibility, yet not valued enough for them to afford the resources they need. "Maybe it's the neighborhood we're in? All those parents have remote jobs, and we're the only ones who have to work in person? I don't know. But I started to feel like, I went to school and got all these master's degrees and I still didn't make it." She always knew that class mattered, but nothing in her education prepared her for the way it affected her family now.

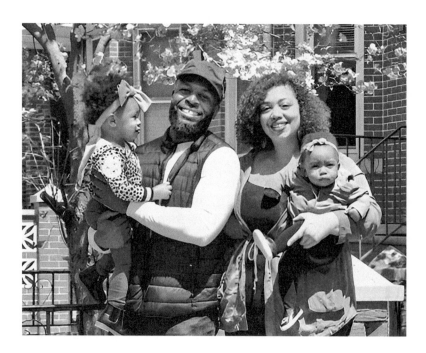

CHAPTER 8

The Problem of Distancing

Face masks are not the only tools for reducing the spread of a coronavirus when there's no vaccine or medications available. In early 2020, health agencies around the world began to recommend a battery of everyday "nonpharmaceutical interventions," such as washing hands, covering coughs and sneezes, avoiding hugs and handshakes, and staying home when sick. They also called for a more extraordinary measure, "social distancing," that proved especially challenging. The concept was capacious, and included, among many restrictions: closing schools, libraries, parks, beaches, gyms, and restaurants; limiting the number of people in grocery stores and stadiums; prohibiting home visits from neighbors, friends, and family; shuttering offices; and, in some places, sequestering entire states, cities, or neighborhoods, to keep the virus contained.

Isolating people who are perceived as contagious, dirty, or dangerous is an ancient social practice, used commonly during infectious disease outbreaks but also in more routine situations, and often applied against stigmatized groups. The Old Testament instructs women to separate from their husbands for several days after menstruation, a practice that is maintained today not only among some observant Jews but also in parts of India, where menstruating women must leave the village and move into basic huts.[1] The idea of quarantining for public health began in the fourteenth century, to prevent the spread of plague by contaminated people, rodents, and objects. "Some city-states prevented strangers from entering their cities, particularly, merchants and minority groups, such as Jews and persons with leprosy," writes the medical historian Eugenia Tognotti. "A sanitary cordon—not to be broken on pain of death—was imposed by armed guards along transit routes and at access points to cities. Implementation of these measures required rapid, firm action by authorities, including prompt mobilization of repressive police forces. A rigid separation between healthy and infected persons was initially accomplished through the use of makeshift camps."[2]

The social distancing policies that nations throughout the world adopted in the COVID-19 pandemic penetrated into the daily lives of ordinary people, extending to the classroom, the workplace, the public realm, and the family home. In some countries, the constraints on mobility and interaction were severe. The Chinese government enforced periodic lockdown orders in regions where COVID was surging, forcing residents to remain inside their apartments at all times, with only brief exceptions for essential shopping and physical activity. Strict measures like this were not unique to authoritarian societies with limited civil rights and liberties. In early March, the Italian government imposed what observers called "the most draconian lockdown measures outside mainland China," with bans on trips outside the home for some 10 million residents in northern regions with clusters of COVID. Within weeks, the entire population was subjected to these rules.[3] France followed suit. From mid-March to early May, the French national government instituted a policy locals called "Confinement," which required everyone who ventured outside to carry an official form justifying the reason, and involved deploying some 100,000 police officers to ensure compliance. "Stay Home," the state implored. Those who refused paid a fine of up to 375 euros.[4]

In the U.S., where individual freedom is sacrosanct, restrictions on mobility were far less strict. American pandemic policies, most of which were developed and enforced at the state level, were shaped by both deep-seated concerns about the importance of freedom and by new scientific discoveries about the value of social regulations during infectious disease outbreaks. Much of this science came from researchers working with the White House in the years after September 11, 2001, when President George W. Bush grew concerned about a range of domestic security threats, including pandemic disease. In one project, Laura Glass, a public high school student in Albuquerque, New Mexico, and her father, Bob Glass, a scientist at the Sandia National Laboratories, led a team that simulated the spread of influenza through a small American community, varying levels of school closures and other behavioral restrictions. Their findings, published in 2006 in the influential paper "Targeted Social Distance Designs for Pandemic Influenza," show that "targeted social distancing strategies can be designed to effectively mitigate the local progression of pandemic influenza without the use of vaccine or antiviral drugs." The authors caution that "implementation of social distancing strategies is challenging. They likely must be imposed for the duration of the local epidemic and possibly until a strain-specific vaccine is developed and distributed." But the payoff of compliance is potentially massive, allowing a community to avoid the epidemic altogether.[5]

In 2007, another important study, led by the eminent medical historian Howard Markel, added empirical evidence to the case for social distancing in pandemic prevention efforts. Markel and his collaborators built a massive dataset that included weekly mortality records and the timing of a variety of nonpharmaceutical interventions, including school closures and bans on public gatherings, from forty-three U.S. cities during the Great Influenza pandemic. The data allowed them to assess whether and to what extent distancing measures protected people from one of the great public health crises of the modern age. Before the study, Markel and his coauthors write, "Most pandemic influenza policy makers agree[d] that even the most rigorous nonpharmaceutical interventions are unlikely either to prevent a pandemic or change a population's underlying biological susceptibility to the pandemic virus." But their findings established the opposite: "a strong association between early, sustained, and layered application of nonpharmaceutical interventions and mitigating the consequences of the 1918–1919 influenza pandemic." Although Markel and his team warn that "history is not a predictive science," when COVID arrived in America, the lesson was hard to ignore.[6]

The U.S. Centers for Disease Control and Prevention introduced its first COVID-related quarantine order in January 2020 when it repatriated 195 Americans in Wuhan to the March Air Reserve Base in Riverside County, California. At a press conference on January 31, Dr. Nancy Messonier, director of the CDC's National Center for Immunization and Respiratory Disease, announced that "CDC, under statutory authority of the HHS Secretary, has issued federal quarantine orders for all 195 passengers." The legal order, which was imposed after one of the passengers tried to leave the quarantine, allowed the government to detain the entire group of Americans at the military base for fourteen days. It was "an unprecedented action . . . part of an aggressive public health response, the goal of which is to prevent, as much as possible, community spread of this novel virus in the United States." Messonier assured the public that this strategy came from "evidence-based recommendations from CDC experts who have been working on exactly these kinds of issues for many years," and that "the actions that the federal government is taking are science-based, with the aim of protecting the health and safety of all Americans."[7] Journalists at the conference did not question her assertion. Instead, they wanted to know whether every American who returned from China would be detained by the military, and if not, how the quarantine would be enforced. "The best way to enforce a quarantine is to educate people on its purpose and educate what the benefits are for the individuals who cooperate," said Messonier's colleague, Dr. Marty Cetron. "These are American citizens who clearly want to do the right thing."[8]

It did not take long to see that the medical experts had overestimated both the effectiveness of educating the American public about the benefits of distancing and the extent to which American people would accept their "science-based" views on what it meant to "do the right thing." By late March, when cases were popping up throughout the U.S., city and state governments began to impose their own restrictions: a "shelter-in-place" order in San Francisco and New York City; an executive order to shut down "nonessential businesses" in New Jersey; a statewide "stay-at-home" order in Illinois; a ban on gatherings of more than fifty people in Seattle; a mandatory two-week quarantine for all out-of-state visitors to Vermont.[9] In Florida, Republican governor Ron DeSantis set up checkpoints on major highways to turn away people from states with high COVID-19 caseloads; in Rhode Island, Democratic governor Gina Raimondo ordered police to do the same.[10] Soon, nearly every state and local government had implemented its own set of "social distancing" measures, and with great effect. Statistical models that estimate early COVID cases and mortality with and without various distancing policies leave little doubt that shutdowns prevented millions, and perhaps tens of millions, of cases, and tens of thousands of deaths.[11] But other research has established that distancing is a double-edged sword, with potentially dangerous consequences for some people and institutions.[12] Millions of Americans objected to them, some fiercely, and it did not take long for them to push back.

That shouldn't have been surprising. Distancing slows down market activity, particularly in sectors that rely on customers being there in person, such as retail, restaurants, entertainment, and tourism. Staying at home deprives us of connections we need. "Human beings are social animals," as the Roman emperor and Stoic philosopher Marcus Aurelius put it. Our drive to engage in collective life is primal. The will to do things together cuts against what the sociologist Émile Durkheim called the modern "cult of individualism," especially during difficult times.

In many nations, the refusal to respect distancing policies became associated with groups that rejected government regulations, including those around COVID, more generally. Conservatives, and conservative religious groups, openly defied and aggressively challenged them. In Israel, and New York City as well, Orthodox Jews flouted distancing rules, even when the initial spike in cases and deaths overwhelmed the medical system and officials were pleading for compliance; conservative evangelical

Christian churches, some with substantial and politically influential followers, acted similarly throughout the United States.[13] In Ontario, Canada, protesters expressing skepticism about the mainstream media and professional science began demanding that the government "End the shutdown!" and "Free the healthy," as early as April 2020. In the U.S., an antigovernment group that opposed Michigan governor Gretchen Whitmer's restrictions on social and economic life during the first year of the pandemic plotted to kidnap her, and some entered the statehouse carrying long guns in hope of executing the plan.[14]

If direct opposition to distancing was more common among conservatives, ambivalence was nearly ubiquitous. Everyone, including liberals, progressives, and strong advocates of public health interventions, struggled to comply with tight restrictions on social activity, because following them caused real distress. Consider the confessional column from the *New York Times* essayist Farhad Manjoo, who shared his tortured thought process for considering whether his family should visit his older parents over the holidays, despite ample official and scientific warnings to stay home. Manjoo goes to great lengths to assess the risks. He measures the size of his contact circle, or social network, by counting the number of kids whom his kids saw daily in an in-person "learning pod," then adding the people in the bubbles of those kids and their families, as well as the teachers and their bubbles, too. "Once I had counted everyone, I realized that visiting my parents for Thanksgiving would be like asking them to sit down to dinner with more than 100 people," he writes. "So that sealed the deal, then, right—we're staying home for Thanksgiving?" Well, no! Instead, they come up with an elaborate plan: quarantining before the visit; driving instead of flying; limiting the number of family members at the meal; eating outdoors; trying not to hug. Manjoo recognizes the potential for disaster but also the benefits of being with loved ones during a time of stress. "It's all so much work—the worrying, the double-checking, the uncertainty, the constant specter of death. But for family, it's worth it."[15]

In the first year of the pandemic, there was, indeed, good reason to wonder whether distancing was worth it. It was by no means clear how distancing policies would affect children, for whom social interaction is necessary for personal development. For young people, remote schooling meant less learning and more cognitive and emotional struggles. It also increased inequality, leaving poor families in districts like May Lee's on their own, unable to pay for extra tutoring and ill-equipped to take over the work on their own. Forcibly separating infected young children from parents, as China did during one severe outbreak, was traumatic for everyone. Old people, for whom isolation can be physically and mentally devastating, were certain to suffer from a loss of intimate contact with friends and relatives. Of course, governments have good reason to discourage close interaction during an infectious disease outbreak, because proximity to a person carrying a contagious virus is what allows it to spread. But there is a crucial difference between "physical distancing," which involves reducing the risks of catching a disease through aerosols or droplets, and "social distancing," which implies a more dramatic reduction of interaction. In the pandemic, health agencies around the world got the messaging wrong.

"Social distancing" turned out to be the very opposite of what people needed to maintain health and vitality. The concept conveyed a strong message: Sever ties and limit contact with friends and neighbors. Seal your domestic space. Create a bubble for the members of your nuclear family. Stay inside of it until the emergency ends. In a crisis, however, social closeness protects people. Social solidarity, the bonds of mutual obligation and linked fate between people who share a neighborhood, city, or nation, can be a crucial resource—but only if states and societies are capable of producing it. Solidarity means actively communicating with old, sick, and frail people, to see if they need help getting things like medications or groceries. It means reaching out to people who live alone and asking if they need companionship, whether virtual or in person if it's safe. It means not hoarding food or medicine when there's scarcity. It means considering how your own personal behavior may affect those around you, so that you don't go out when you're having flulike symptoms, that you wear a mask in the grocery store.

The call for social distancing was rooted in good epidemiological science. Sociologically, though, it was destined to fail.

.   .   .

Distancing during a pandemic is a luxury. Some can afford to go remote with relatively few negative consequences; some cannot imagine what distancing would mean. Postal service data show that some eighty thousand people submitted change-of-address requests in New York City during March 2020, for instance, and more than 333,000 people moved out of the city that year. We don't know exactly who moved, but we know which neighborhoods they occupied before the coronavirus arrived, and where they went. The patterns have everything to do with social class. "The higher-earning a neighborhood is, the more likely it is to have emptied out," *The New York Times* reported, after analyzing geolocated mobile phone data. "In the city's very wealthiest blocks . . . population decreased by 40 percent or more, while the rest of the city saw comparably modest changes."[16] Sharp declines in the weight of garbage collected by the Sanitation Department in affluent residential areas confirm these trends. Meanwhile, real estate prices spiked in the Hamptons, the Hudson Valley, and the suburbs of Westchester County and New Jersey.[17] Wealth, income, education, and professional jobs that allowed workers to "go remote" facilitated immediate relocation to a place that afforded more physical space, and more protection from COVID-19 as well.

Class also mattered when it came to maintaining distance at work. In theory, one might expect that people whose jobs are considered necessary and vital would get extra protection. During the pandemic, however, governments around the world applied a rarely used policy concept, "essential worker," that allowed employers to ask people like Persol, who worked at Rikers, to do their jobs in person if they were in a select few fields, including health care, criminal justice, agriculture, food preparation, transit, delivery, and retail. At first glance, the essential worker designation looks like an honorific, a sign of recognition and respect for people whose labor a society depends on and whose wellbeing it is determined to protect. In practice, the classification effectively imperiled those it covered, eliminating the possibility of physical or social distancing for those who wanted to keep their jobs, even when working conditions were manifestly dangerous. In other words, being called essential meant being treated as disposable.

Official declarations that some people were "essential workers" and had no choice but to work in the pandemic or lose their jobs came early in the crisis, and the term became so common, so quickly, that there was little public debate about where it came from or what it meant. It's no small matter, determining which jobs are necessary for an economy and society to function. And it's worth pausing to consider the discrepancy between the occupational sectors that are valued most by the market economy, such as law and finance, and those that the government deemed most valuable when the foundations of modern life were threatened, such as agriculture, meatpacking, transit, and care work. It's worth asking: Who makes that decision? What are the criteria? What protections and how much compensation should we give to those who put themselves at risk so that the rest of us can consume as we are accustomed to and get the kind of care we need? There are a number of ways that a state or society could answer these questions. When the coronavirus outbreak started, however, few political officials were demanding explanations, and most governments offered little justification at all.

The idea of essential workers adopted by the U.S. government, as the anthropologist Andrew Lakoff explains, comes from Cold War national security planning, when defense strategists defined a set of industries and services as elements of the "critical infrastructure," and established provisions to keep them operating after a military attack. In March 2020, the Department of Homeland Security issued guidance on how local officials could identify "essential critical infrastructure workers" who had "a special responsibility to continue operations" even when the government ordered others to stay at home.[18] Highly trained, and in some cases highly compensated, health care professionals were the most publicly visible essential workers during the pandemic. But they were the exceptions—even in their own industry, where janitors and home care providers worked outside the limelight and at real risk. Essential workers were disproportionately Black and Latino and in blue-collar positions. Many toiled in the context of job insecurity, low status, and low wages as well.

The hazards of doing essential work were apparent immediately in New York City, where COVID hit early and hard. In
a survey conducted by epidemiologists at the City University of
New York, 39 percent of Black respondents and 38 percent of
Latino respondents said that there was an essential worker in
their household, compared to just 28 percent of whites. Moreover, only 44 percent of Latino workers said they could work
remotely, compared to 69 percent of Blacks and 81 percent of
whites. These patterns help explain why, during the first three
months of pandemic, COVID mortality rates for Blacks and Latinos were more than two times higher than they were for whites
and Asians.[19]

New York City was not the only place where low-wage essential workers faced the gravest COVID risks. A study by a team
of epidemiologists from the University of California, San Francisco, published in *PLOS ONE*, examined levels of excess mortality in California during the first nine months of the pandemic,
comparing death rates across occupational sectors and occupations, and also considering ethnicity and race. The sectors with
the highest relative and per capita excess mortality were, in order:
food/agriculture, transportation/logistics, manufacturing, and
facilities. Working-age Latinos, the paper reports, "experienced
the highest relative excess-mortality" in the state, with food
and agriculture workers most likely to die. Working-age Black
Californians had the highest per capita mortality, with those in
transportation and logistics jobs most at risk. The epidemiologists recognize the reasons that the state deemed some industries
and occupations so important that they had to continue, despite
the threat of COVID. But they condemn the practice of forcing people to work in person when basic protective gear, such as
masks and gloves, was unavailable, or when labor conditions, such
as indoor settings with poor air circulation, facilitated viral transmission. "If indeed these workers are essential," they conclude,
"we must be swift and decisive in enacting measures that will treat
their lives as such."[20]

The United Farm Workers (UFW), America's largest agriculture labor union, made this point as soon as the federal government issued its guidelines. There are more than one million

hired farmworkers in the U.S., roughly three fourths of whom are immigrants, two thirds of them Mexican, and about half not "work-authorized."[21] In the years preceding the coronavirus outbreak, the federal government had been treating undocumented Mexican immigrants as the very opposite of essential. During his campaign and his presidency, Trump had referred to them as "animals" and "rapists" engaged in an "invasion" of America, and he treated them accordingly.[22] In March 2020, his administration was not only building a wall on the Mexican border, but also holding undocumented immigrants in crowded, squalid detention centers where the risk of contracting COVID-19 and a host of other health problems was dangerously high. Children were separated from their parents, and in many cases their location records were lost. "Detention is a black box, with no way out," a report called "Justice-Free Zones" by the American Civil Liberties Union, Human Rights Watch, and National Immigrant Justice Center explained. Conditions, they said, are "inhumane."[23]

Conditions for immigrants who got hired as farmworkers were significantly better than for those detained by the Department of Homeland Security, of course. The Trump administration, despite its public campaign to demonize and deport the people it called "aliens," understood the value that low-wage agricultural laborers brought to the U.S. But when COVID hit, arrangements that had become standard practice in the industry—including crowded, employee-sponsored housing quarters and long bus rides to the fields—made farmworkers especially vulnerable to the virus. "Physical distancing was not a possibility," said Giev Kashkooli, the UFW's political and legislative director. "The idea that you should stay home and only be with your family, that was something that no one had been grappling with, and it was literally about life and death." In the first weeks of the pandemic, he told me, the union was concerned that plants would shut down, leaving immigrant workers with no access to government benefits in dire poverty. At that time, organizers were fighting for paid sick leave and eligibility for public benefits. But when states like California and Washington deemed farmworkers "essential," the challenge shifted. Now they needed masks and other basic PPE for the workers, things to protect them in cramped buses and dense residential communities. They needed tests, not only for workers and their families, but for the new recruits coming in from Mexico on special visas that the Trump administration, under pressure from agribusiness, was processing quickly. "The pandemic was raging, raging in the U.S., raging in Mexico," Kashkooli recalled. "And we had to make sure everyone was healthy and safe."

Agriculture is always critical for America's health and economy, but in most parts of the country, farmworkers are invisible. During the pandemic, their significance—and the value of the industry—became visible. Demand was surging, but also shifting. "For farmers, business was cranking," Kashkooli explained. "But things were unstable. The farms that supply restaurants, universities, food service companies, they had to regroup. But supermarket sales went through the roof, and the workers were shuffling." The spike in activity created new risks. People were moving around, mixing with new coworkers, getting exposed in countless ways. Kashkooli, whose children were teenagers at the time, couldn't help but feel strange about the situation in his family and at the farms. "I remember when my kids' school closed. We were taking all these precautions. Around then we had a UFW member meeting. We handed out masks. We told people we weren't going to shake hands. We separated the chairs six feet. It was everybody's first experience doing that. It had not been happening at the companies where they worked." It also hadn't been happening in the places where farmworkers lived, employer-sponsored or not. "We're talking about three or four families sharing a three-bedroom house," Kashkooli said. "People living in garages. Distancing wasn't an option."

"Pretty immediately, we started learning about deaths," Kashkooli told me. "At first, it wasn't happening at the union contract companies. I think it's partly because we were more attentive and cautious. But there were exceptions." The biggest, he said, were at poultry plants, places where only a small fraction of the workforce belonged to the UFW, and their negotiating power was limited. At Foster Poultry Farms, the largest employer in Livingston, California, at least four hundred farm workers caught COVID, and nine of them died, during the first nine months of the pandemic. In December 2020, the UFW sued the company, charging that "in naked disregard of both national and local guidelines, Foster Farms requires employees to work substantially less than six feet apart from each other for prolonged periods of time with no plastic divider or similar protection between them, fails to rigorously or effectively enforce social distancing or even to supply masks, and fails to keep its workforce adequately informed of safety and sick leave protocol, including access to COVID leave pay."[24]

In January 2021, the Superior Court of California in Merced County granted the UFW's request for a preliminary injunction that required Foster Farms to implement COVID safety protocols. By then, it was already clear that major companies throughout the industry had been treating their workers as disposable, failing to provide testing and other health screens, refusing to invest in safer housing or transportation, or neglecting to provide face masks and PPE. According to a report by the House Select Subcommittee on the Coronavirus Pandemic, more than 59,000 American meatpackers got COVID during 2020, and at least 269 died. Foster Farms was hardly an outlier. The House found that 54 percent of the workforce at a JBS plant in Hyrum, Utah, contracted the virus, as did nearly 50 percent of workers at a Tyson plant in Amarillo, Texas, and 44 percent of employees at National Beef's plant in Tama, Iowa.[25] Although those who did agricultural work outdoors fared relatively better, they, too, were among the most vulnerable occupational groups in the pandemic. In California, for instance, the food/agriculture sector had the highest relative and per capita excess mortality during the first nine months of the pandemic.[26] Counties where farmworkers were concentrated consistently ranked among the deadliest places in America, because—in a social context where distancing was impossible—the virus did not only reach those who labored in the plant or the field; it spread to their housemates, friends, and families as well.[27]

The impossibility of distancing for another group of essential workers, health aides and nurses in long-term-care facilities for older people, played a major role in the transmission of COVID-19 in nursing homes, which were the deadliest places to be during the pandemic. Nursing homes were bound to be among the most lethal sites in the health crisis, because the population is composed almost entirely of old people whose physical ailments or mental illnesses require special attention and support. A *Wall Street Journal* analysis of data from more than two dozen nations with significant elder care facilities shows that, by the end of 2020, "such institutions are tied to more than a third of COVID-19 deaths, though they typically house less than 2% of the population."[28]

It's not surprising that long-term-care residents were far more likely to die of COVID-19 than older people who lived at home.[29] But the size of the disparity was not inevitable; in fact, it varied considerably across nations, based largely on how well they kept nursing home residents distanced from those who were sick. If, as Mahatma Gandhi said, "the true measure of any society can be found in how it treats its most vulnerable members," the way different countries protected people who needed long-term care is a vital indicator of what they value and who they are.

In some places, such as South Korea, Hong Kong, and Germany, aggressive COVID-control policies at the community level, such as testing, tracing, masking, and isolation protocols for positive cases, resulted in relatively low levels of transmission during the first stage of the pandemic. Reducing the amount of COVID in the general population is just the first step in protecting residents in long-term-care facilities, however. The second step was to implement a set of special protocols in the nursing homes themselves. Screening all workers, including nurses, health aides, physical therapists, administrators, cooks, and cleaning crews. Ensuring that face masks and PPE were easily available and used where necessary. Maintaining physical distance when possible and eliminating crowded environments, including ordinary gathering places such as dining rooms and exercise areas, as well as bedrooms and bathing areas. Improving air circulation and ventilation. Testing residents and workers often, and expeditiously sending positive cases to local hospitals, before they infect other vulnerable people in the home.

Health agencies and nursing home managers had long understood the risks that an airborne virus could pose for their physically fragile residents, and the ways to mitigate the threat as well. In some nations, particularly those where old people had suffered acutely in prior infectious disease outbreaks, health agencies had developed special plans to protect residential centers for the elderly during epidemics, and their efforts often made a difference. In 2003, *The Wall Street Journal* reported, residents of elder care facilities in Hong Kong were "five times more likely to catch SARS than the general public, and 57 died."[30] The government responded by creating a new regimen of infection-control measures, including stocks of masks and other PPE for staff and occupants, and better ventilation. In January 2020, when China acknowledged the emergence of a new coronavirus, Hong Kong immediately barred most visitors from nursing homes, announced that all infected nursing home residents would be moved to hospitals, and that residents or staff exposed to the virus would be forced to quarantine. At the end of November 2020, the *Journal* investigation found, "Hong Kong, with more than 76,000 nursing-home beds, had seen 30 resident COVID-19 deaths."[31]

South Korea waited slightly longer to introduce special COVID-control measures, prohibiting visitors in mid-February. This proved too late to prevent a spike in cases in the city of Daegu, where at least five nursing homes reported clusters of the disease. The government reacted with a sweeping set of screening measures, removing caretakers who had recently traveled to China, and testing and tracing employees at the nation's 1,470 nursing homes—even in regions where the virus had not yet arrived. When a new COVID cluster emerged in a church or nightclub, South Korea responded by testing residents in nearby long-term-care facilities, since every local case increased their risk of exposure, and by using GPS records to track the movements of nursing home staff. In fall 2020, nursing home employees were explicitly prohibited from attending large social gatherings. Not everyone approved such sweeping restrictions in the private lives of South Korean caretakers, but the government's protective policies were strikingly effective.[32]

In Canada, by contrast, some estimate that nearly 70 percent of all COVID deaths during the first year of the pandemic took place in nursing homes—a clear sign that not every nation that experienced a major scare during the SARS crisis had prepared its long-term-care facilities for the next infectious disease outbreak.[33] Like Hong Kong and South Korea, Canada did well limiting cases in the general population when the coronavirus first arrived, but it did far less to protect those who lived and worked in its notoriously short-staffed and underfunded nursing homes. Although Canada has a strong national health system, long-term-care facilities are excluded from its public health network, and more than half of its nursing homes are privately owned, profit-seeking corporations. Nathan Stall, a geriatrician in Toronto's Sinai Health Network, led a comparative study of all 623 nursing homes (360 for-profit, 162 nonprofit, and 101 municipally controlled) in Ontario from March 29 to May 20, 2020. His team found that COVID outbreaks were equally likely to occur in all three types of facilities, but the size of the outbreaks and the concentration of deaths were significantly higher in for-profit homes.[34]

What made for-profit nursing homes so much more dangerous? Stall and his colleagues analyzed the physical environments across the residential facilities, and discovered that for-profit institutions, which run on slim margins, were more likely to have "outdated design standards," with denser, more crowded spaces that fostered transmission of the disease. "Thirteen of the fifteen homes with the highest infection rates were for-profit-homes with older design standards," the authors report.[35] Demand for beds, the Canadian geriatrician Samir Sinha told me, is so high that the owners had little incentive to invest in renovations and upgrades that would bring living conditions up to current standards, with far more private rooms. "A lot of the for-profit homes are in older facilities that have three- and four-bedded rooms. And frankly, if you're just running a business with 40,000 people on your waitlist, why would you upgrade your beds? You don't have to attract customers, because there's always a captive audience ready to move into whatever bed you're willing to offer."

Physical crowding was only one part of the problem. The

other was the industry's reliance on part-time employees, poorly paid nursing assistants, cooks, and cleaning crews that circulated from one perilous environment to another, becoming unwitting carriers of disease in the communities they were trying to serve. These practices, the data show, are far more common in Canada's for-profit homes.

The challenge of providing care in Canada's virus-ridden nursing homes overwhelmed workers, prompting the largest labor union representing long-term-care employees in Ontario and Quebec to call for assistance from the Canadian Army. The soldiers who were deployed to these facilities were horrified by the conditions, and their daily assessments depicted nursing homes as, to use the CBC's descriptions, a "shocking catalogue of abuse, neglect and cruelty." One report found "cockroaches and flies present"; others "noted unsafe conditions that could help spread COVID-19, including instances where patients who had tested positive for the virus 'were allowed to wander' and staff members left with inadequate personal protective equipment."[36] Canadian observers noted similar problems in other provinces. In Montreal, for instance, the local health authority took control of a private nursing home where thirty-one residents died in less than a month and investigators "found dehydrated residents lying listless in bed, unfed for days, with excrement seeping out of their diapers," because staff could not handle the surge of death and disease.[37]

In June 2020, Canada's national health data agency reported that during the first months of the pandemic it had "the worst record among wealthy nations for COVID-19-related deaths in long-term care facilities for older people."[38] Prime Minister Justin Trudeau acknowledged the nation's sense of shame over the situation: "We are failing our parents, our grandparents, our elders—the greatest generation who built this country. We need to care for them properly."[39]

Nursing homes in the U.S. also failed to provide proper care for their residents, and their workers suffered greatly as well. During the first wave of the pandemic, roughly 40 percent of all American COVID deaths took place in nursing homes, a far smaller proportion than in Canada. But that's not a sign of successful COVID containment policies in American long-term-care facilities; on the contrary, the U.S. had a higher nursing home COVID mortality rate than Canada, and more overall nursing home deaths than any other nation.[40] Instead, it reflects the fact that, unlike Canada, the coronavirus was rampant in the larger community as well as in long-term-care facilities.

American workers were more likely than Canadian workers to catch COVID, simply by virtue of the fact that they lived in a country where the virus was rampant. That also meant that American workers were more likely to carry the illness into nursing homes and infect the vulnerable residents who lived in them. The compounded risks added up to a staggering level of death and disease. For perspective, that means the overall death toll among the 1.5 million or so Americans living in nursing homes was greater than the entire national mortality numbers during 2020 in all but six countries: Brazil, Britain, India, Russia, Mexico, and Peru.[41]

As in Canada, the crisis in American nursing homes stemmed from both physical conditions in residential facilities, some 70 percent of which are owned by private and for-profit corporations, and heavy use of low-wage contract labor, with workers who held multiple jobs. It was also rooted in the long-term-care industry's sustained opposition to federal regulations that required them to plan for disasters such as epidemics. According to an investigation by *ProPublica*, nearly half of U.S. nursing homes had emergency plans for an infectious disease outbreak that failed to meet federal guidelines, despite a mandate dating back to the Obama administration and an official clarification, in 2019, that they must train all staff for handling new and emerging infectious diseases.[42]

The perilous state of care workers was apparent long before the COVID-19 pandemic. In 2016, for instance, a study by researchers at the University of Massachusetts reported that the long-term-care occupational sector ranked second in work-related injuries and illnesses.[43] Jobs in nursing homes are both physically demanding and psychologically taxing, with daily stressors high enough to affect resident health and safety. Compensation in the industry is notoriously low, particularly for health aides, housekeepers, and facilities workers, positions that paid a median hourly wage of $16, $12, and $19, respectively, in 2018.[44] Compared to care workers in other affluent nations, those in the U.S. are more likely to work on part-time contracts, and to hold jobs in multiple nursing homes.[45] Residents, of course, were not the only ones affected by these conditions. In the first year of the pandemic, COVID mortality rates for nursing home staffs ranked among the highest of any occupation in the U.S.[46]

To understand the nature of pandemic life and labor in long-term-care facilities, in July 2020, the labor historian Gabriel Winant interviewed Shantonia Jackson, a certified nursing assistant (CNA) in Chicago who worked at both City View Multicare Center in Cicero, Illinois, and Berkeley Nursing in Oak Park. At City View, she works with both old residents and people with severe psychiatric illnesses. "Me and my coworker had thirty-five residents apiece," Jackson explained. "City View was one of the nursing homes that made the news for the outbreak. We had 253 residents that had the corona out of around 315. My coworker who worked on the unit with me passed away from the corona. Now I work with seventy men in an all-men's unit. It's rough, because it's seventy brains on one brain. I'm the only CNA."[47]

Jackson had started working at City View eight years before, at $9.20 an hour. By 2020, she had six years on the job and union membership in the Service Employees International Union, and her hourly wage was $14.30. "Do you think that's enough? To properly take care of your family members? No. It's not. $14.30. I have a daughter in college. That's why I have to work two jobs." She told Winant that the demands on her time made it impossible to provide the level of care that the residents needed or, by virtue of their humanity, deserved. During the pandemic, "management never came upstairs on the floor with me to see what I was dealing with. They would come upstairs and yell at me, 'Well, you need to give a shower.' I already gave thirty showers out of seventy people. I can't make sure seventy take a shower. Because I've got to still pass trays. I've got to still make beds. It's hard."[48]

When COVID tore through City View, Jackson called her

managers at Berkeley, which has only old residents, and told them she needed to take a leave. "I felt like I didn't want to take the virus from City View, with 253 infections, to Berkeley, which didn't have one case." She anticipated that her employers would be grateful; instead, they were incensed. "The nursing home industry is so fickle, and selfish, and disrespectful, because they were actually angry at me for leaving. I thought my director of nursing would be appreciative, because what if I came over here and I transmitted to all these elderly people? They all would have died. And they have the nerve to be mad at me, and calling me, saying, 'You're not going to come back?'" Jackson couldn't help but feel like the institutions that were charged with providing care lost sight of their mission, and refused to implement the changes that would have saved people's lives. "In America, we don't care about the elderly," she lamented. "They're about to die anyway, we don't care."[49]

Of course, both long-term-care managers and policymakers in the U.S. could have imposed special regulations limiting the job mobility of care workers during the pandemic, as officials did in South Korea. They could have implemented emergency screening and testing requirements for staff and residents, and offered clear guidelines about when to move infected people to hospitals. They could have prioritized long-term-care facilities for delivery of face masks and PPE. Instead, they allowed residential care operators to go about their business. On March 24, 2020, the CDC, working closely with the White House COVID-19 Response Team, issued national COVID testing guidelines, but chose not to include nursing homes in the top-priority group for testing. "Long-term care facility residents with symptoms didn't get into the top testing tier until April 27," *The Wall Street Journal* reported. "Even then, asymptomatic nursing home residents weren't mentioned in the priority groups. Ultimately, federal regulators didn't mandate testing of nursing home staff until August." And they never prohibited workers from moving between long-term-care homes.[50]

Working conditions in nursing homes were only one part of the equation; living conditions were another. As in Canada, long-term-care facilities with crowded bedrooms and common quarters were especially dangerous; so were facilities that had higher levels of poor, Black, and brown residents. In fact, the two trends are related, because impoverished people of color in the U.S. are more likely than others to wind up in crowded long-term-care institutions, the lower part of what public health scholars call the "two-tiered system" of homes for the elderly and frail. As a team led by the Brown University gerontologist Vincent Mor reports, in their analysis of socioeconomic and racial disparities in American nursing home care, during ordinary times, "poor, frail, and minority residents served by 'lower tier' providers are particularly likely to receive substandard care."[51] In an infectious disease outbreak, they're also particularly likely to die.

In Illinois, for instance, a report by the Department of Healthcare and Family Services found that Black and Latino nursing home residents were overrepresented among those who lived in a bedroom with three or four people.[52] "Over-bedding," as the industry calls this practice, is a clear risk factor for COVID mortality, and it's more common in homes with high proportions of Medicaid recipients, because Medicaid (the highly stigmatized public health care program for low-income Americans) pays providers lower rates for nursing home care than most private insurance companies. Although stingy public funding for poor people's programs, rather than observable racial discrimination, may be responsible for these conditions, it's both notable and disturbing that Black and Latino nursing home residents in Illinois had higher COVID mortality rates during the pandemic. Nationally, as a study in *JAMA Network Open* reports, "nursing homes with the highest proportions of non-White residents experienced COVID-19 death counts that were 3.3-fold higher than those of facilities with the highest proportions of White residents."[53] These disparities are not solely due to crowding; concentrations of COVID in Black and brown communities, pre-existing medical conditions, and racial discrimination in the health care system also contributed to the problem. But poor conditions in nursing homes vastly increased the vulnerability of people confined in them, as did America's indifference to their plight.

Tragically, old people who lived in one of America's higher-quality nursing homes faced a different kind of problem during the pandemic: social isolation so extreme that it contributed to emotional suffering, physical illness, and in the long run a surprisingly sharp spike in deaths. Although distancing is important for protecting the frail and elderly from an infectious disease outbreak, it takes a toll on their bodies and minds. In recent decades, epidemiologists have established that social isolation is a major risk factor for a variety of health problems, from heart disease to depression and mental illness.[54] When COVID hit, the highest-rated long-term-care facilities imposed strict restrictions on visitors, made sure nurses and health aides wore masks and other protective equipment, and limited social gatherings among residents. The measures dramatically reduced the death toll from COVID during the first six months of the crisis. But did the social isolation make other health problems worse?

Christopher Cronin and William Evans, economists at the University of Notre Dame, found a novel way to answer this question. They found that although higher-rated nursing homes were no more successful at limiting COVID cases than lower-rated institutions, they were far better at preventing deaths. From May 24 to September 13, 2020, five-star nursing homes had 15 percent fewer reported COVID deaths than one-star homes—a significant difference. Yet during that same period, five-star homes had 11 percent more non-COVID deaths than one-star homes, and by April 15, 2021, the figure was nearly 15 percent.[55]

The data, as the economists acknowledge, are hardly perfect. It's possible that some deaths classified as "non-COVID" were actually COVID-related, and there are likely lots of missing data. That said, other research confirms that, in general, even nursing home residents who avoided COVID experienced a loss of mental and physical health during the pandemic, with symptoms including depression, unplanned substantial weight loss, and incontinence.[56]

The findings also point to another essential lesson: distancing can save lives, but only if it's done carefully, without severing the bonds that preserve us. Even in pandemics, people need a way to remain socially close.

. . .

Severing social bonds is a core objective of detention facilities, such as jails and prisons, which exist to discipline and punish people accused or convicted of serious crimes. Paradoxically, however, detention facilities also congregate those confined within them, and in societies with high incarceration levels, living conditions are often dangerously crowded, with over-bedded cells, overused washrooms, densely packed cafeterias, and common areas so busy it's hard to find personal space. There is no distancing in these harsh places, with one major exception: those who are condemned to solitary confinement, a torturous punishment whose only virtue may be a dose of protection from infectious disease.

Like nursing homes, jails and prisons rely on a large number and wide variety of workers who move between the community and the compound. Corrections officers. Cleaners. Counselors. Cooks. Clerks. Nurses. Health aides. Drivers. People like Persol, who are busy parenting and spending time with family when they're not on the job, mixing it up with people who may well be exposed. Jails and prisons are also highly trafficked sites for visitors, from attorneys to investigators to family and friends of the people who are detained. The detainees themselves move in and out on a frequent basis, with new people being locked up or released every day. Places that had high rates of COVID in the community had to take extraordinary measures to limit transmission into jails and prisons. Testing and screening workers, visitors, and detainees. Issuing and enforcing mask mandates. Reducing crowding by giving early parole to nonviolent offenders and to older people who were most threatened by COVID. In the United States, which had both more cases of COVID and more incarcerated people than any other nation, few institutions were willing or able to implement these changes. The results were lethal.

We will never know exactly how many incarcerated people or corrections workers in the U.S. contracted COVID, because for much of the crisis the criminal justice system lacked a sufficient number of tests to find out. A research article in the *American Journal of Preventive Medicine* reports that, from March 31 to November 4, 2020, the confirmed COVID rate for corrections workers in state and federal prisons ranged between three and five times higher than the rate for the general population.[57] Another paper, in the prestigious medical journal *JAMA*, shows that by June 6, 2020, there were 42,107 confirmed COVID cases and 510 COVID deaths among the 1,295,285 detainees in American prisons. The case rate, 3,251 per 100,000 incarcerated people, was more than five times higher than it was for the general U.S. population. The crude death rate for that period, 39 per 100,000 incarcerated people, was significantly higher than the overall U.S. mortality rate, 29 per 100,000. But, as the *JAMA* paper explains, old people, who are most vulnerable to death from COVID, represent just 3 percent of the prison population, compared to 16 percent of the U.S. population. When the authors calculated the age-adjusted mortality rate, they discovered that the people in prison were three times more likely to die of COVID than people their age who were free.[58]

Even this adjusted death rate is an understatement of the actual mortality, in part because so many people who died from COVID in jails and prisons were never formally diagnosed with the disease. Although we don't have excess death figures for every state system, the available data suggest that mortality in detention centers was far higher than the official record shows. In Florida, for instance, a team of researchers from the UCLA Law COVID Behind Bars Data Project found that there were 42 percent more deaths than expected in the population of incarcerated people during 2020, and from 2019 to 2020, the life expectancy of people detained in the state at age twenty dropped by four years.[59]

When investigative journalists at *The New York Times* scrutinized the mortality records of select state prison systems throughout the U.S., from New York to California, Texas to Ohio, they found dozens of cases where incarcerated people who died of COVID were not listed in the official tally. In some instances, prison wardens sent incarcerated people to hospitals when they became ill, then refused to include their deaths in the prison count.[60] Officials defended this policy. "It is unfair to expect jails to somehow take ownership of what happens to people once they are released from our custody," said a spokeswoman for the Virginia Beach Sheriff's Office. "It is asinine to think that we could somehow keep tabs on those thousands of people and take responsibility for them." But the family members of those who died saw things differently. As the son of a man who caught COVID while awaiting trial in a Florida jail and died soon after told the *Times*, "Maybe no one's actually died inside of the jail with COVID-19—because they sent him to the hospital to die."[61]

At Rikers Island, where Persol works, the connection between detention and death was harder to question. In July 2021, Vincent Mercado, a sixty-four-year-old who was overweight and suffered from circulatory problems, was arrested for illegal possession of a firearm and drugs that police found in a parked vehicle. Although Mercado insisted that the contraband belonged to his partner, a judge ordered that he be placed in Rikers and set bail at $100,000, far more than he could pay. Mercado wound up in the infirmary, where he faced an elevated risk of exposure to the coronavirus. "Turned out it was the worst place he could have been," said James Kilduff, his attorney. Kilduff pleaded for the court to lower the bail, citing Mercado's advanced age and precarious health. The judge refused. Predictably, Mercado caught COVID, and his symptoms quickly became so serious that the jail transferred him to Elmhurst Hospital Center, in Queens. On the day he was transferred, the judge finally granted Mercado emergency release. At that point, it was irrelevant. Hours later, Mercado died.[62]

In June 2020, researchers from the Prison Policy Initiative (PPI), a nonprofit, nonpartisan organization dedicated to criminal justice reform, and the American Civil Liberties Union assessed the actions that each state took to protect incarcerated people and corrections workers during the first months of the pandemic. Their findings are disheartening. "Despite all of the information, voices calling for action, and the obvious need, state responses ranged from disorganized or ineffective, at best, to callously nonexistent at worst," they reported.[63] Not every state handled COVID identically, however, and some were more considerate, or cruel, than others. California, for instance, provided free phone calls to detainees during the first year of the crisis to ease the pain of social isolation, and offered free hygiene products to curb the risk of infection. It curbed crowding by reducing the overall population of incarcerated people by nearly 20 percent through early release and delayed induction (though, as the researchers note, its facilities were so overfilled before the pandemic that they remained above design capacity even after these efforts).[64] In Texas, officials refused these reforms. No free calls. No accelerated paroles or medical releases. No plans to give incarcerated people priority access to vaccinations. No policies to improve access to hand sanitizer and soap.[65]

These differences mattered, but only at the margins. Both Texas and California have enormous numbers of people incarcerated in their chronically crowded, understaffed, and unsanitary jails and prisons, and they ranked first and second among all U.S. states in the number of confirmed COVID-19 prison deaths. As the PPI and ACLU report concluded, "No state had close to adequate prison population reductions, despite some governors issuing orders or guidance that, on their face, were intended to release more people quickly."[66] No state did universal testing of detainees and staff, nor did many make major improvements to their ventilation systems or enforce the kind of physical distancing protocols that could have reduced viral spread. It's unclear exactly how many lives states could have saved if they had made more substantial changes to protect the men and women they kept in detention, but it's worth noting that France, which was far more aggressive about releasing prisoners in the early stage of the pandemic, reported only one death from COVID among detainees from the initial outbreak until June 1, 2020. The U.S., by comparison, reported 510.[67]

The range of grades that the PPI and ACLU issued for state prison performance in the pandemic ranged from F to C-, with one state, Illinois, going ungraded because its data were subject to pending litigation. The truth is, nearly every jail and state prison system in America deserves scrutiny for the way they treated incarcerated people and corrections workers in the pandemic. They isolated those who needed connection, and concentrated those who needed safe space.

In this, at least, the U.S. was in good company. Nations everywhere struggled to find the right balance between physical distance and social connection, both of which were essential for getting through the first pandemic year. But the U.S., more than other affluent democratic societies, relies on mass incarceration for those it wants to punish and low-wage labor for those who are old and require residential care. These basic features of its social system make millions of Americans far more vulnerable than is necessary, not only during crises, but every day.

CHAPTER 9

"The Bridge"

NUALA O'DOHERTY

Nuala O'Doherty was fuming. "Honestly," she thought. "Don't these people understand how Queens works?"

It was December 31, 2019. O'Doherty, a fifty-one-year-old, first-generation Irish American married to an immigrant Ecuadoran auto mechanic, was home in Jackson Heights for the holidays—not quite resting, but home, at least, with her five children, a grandchild, and the family of five, dear friends, who lived on the first floor. Earlier that year, O'Doherty, who's five feet in heels with the energy of a hand grenade, had retired from a twenty-three-year career as a prosecutor in the Manhattan District Attorney's Office. But retirement, she told me, was really just a way to do more meaningful work. That fall, neighbors had drafted O'Doherty into an unexpected project, running for the State Assembly. Now here she was, fresh off of Christmas and a day from New Year's Eve, down in the basement, her campaign headquarters, brainstorming solutions for local problems. She just wasn't expecting the transportation system to be one of them.

That day, the Metropolitan Transit Agency (MTA), aiming to improve efficiency and reduce operating costs, had released a draft plan, the Queens Bus Redesign, that eliminated bus stops across the city's largest and most diverse borough. "This is a result of totally wiping the existing map clean and redrawing the network," said Mark Holmes, chief officer of MTA Bus.[1] Once implemented, Holmes promised, travel times would be faster for nearly all passengers. That sounded good, too, because Queens, whose population of 2.3 million is nearly half foreign-born, is a borough of hardworking people, and their jobs take them all over the region, as far as public transit allows. Everyone in Queens is used to crowded subway cars, to packed buses, trapped in thick city traffic. It's part of daily life here, as predictable as the seasons. You get to work on time by leaving a little earlier, sacrificing some sleep. You elbow your way to a seat. You carve out a few inches of breathing room. You wait.

O'Doherty was all for faster buses. The issue, she learned, was that the MTA wanted to speed things up by making buses less accessible. Shorter routes. Sending riders to the subway system rather than letting them travel where they used to go. The plan eliminated the crowded Q49 bus, which wiggled through East Elmhurst and Jackson Heights, ending at the modern, accessible express subway hub. It also involved expanding the average distance between bus stops from 850 to 1,400 feet, which would dramatically increase walking time, and cutting service between Queens neighborhoods.[2] "They can't possibly have talked to current bus riders in Jackson Heights," wrote Jim Burke, a transit advocate who lives a few blocks from O'Doherty and helped run her campaign. "I can't imagine anyone demanding *less* service, fewer destinations and less access."[3] O'Doherty considered the plan—and the process for creating it—an insult to her community. "It was," she said, "totally dumb."

It was also clarifying. As O'Doherty saw it, the plan showed everyone in Jackson Heights just how little their wellbeing mattered to the people who ran New York City, how easy it was to ignore their voices, how much they stood to lose—job opportunities, mobility, access to services, basic health and security in the event of a crisis—unless they could put up a fight.

Not that they would be easy to organize. Doing collective work is always complicated in Jackson Heights, where residents speak 167 languages, making it, as *The New York Times* put it, "the most culturally diverse neighborhood in New York, if not on the planet."[4] But she had lived in the neighborhood for nearly twenty years already, and from the beginning she'd been struck by how few basic public goods the city offered there. With less than two square feet of park space per resident, compared to 140 square feet per resident in more verdant areas, Jackson Heights is a green desert.[5] Schools typically lack fields. Some don't have playgrounds, even for the youngest kids.

It would be hard to find a place in New York City where residents need access to good public spaces more than they do in Jackson Heights. With one in four apartments designated as "overcrowded" (meaning it has more than one person per room), Jackson Heights is among the most residentially congested areas in New York City.[6] "Families live together here," O'Doherty explained. "They chop up apartments, make a bunch of new bedrooms. They'll have eight, ten people in one unit. That gives them the ultimate security. One person can lose their job and they'll all be okay." Conditions like this, and the neighborhood's booming restaurants and street markets, make sanitation a constant challenge. The city invariably fails to keep the place clean, which means that, as in most other aspects of their lives, Jackson Heights residents get stuck with the work.

"That's how I got to know the neighborhood," O'Doherty told me. "I found out about the Jackson Heights Beautification Group. They did a community cleanup on Saturday mornings at 8 a.m., wore these orange shirts and went up and down the avenues. I said I'm gonna do it!" She was especially excited about the group's gardening projects. "I grew up in this immigrant family that moved around from place to place," she explained. "I never felt that I was from somewhere, and I wanted that for my kids. When I moved here, I wanted them to create a place for themselves. And if you plant a flower somewhere, that's your place." Her husband, who slept in on Saturdays, insisted that O'Doherty take their three youngest children with her so he could rest. "He thought I wouldn't go," she recalled. Soon, though, it became a family ritual. Dress the kids. Throw together breakfast. Race out the door and find the congregation of cleaners. "Like some people go to church, I wanted to do community service," she said. "It's how I cleanse my soul."

O'Doherty had been doing community service since she fin-

ished college. First in Rochester, where she interned at Eastman
Kodak and felt called to help out in a homeless shelter. Next, in
law school at St. Johns, and in her apartment in the neighborhood
of Astoria, where she became a regular in the local bodega that
functioned like a community center for Latino immigrants. The
place was buzzing with drama and activity, and O'Doherty discovered that she could help her friends register for school, enroll
in public programs, and solve problems with housing and rent.
She volunteered at Legal Aid, and for most of her time in graduate school she thought she'd pursue a legal career in an organization that fought poverty. "But then I found out how hard it was to
get an actual job in that," O'Doherty said. "I got an internship at
the Bronx DA's office, working homicide. And I loved it. I mean,
wow! It was better than *Law & Order.* I did cases there that will be
with me forever, things I'll never forget." When she graduated,
the Manhattan DA's office, a prestigious bureau known for pursu-
ing high-profile cases, offered her a full-time position. "I couldn't
believe it," she recalled. "They had turned me down for intern-
ships every year." She had developed new skills, though. Not just
in law school, where she'd earned a recommendation (and a job
offer) from the legendary Brooklyn DA Charlie Hynes; in the
bodega, as well. "If you want to be a good prosecutor," she told
me, "the best thing you can do is get to know bodega life."

O'Doherty is from a family of driven, disciplined workers.
Her parents had doctorates in chemistry—that's what got them
from Ireland to Indiana, where they worked in pharmaceuticals
and pushed their children to study like their lives depended on it.
Her sister is now a professor of medicine, her brother a professor
of chemistry. None of them, O'Doherty said, "work as much as
the people in the bodega. I'd never seen such hard lives." Some
of her friends there were manual laborers. She got close to a kid
from Mexico whose job was to lug boxes from the overheated
basement storage room to the shelves upstairs. "He'd carry
these heavy containers of soda when it was, like, 120 degrees. He
worked ten times harder than I did. I had huge respect for that."
Most people she knew worked off the books. No insurance. No
Social Security. No vacations or sick days. You work or you can't
pay rent. When she fell in love with Marcelino, the man who

would become her husband, she saw what it took to work as a car mechanic in New York City. "Later, when I became a prosecutor, I'd meet drug dealers. And you know, they work really hard. Like, you have to be on that spot, day in, day out. It's a job. You had to do it. I always tried to see their perspective, where they saw their lives going. A lot of my colleagues looked down on them, treated them like they were dumb. Maybe they made bad choices, but they were always in difficult positions. And I always treated them with respect."

Respect for hard work and hard workers served O'Doherty well in Queens. It helped her build a life as a young adult in Astoria, but it really paid off when she moved to Jackson Heights with Marcelino and their kids in 2002. "We bought a huge house," she said. "I had gotten some money from my father, and a little more from my brother-in-law, because his wife died in the World Trade Center on September 11 and I handled everything for the Victim Compensation Fund, dealing with the police, identifying the body, you know, horrible stuff." It's a semi-detached brick house with two legal apartments, a basement, a garage, and a small side garden, just a few blocks from a subway station, and an easy commute to Manhattan. In a neighborhood where people live cheek-to-jowl, O'Doherty now had nearly 3,800 square feet. "But it was a complete wreck," she reported. "There had been a fire, and the roof leaked like a sieve. That's why we could afford it." The place needed a total renovation. It would take years to do it, and her family, led by Marcelino, would be the crew.

It didn't take long for the neighbors to figure out that O'Doherty had a lot to offer. A Chilean woman named Beatrice organized the Saturday cleanups, and when she found out her new volunteer was an attorney, she enlisted her to write a grant for their work. When they got it, they used the funds to buy new T-shirts, posters, and launch a recruitment effort. O'Doherty looked into the group's strategy, and noticed that they had been cleaning up a commercial street where the proprietors of local businesses were legally responsible for sanitation. O'Doherty informed them, perhaps not politely, that from now on they would be living up to their obligations or facing, in her words, "enforcement." She and Beatrice redirected the volunteers to parts of the neighborhood that really needed their help. The boulevards, for instance. Small unkempt gardens. Patches of land near the BQE, the Brooklyn-Queens Expressway, where people had been illegally dumping because, apparently, no one really owned them. Suddenly, they'd found more places to clean than they could manage. O'Doherty, whose children were now in local public schools, had a solution for that, too.

The martial arts studio. The parents group. The dog owners. The gardeners. The religious groups. Jackson Heights was chock-full of active people and small but busy organizations. Wouldn't they pitch in? By then, O'Doherty had gotten active in the school leadership team. She couldn't help it. She'd befriended lots of well-educated professionals in Jackson Heights, people who lived in beautiful old apartment buildings and commuted into Manhattan. "Most of them sent their kids to private schools, Catholic schools," she reported. "I had five kids and was putting every dollar I made into the house. We had to use the public schools, and I had to make sure they were great." Each little project O'Doherty took on involved creating a team of allies. Partners. Sometimes friends. She couldn't feel it happening, but before long she had roots everywhere in the neighborhood, tangled up with others, feeding into all kinds of small worlds. There were cleaning projects. Gardening projects. School projects. Safety projects. O'Doherty was a connector. She could get her neighbors where they needed to be.

In the first days of 2020, O'Doherty could see that the MTA's bus plan was going to be an obstacle and an opportunity. On the one hand, it threatened to break up the neighborhood routines and complicate everyone's commute to work; on the other, it was a way to unite the community—to create one, even, because suddenly, despite all their ethnic differences, the people of Jackson Heights had something in common: they were furious with the MTA. O'Doherty had never run for public office before. She'd never imagined being a politician, never thought she could win. But she knew a political opening when she saw one. "I converted my whole campaign to the bus issue," she remembered. "We'd go to every bus stop and hand out these flyers. 'Nuala for 34! Stop the bus cuts! Stop the bus cuts!'" They knocked on doors, worked the street markets, held rallies, got coverage in local media, started a petition, whipped up lots of outrage and support.

"It was a great campaign," she said. "And then, in February, there was this big rally planned near Elmhurst Hospital. People started saying to me, 'I don't want to go near the hospital. I hear there's this virus.' I was like, 'You're crazy! Come!' We're still at the markets, trying to get on the ballot. Everything's fine." By early March, she could tell that it wasn't. "It was like a storm was coming," she recalled. "My basement was a war room. My family had all come in to help me get the signatures. We had all these printers going. We were racing. Everyone was like, 'Hurry up! Hurry up!'" They didn't want to lose momentum if the city shut down.

In early March, her friend Jim Burke, the transit advocate, told her he was going to a fundraiser for Carlina Rivera, who was running for City Council in Manhattan. "It was in a crowded bar," she told me. "I had been in a bar the night before. We were spitting all over each other, and I started thinking, 'I'm gonna get sick here. I gotta go!' A few days later, Jim called me and said, 'You know, I don't feel great.' I didn't see him for, like, two weeks, and when I did he said, 'It's so weird, I can't taste any-thing.' Everyone knows that Jim's a big eater. He loves peanut butter! And he was like, 'I don't even want it. It tastes like muck.' It was the very beginning. We didn't know that was a thing. But we realized something was happening. It was just like, whoa."

Before she knew it, the sickness was everywhere. Her cam-paign was sputtering; everything else was, too. On March 14, Governor Cuomo issued an executive order cutting the signature requirement for getting on the ballot to 30 percent of the original threshold, and ending all petitioning on March 17. O'Doherty had already qualified, so she and her daughter drove to the Board of Elections to submit the paperwork. "My daughter went in with the lawyer," she recalled. "I stayed outside and parked ille-gally. People from all over the city were coming in, handing in the petitions, everyone in these small rooms." Hundreds of can-didates submitted their petitions that week, right on schedule. O'Doherty was on the ballot, and the coronavirus was on the march. Jim recovered. But by April, a dozen Board of Elections staff members had tested positive for COVID-19, and two were dead.[7] Suddenly, the race was different. Everything was different. Especially in Jackson Heights.

"I remember the sound of the birds chirping," O'Doherty told me. "It was the beginning of spring, all this life blooming. And it was silent. Absolutely quiet. No one was driving. No one was playing in the street. Hardly a sound. It was just the birds. The birds and the sirens. It felt like there were ambulances on every block."

From March to May, when New York City became the global hot spot for the coronavirus, Jackson Heights was its fiery core. Along with the adjacent, similarly crowded immigrant neighborhoods of Elmhurst, East Elmhurst, and Corona, Jackson Heights was part of a cluster in central Queens that experienced more cases, more hospitalizations, and more deaths than any part of the city, and any part of the world. "We're the epicenter of the epicenter," said Daniel Dromm, the city councilman representing Elmhurst and Jackson Heights. "This has shaken the whole neighborhood."[8]

Pummeled is more like it. One way to measure the impact is to consider the official mortality figures issued by New York City's Department of Health and Mental Hygiene. For the week ending March 21, the COVID-19 mortality rate for Jackson Heights was 8 per 100,000 residents, compared to zero in adjacent neighborhoods like Corona and Flushing, and 0.13 for the entire city. The next week, the mortality rate shot up to 40 per 100,000 in Jackson Heights, compared to 9 in New York City. By April, when cases were spreading quickly, the people in Jackson Heights and the neighborhoods around it were dying at roughly two times the overall city rate.

It's hard to know precisely how many cases there were in central Queens, because case counts require testing, and at that time tests were scarce. On April 9, 2020, *The New York Times* reported more than seven thousand cases in the "seven-square-mile patch of densely packed immigrant enclaves" of central Queens.[9] Elmhurst Hospital Center, a 545-bed public facility located in the heart of the area, got so crowded, so quickly, that patients packed the halls and admission rooms, while those needing a test waited hours outdoors, in long, snaking lines, and were often turned away when they ran out of kits. Some died before they could get care. Administrators there had no choice but to divert some patients to other hospitals, and to store those who died in a fleet of refrigerated trucks parked outside. One staff member described feeling that the hospital was "under siege."[10]

O'Doherty didn't need to see the hospital to know how dire things were in her neighborhood. "My brother-in-law got sick early on," she told me. "Very sick. He was on the ventilator, first for a day and then he came off. And then he was back on it for fourteen days. He was literally one of the first people I heard of who went to the hospital for this. And when I went to help his family, they were so scared that they didn't even want to open the door." Their anxiety was understandable. Entire households, filled with people, were falling to the virus. O'Doherty described seeing ambulances line up on the streets near her: "If the ambulance came and left it was okay. It was when they stayed it was a problem. They'd try to revive people. Then another ambulance would come. Then the medical examiner would come. He would come in a moon suit. This big white suit, and all the people in the building would come out in T-shirts and shorts. No masks. No protection. And we'd look at each other and say, oh man, everybody in that house has it. It was so weird. It just didn't seem real."

Her brother-in-law survived and got out of the hospital. The two people in the house in front of O'Doherty's didn't. Soon, people in Jackson Heights were telling each other to avoid Elmhurst Hospital Center at any cost. "There were horror stories about Elmhurst Hospital and how bad things were there," O'Doherty told me. "One of my neighbors called for help because her husband was sick but they would not call 911 because they knew he would be brought to Elmhurst." It wasn't just the hospital. O'Doherty started hearing about people who were avoiding grocery stores, pharmacies, bodegas, even. Everyone in the neighborhood heard the sirens, saw the men in moon suits carrying away the dead. They couldn't get masks, couldn't even get sanitizer, paper towels, or soap. They were hunkering down, unsure how to protect themselves in public, uncertain how to get the basic things they needed to survive. O'Doherty realized that the neighborhood was likely full of people in this situation. Her basement was still a war room, but the stakes of her campaign had changed dramatically. Life was on the line.

Her primary instrument was a Post-it note. "That's what made me famous," O'Doherty joked. "Never do that!" In fact, she meant the opposite. The Post-it notes marked the beginning of a transformative collective project, one that would weave her neighbors together in ways she had never imagined, maybe for good. Governments around the world were advising people to maintain "social distance" as a survival strategy. But that didn't make sense to O'Doherty, and it didn't work in places like Jackson Heights. In fact, people there needed the opposite. Social closeness. Support. They had never depended on their neighbors more.

Physical distance. That was sensible. That kept people from getting sick.

Social solidarity. That was essential. And the way to produce it was mutual aid.

On March 13, O'Doherty reached out to the volunteers on her campaign team.[11] "I said, 'Put a Post-it note on your neighbors' door. Give them my phone number.' For me it wasn't a big thing. Like, the world has my phone number. I don't care. I took a picture of a Post-it note with my number, and we made a flyer with it. We told people to give them to their neighbors, and then we went to the same places where we did the bus flyers and gave them out there, too." Soon, thousands of flyers with her phone number and the message "Call me if you need any help" were circulating in the neighborhood. O'Doherty's goal was simple: she wanted everyone in Jackson Heights to be connected to someone who could support them, an ear, a voice, a hand. She hadn't realized how much help people would need as the pandemic dragged on. But neither had she understood how much her neighbors would give.

It was extraordinary, how many people wanted to participate. "Right away, I had about one hundred people offer to volunteer," she told me. "That was the beginning of COVID Care," the mutual aid network she organized. (Its formal name was COVID Care Neighbor Network.) "But we didn't know what the problems were, what people needed." O'Doherty thinks of this initial stage as the "Time of Confusion," followed by a brief period she calls "Life Interrupted." Neighbors called to ask if someone could pick up their laundry, get cleaning supplies, deliver groceries. They were small, stopgap measures, and they were easy to do. By the second week, though, the calls became scary. "One morning, someone called and asked for a hot meal. My daughter loves to cook and made something. We brought this meal, and found an elderly woman sitting on a chair. She was waiting for us, propping open the door. She could barely stand. Her husband was worse. She called the next morning to say that her husband had died. We had made him his last meal." Not long after, a woman whose husband died at home asked if someone could come and sanitize her apartment. Then O'Doherty fielded a call from a Nepalese woman, a mother with two young children at home. "Her husband had just gone to the hospital with COVID," she recalled. "She was also really sick, and the EMTs wanted to take her, too. She wouldn't go because of the kids. No one else would go inside the apartment and help, so I personally went over. It was just the kind of thing you couldn't ask anyone else to do."

O'Doherty has a catalogue of stories from the "Scary" period, each with its own particular horrors. In retrospect, she told me, this was still a relatively quiet time for the COVID Care Network. Dangerous. Stressful. But quiet. It wasn't until the beginning of April that her phone started ringing constantly. "I call this the Crash stage," O'Doherty said. "The economic crash. It came after the shutdowns. People had enough food to get themselves through the first few weeks. But the restaurants were closed. The street vendors couldn't operate. Not many calls for drivers. There were no more cleaning jobs. No more nannies working off the books. We had all these immigrant families living paycheck to paycheck. Now there's no more paychecks. No stimulus coming. People were like, 'What are we going to do?'"

"That's when we started the food pantry in my garage," O'Doherty recounted. "Food. Diapers. Formula. Those were the fundamentals. Rice. Oil. Beans. Spaghetti. Canned goods. We had, like, gringo bags, Hispanic bags, and Indian bags. We'd do one emergency delivery per family, and then try to set them up with city services so they could survive." The demand seemed endless. "There were times when you couldn't even walk in here, we had so many boxes of diapers." On Tuesdays and Fridays, roughly fifteen volunteers would come to her home to pack bags and prepare them for pickup. Her house could not contain all the activity. COVID Care set up a leadership team, people who could help with fielding calls, match volunteers with jobs, raise funds from donors, and apply for government grants. They set up a Facebook Group page and a WhatsApp chat to facilitate communication, started a Google phone service to handle calls, organized a schedule with regular workers, and developed a system for managing more serious problems, cases that required more than a bag of food. The ranks of volunteers kept growing. At first it was mainly women, but as the pandemic wore on more men showed up. "There were no jobs!" O'Doherty exclaimed. "They had nothing to do." One family I met signed up for a weekly food delivery, which they did with their son in the backseat. Another, where the father had lost his job in a restaurant, made sandwiches for one hundred unemployed day laborers every Monday.

Food is the heart of Jackson Heights culture, and when restaurants closed because of the virus, pantries popped up throughout the neighborhood. Churches. Community centers. Restaurants. It seemed like every week another organization jumped in to help. O'Doherty's garage was no longer big enough for the effort. Friends of hers who had been volunteering were close with the proprietors of a local restaurant, the Queensboro, who were looking for a way to contribute. Soon they took over the operation, relieving O'Doherty's family, at least temporarily. The diaper boxes kept coming, as did a daily stream of people looking for help or a visit with the woman who some members of the mutual aid network were calling "the mayor" of Jackson Heights. O'Doherty rejected the label. "I'm not the mayor," she told me. "I'm the bridge."

. . .

By May the surge of illness and death in Queens had subsided.
The death rate was still more than twice as high as the city average, but the numbers were declining, the air was warming. New
Yorkers were eager to return to life. Now the mutual aid group
had new problems to tackle. Families throughout the neighborhood had been unable to hold funerals for relatives who died of
the virus in March and April. COVID Care could help make
arrangements. New York State had issued a moratorium on evic-
tions, but landlords in immigrant neighborhoods knew that their
tenants were scared and vulnerable. Some were demanding rent
and making threats. "There's a new sense of fear," O'Doherty
told me. "We're not as worried about dying, but everyone's terrified of being evicted." O'Doherty had spent her career as a prosecutor, but she also knew how to defend her neighbors. "I told
everyone: Your landlord is not with you in the food line. They're
going to be okay. If you have money, use it to take care of your
family. You're not losing your home." Now she was effectively
running a legal clinic, too.

Since March, O'Doherty and her partners at COVID Care
had been trying to ward off dangers. Hunger. Eviction. Stress.
Isolation. Keeping each other alive. Now it was nearly summer.
The sirens were quiet. Restaurants would soon open. The whole
neighborhood, O'Doherty told me, was "itching to get outside."
She was eager to do something positive, and she had an idea.

For years, O'Doherty and Jim Burke, the transit activist, had
been pushing the city government to do something about the traffic hazards on 34th Avenue, a long boulevard lined with apartment
buildings and nine schools that runs through the heart of Jackson Heights. Burke, a youthful fifty-five-year-old with cropped
gray hair and a muscular build, is a consultant for e-commerce
and social media companies. He knows how to craft a message,
and also how to make it stick. Burke lives on 34th Avenue, and
although he has fond memories of playing on the streets as a child
in New York City, he rarely saw kids do anything but dodge traffic in Jackson Heights. "Unfortunately cars kind of took over,"
he said, and not without doing real damage.[12] It went beyond the

typical problems: air pollution, noise pollution, the sudden chaos when apps like Google Maps and Waze diverted vehicles onto the boulevard because the highway nearby filled up. There were accidents. Sometimes, O'Doherty told me, "the apps would send cars here right when all the schools let out—all nine of them! The traffic would literally stop. Drivers would get irate. They'd literally jump out and curse at the principal in front of the students.

"Other countries do incredible things with their streets," O'Doherty explained. "Look at European cities, where they've expanded the medians and created little playgrounds where the cars used to be. They've got these little bollards that go up or down with the push of a button, so they can quickly turn a roadway into a park." She and Burke wanted the city to do something similar in Jackson Heights. In March 2019, the issue took on new urgency when a twelve-year-old student at I.S. 145 Joseph Pulitzer Magnet School, on 34th Avenue, got pinned under a Jeep as he was leaving school.[13] He was hospitalized with serious injuries, and local media rushed to the street to cover the tragedy. "It was really unfortunate," O'Doherty said. "But in a way it was also fortunate, because now everyone is saying 'How can we help?'" The boy survived, and after he was discharged from the hospital, community leaders set up a series of meetings with the Department of Transportation, school officials, and parents' groups. "I told them we wanted the streets closed around the schools at drop-off and dismissal," O'Doherty recalled. "All nine of them." In Manhattan, the city had gotten favorable press for closing major streets, like Broadway, to car traffic. "They had millions of dollars for these kinds of projects," O'Doherty said. "But not everybody was on board."

The pandemic changed things, and created new possibilities. In April 2020, as city residents accustomed to being in public grew stressed and tired of life in claustrophobic apartments, neighborhood groups throughout New York City pressured local leaders to close streets to automobile traffic and expand sidewalks for pedestrians. They wanted more space for recreation, more places for kids to play, better green space, new options for outdoor dining, anything that could revive collective life. On April 27, Mayor de Blasio and the City Council announced that they planned to open forty miles of city streets in the next month, with an ultimate goal of one hundred miles.[14] O'Doherty and Burke were excited about the announcement, but they knew how power politics works. The affluent professionals in brownstone Brooklyn were clamoring for open streets. So were the wealthy families in Tribeca, Greenwich Village, and the Upper West Side. They doubted that Queens, or Jackson Heights, would be prioritized. When did that ever happen? So instead of waiting to find out where the mayor wanted to invest first, they decided to force the issue.

The next day, April 28, Burke and O'Doherty led a group of local activists onto 34th Avenue for a political demonstration and a citizen-led, do-it-yourself street closure that lasted just a few hours.[15] The organizers wore fluorescent construction vests, brought bright yellow tape, orange cones, and sandwich boards marked "Emergency Vehicles Only" to block traffic, and protesters carried small signs with messages like "Hey Simple Minds Don't You Forget About Queens." They were a small group at first, maybe thirty or forty. But once they set up and invited people to claim the boulevard, onlookers turned into participants, and the asphalt blossomed. O'Doherty, in a black coat with white polka dots, black pants, a sign that said "Open Streets," and a mask pulled down below her chin, grabbed a megaphone and called out to the neighborhood.

"Who here has a backyard to play in?"

"Nobody!"

"Who here has a yard to play in?"

"Nobody!"

"Who here is stuck in a tiny apartment?"

"Me!!" the crowd screamed. Residents of the congested brick apartment buildings that face the avenue poked their heads out of the windows, banging pots and pans and voicing their support.

"Who here wants some sunshine?"

"Me!"

"Who here wants some fresh air?"

This time a group of small children sitting on the street and making chalk drawings chimes in: "Me! Me!"

"Who wants their kids to be able to run again?"

"Me!"

A chant begins: "Open our streets! Open our streets! Open our streets!"

Burke and O'Doherty decided to roll with the momentum. They contacted neighborhood organizations and got support for a group they called the 34th Avenue Open Streets Coalition. O'Doherty's teenage son set up a website so that it looked official and strong. "Then we got lucky," O'Doherty reported. "One day Jim and I were in my basement, the campaign headquarters, and my friend Leslie Ramos, who ran the local business improvement district [BID], came by to drop off donations for COVID Care. Well, just then she gets a phone call from the mayor's office. They asked the BID to host the new open street and she said, 'No, that's too much work.' We were astounded. We looked at her and we asked, 'Who will they call next?' She said, 'The precinct.' So we called Lillian, who ran the local precinct council. We told her, 'Just say yes!' Jim and I knew this was it." They told the city about the congestion in Jackson Heights, the traffic hazards around the schools, the horrible toll from COVID, and their need for local parks. They said they had volunteers lined up for the project, and endorsements from local leaders, too. "They were like, 'Well, how are you going to do it?'" O'Doherty recalled. "And we said, 'Just give us the barricades. We'll do it ourselves.'"

That night Burke got on Twitter. "He was relentless," O'Doherty said. "He just pushed and pushed." They called their local political leaders, and after some initial hesitation, they agreed to back them, too. Then something unexpected happened. "We got a call from the city," O'Doherty remembered. "They said yes!"

This time, the open street would last more than a few hours. The city offered them a 1.3 mile stretch of 34th Avenue from 8 a.m. to 8 p.m., daily, but with strict conditions: the coalition would have to set up and take down the barriers, post the right signage, and keep the area clean. They could raise money independently, but they wouldn't get much support from the government. "Basically," O'Doherty said, "we were on our own." The work required real organization. "We needed ten volunteers every morning and every night, and they'd have to set up forty barricades at exactly the right time. Honestly, I think they expected us to fail."

Instead, the avenue blossomed. When I met O'Doherty there, on a sunny spring morning, the open street was bursting with activity. There were walkers, runners, cyclists, and street artists—people of all ages and groups. There were dawdlers, dancers, parents walking their children to school or sitting on portable chairs, drinking coffee as their toddlers played. O'Doherty, wearing a red baseball cap, a light purple jacket, and heavily used shoes, walked with me along the corridor, pausing every few blocks to show me plantings that she had installed on the median, or to introduce me to volunteers and staff members they had raised funds to pay. It was impossible to miss the pride she felt in the project. She gushed about the nightly pickup soccer matches there, the salsa classes, the arts and crafts sessions, the kids' races, the dominoes, the chess. She pointed out the blocks where the coalition helps set up food pantries, the immigrant proprietors of a food truck who live on the avenue and, having lost their customers in Midtown when offices closed down there, set up shop near their apartment, and got back on their feet. But in truth, she didn't need to say anything; the street spoke for itself.

Within months of opening, 34th Avenue became the city's showpiece for renewal and resilience. Mayor de Blasio came for photo ops. Political officials who had refused to endorse the initial idea now claimed it as their own. People from adjacent neighborhoods visited regularly, wondering whether they could get something similar where they live. It became, as *The New York Times* described it, "the gold standard of what a modern street should look like in a sustainable and equitable city that has fewer polluting cars and more space for people."[16]

Predictably, there was some backlash. Commuters complained about traffic problems building up in other areas. Some people who lived on the avenue were upset about music, garbage, change. But most residents were thrilled about the transformation. "It's changed our lives," a mother told me after O'Doherty introduced us. Another called it "a little miracle."[17]

I couldn't help thinking how much work a miracle takes.

. . .

In June, O'Doherty lost the primary election. "I got trounced," she said, her eyes rolling upward, like she couldn't believe how badly she had flubbed things. "I never should have run." I asked some people involved in local politics if they could explain what happened. "White woman, trying to beat a Latina in a district full of immigrants," someone told me. "A career prosecutor, from the DA's office, running as a progressive? It makes sense if you know Nuala. But she doesn't really tick the boxes. In this city, it's a tough sell."

Losing meant that O'Doherty could spend even more time on COVID Care and 34th Avenue. The health crisis abated, but the pandemic brought new challenges. An education and vaccination campaign for people who were worried about the risks of inoculation. A push to get children and teenagers ready for school in the fall. Hunger remained a problem, and O'Doherty worked with La Jornada, a food pantry run by evangelical Christians, in Flushing and in Woodside, where a project called Manos Que Dan gave away a thousand bags of groceries each weekend. Sometimes more. On the COVID Care Neighbor Network Facebook Group, more than 1,100 members communicated regularly, some offering services, others requesting help. In fall 2021, a cooperative of Jackson Heights women who lost their jobs during the pandemic announced that they had created NYC Green Clean, an environmentally responsible domestic cleaning service, and asked people for work. People called for volunteers at a neighborhood film festival, asked if anyone had an old laptop for their child to use at school, or a used T-Mobile cell phone they could give to a grandmother who needed one "to call or text with family."

On October 19, 2021, the city's Department of Transportation released a plan for making the 34th Avenue open street permanent. There would be car-free plaza blocks, nine "shared street configurations" with expanded pedestrian areas and spaces for cars during off-hours, and "diverters," which would replace temporary barricades, at the twenty-six intersections to prevent through traffic along the corridor.[18] The arrangement would be a compromise. While a few dozen activists called for a return to regular car traffic, a growing number of residents were pushing for a full-fledged linear park, with far more greenspace and far less room for cars. "Jackson Heights suffers from the least amount of access to public greenspace of any neighborhood in New York City," the creators of the 34avelinearpark.com website wrote. "34th Avenue is a once-in-a-lifetime opportunity." As they saw it, the future park would be akin to the High Line, the celebrated park and tourist attraction on the West Side of Manhattan, but for a working-class, immigrant community that rarely gets the best urban amenities. "Who knows what's possible," O'Doherty told me. "All I can say is that things have changed for the better." Not only has the avenue remained open, it has inspired leaders in other crowded neighborhoods to demand that the city give some of their streets to pedestrians, too.

On another walk along 34th Avenue, I asked O'Doherty what she would do when all these fights are settled, and the pandemic ends. "I don't know when that's going to be," she chuckled. "But I'm pretty sure we'll just be dealing with the next crisis. Unemployment. Back rent. Hunger. Fire. Floods. We're not getting past these things. They're just part of life."

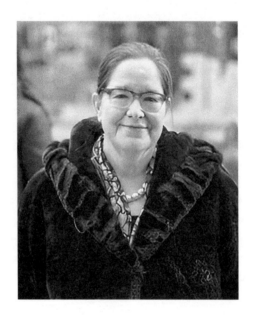

CHAPTER 10

Neighborhoods

No one really lives in New York City. It's true that more than eight million people tell the Census otherwise, but push a little and they'll say something different: it's the neighborhood—Harlem, Greenwich Village, Tottenville, Hunts Point, Astoria, or any of the residential areas where people hunker down together—that they call home. Think of New York City and you see a skyline, a panorama, a bird's-eye view that daily life never affords. Think of a neighborhood and you envision people in their habitat: an apartment building, a pizza joint, a playground, a bodega, a stoopful of characters, each making and marking the place as their own.

The story of where people died in the pandemic is similar. The numbers leave little doubt that New York City suffered more COVID deaths—at least twenty thousand—than any city in the world during 2020. On a planet full of hot spots, Gotham, with its blaring sirens, overcrowded hospitals, and fleets of storage trucks holding dead bodies, was a hellscape like no other. Look closer, however, and a different picture emerges. Some of the city's neighborhoods proved remarkably healthy and resilient, even during the darkest days of the disaster, while others were utterly devastated, with levels of death and disease so high nearly every household was touched. The pattern, which runs quite neatly along class lines and bears marks of the city's ethnic and racial divisions, too, is easily apparent. Consider, for instance, the map of COVID deaths in 2020, which shows the dramatic disparities between Manhattan neighborhoods around and below Central Park and those in the outer boroughs.[1] The demography behind these trends is as plain as the geography: Race and class mattered. "Of the 10 ZIP codes with the highest death rates, eight have populations that are predominantly black or Hispanic," *The New York Times* reported in May 2020. Of those with the lowest death rates, "each has a six-figure median household income."[2]

But the fate of a neighborhood, like the fate of a state or nation, is only partly determined by the characteristics of the people who live in it. In New York City, for example, some areas with high concentrations of Black or Latino residents had exceptionally high COVID death rates while others fared much better. Similarly, there was considerable variation among neighborhoods with clusters of immigrants, and even among those where residents were wealthy and privileged.

There's no question that race, class, and age shaped which areas were hit hardest in New York City, just as they did throughout the United States. But demography is only part of the story. In the U.S., political ideology would shape COVID's fault lines after the first year of the pandemic. As the Harvard public epidemiologist Nancy Krieger discovered, in a study of politics and COVID mortality between April 2021 and March 2022, "the higher the exposure to conservatism" in their congressional district, "the higher the COVID-19 age-standardized mortality rates, even after taking into account the districts' social characteristics, voters' political lean, and vaccination rates."[3] In places like New York City, there's less variation in political ideology. But the physical characteristics of neighborhoods, as well as the social networks that residents relied on to protect each other, helped determine who lived and who died; so, too, did the kinds of labor that people in different localities performed.

To understand how, and why, we have to focus on where residents of a community gather, the built environment of apartments and houses as well as the sites where people work, eat, shop, play, and pray. For the sociologist, that doesn't mean ignoring population statistics, but interpreting them after learning about the

Annual COVID-19 Death Rate By ZIP Code
New York City (2020)

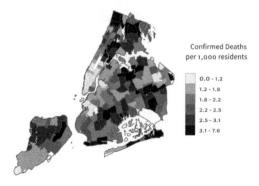

Confirmed Deaths
per 1,000 residents

0.0 - 1.2
1.2 - 1.8
1.8 - 2.2
2.2 - 2.5
2.5 - 3.1
3.1 - 7.6

Sources: New York City Health Department, NYU Furman Center.

places that shape them. It means turning away from screens and spreadsheets, and looking, instead, at sidewalks and streets.

It's no coincidence that the first place I went to make sense of how neighborhoods shaped the pandemic was Corona, Queens, which had the distinct misfortune of being the initial epicenter of cases and deaths in New York City and, perversely, sharing a name with the lethal new virus itself. Corona, which is located in the heart of the borough and tightly linked to the adjacent residential areas of Elmhurst and Jackson Heights, is everything Queens is known for: working-class, ethnically diverse, densely populated with immigrant families, and teeming with social life.

If you travel there by public transit, as most people do, you'll likely arrive at the 103rd Street/Corona Plaza Station, along the busy commercial thoroughfare, Roosevelt Avenue. Since 2012, when a coalition of community organizations led by the Queens Museum got public and private funding to create what they call a "Dignified Public Space for Immigrants,"[4] Corona Plaza has become a hub of social and economic life for the neighborhood. There are outdoor vendors selling everything from phone cases to produce, T-shirts to tamales in the thirteen-thousand-square-foot area. Retail establishments, including a large pharmacy, a martial arts studio, a mobile phone store, a driving school, a bakery, a sneaker shop, a jeweler, a check cashing and money transfer service, and a variety of fast food joints, line the edges. There are benches and portable chairs for people who like to linger and a terraced stage for cultural programs and performances. It's loud, colorful, and bustling. On weekends and summer evenings, it feels busy enough to burst.

That feeling is even more common in Corona's residential areas, which feature a blend of single-family houses (where the single family is likely to include multiple generations, siblings, cousins, and friends) and hulking, multistory apartment buildings where large, extended families pack into relatively small units. When the pandemic began, Corona had roughly 109,000 residents, 60 percent of them immigrants, 75 percent Latino (a mix of Ecuadorans, Colombians, Bolivians, Venezuelans, Guatemalans, Dominicans, and Mexicans), 12 percent Asian, 7 percent Black, and 4 percent white.[5] The median age, thirty-four, was on the younger side for New York City, and the proportion of very old people, aged eighty and above, was only half the rate in the metropolitan area.

The age composition of Corona made the neighborhood far less likely than others to experience a spike in COVID mortality, because the disease was so much more lethal for the old than for the young. Other factors, however, put people there in jeopardy. The poverty rate, 18 percent, was high for New York City. But it was the density of human life inside each domestic unit, not the sheer number of people who live there, that created real vulnerability. According to housing researchers at NYU's Furman Center, Corona and the adjacent Jackson Heights area have more "severe crowding" (the proportion of homes that have more than 1.5 people per room) than any neighborhood in New York City.[6] Such cramped conditions exacerbate a host of problems during normal times, including anxiety, stress, sleeplessness, and relationship strain. During the pandemic, domestic crowding proved far more consequential, transforming the act of hunkering down at home for safety into a potentially perilous move.

It's one thing to live in a crowded home if everyone can stay there, safely distanced from carriers of the coronavirus; it's another to do it with people who have no choice but to go out in public, working and commuting near others who can transmit the disease. Corona, as it happened, was not only one of the

most severely crowded neighborhoods in New York City; it also
had the highest proportion of state-designated essential workers.[7] Cooks. Clerks. Cleaners. Custodians. Care workers. Drivers. Dishwashers. Delivery workers. These rank among the more
common occupations in Corona. This meant that, when the
governor declared that New York was on "Pause" and instructed
most residents to stay home, people in Corona kept on working,
and then brought home whatever they had picked up on the job
or in transit. The city needed them. It just didn't offer much in
return.

Linda Dutan was thirty when the first outbreak hit Corona,
living with her family in the house where she grew up and working at a photography store in Manhattan. "I remember when the
panic hit New York, I was on my way to work and reading all
these things about people getting sick in Spain. I became paranoid. We have tourists coming into our shop, and I just started
cleaning everything with Lysol wipes. I didn't feel comfortable
getting next to people. I went to my coworkers and I was like,
guys, it's really bad." On March 14, she woke up feeling like her
eye was infected. Was that a sign of COVID? She called into
work and told them she wasn't coming in that day. Immediately,
she felt relief. "Then my coworker called and said, 'You don't
have to come in until further notice because we're closing the
store.' So I told myself, okay, this is getting serious."

At first, staying home felt safer than working in Manhattan,
but soon things got complicated, because there were so many
people around. Linda's family had lived together for decades. Her
grandfather came to New York from Ecuador in the 1970s, and in
the 1980s he and his oldest son bought a house in Corona. "We
have a huge family," Linda told me. "We had, like, more than
thirty people in the house. My grandparents. My uncle and his
family. My cousins. In the '80s there were so many people here.
My dad shared a room with, like, five cousins." Linda, along with
her parents and two siblings, lived in the basement unit until their
fortune turned. Their next-door neighbors decided to sell their
house, and her family pounced on the opportunity. "Then it was
just the five of us on one floor," she explained. "My three cousins and their parents on another floor, and we always sheltered

relatives that came from Ecuador or had people who would rent. They'd stay with us until they could pick themselves up."

Most of Linda's family works in the food business. Her father is a cook at an Italian restaurant in Manhattan. Her mother is a food packer. Her aunt owns a restaurant in Queens. "In March, the city started closing restaurants and bars," she remembered. "My father wasn't working, but my mother was working more than ever, because ordering online got crazy. My dad was driving her to work, and then he started helping my aunt—first with deliveries, and then they just started cooking for everybody—my grandma, my grandpa, his sisters who live near us. And then everyone started getting sick around me. My dad's sister got COVID, then her husband and her two daughters. My dad is very thoughtful and nice, and he was bringing food to them. But then he got COVID. My mom got COVID, and my sister got COVID. She just hid from us in her room, but she put her leftover soup in the fridge. I didn't know it was hers, so I ate it. And then I got sick, too."

Suddenly, the virus was everywhere. "Our house is on a street that dead-ends," Linda explained, "and you could hear ambulances coming, like, every hour. It was just one after the other after the other. Cars were unable to leave the block. The ambulances were just, like, covering the street." Fortunately, no one in her immediate family experienced severe symptoms. Elmhurst Hospital Center is just a few blocks away, and on television they saw footage of the grisly scene there. Corona, Elmhurst, and Jackson Heights were registering hundreds of COVID cases per day, far more than other neighborhoods in the area, and the "safety net" hospital was overwhelmed. Long lines for testing and for admission formed around the building, and some people waited hours before being sent home for lack of tests.[8] Thirteen people died of COVID during one twenty-four-hour period, and the hospital experienced so many deaths, so quickly, that the morgue reached capacity. "It's apocalyptic," a general medicine resident said, as refrigerated trucks came to store more bodies.[9] In Manhattan, the high-end hospitals that served affluent neighborhoods largely maintained their standards for caregiving. *The New York Times* reported that there were some 3,500 open hospital beds in New

York, some just twenty minutes from Queens, during the surge of cases in late March.[10] At Elmhurst, however, there were too many sick people, too few doctors and nurses, too little equipment or space. For those who lived in the area, there was nothing more terrifying than the prospect of being taken away in an ambulance, and dying alone in the crowd.

In Corona, the risk of this happening was greater than in nearly any other neighborhood in New York City, and far greater than in any other American community outside New York. For the week ending March 28, the COVID-19 mortality rate for Corona was 32 per 100,000 residents, compared to 9 per 100,000 for the entire city. The next week, the mortality rate rose to 85 per 100,000 in Corona, more than twice the city rate. During its deadliest week, which ended April 11, Corona reached 115 deaths per 100,000, compared to 61 per 100,000 across New York City. (For comparison, during the month of April, the COVID-19 mortality rate was under 10 per 100,000 for the states of California, Texas, and Florida, and no U.S. city other than New Orleans was experiencing COVID rates remotely close to New York City's.[11]) The neighborhood's death toll would remain exceptionally high until summer, when the first wave of cases came to an end.

Fortunately, no one in Linda's immediate family experienced severe symptoms. "I felt scared for my grandparents," she told me. "My grandpa has Parkinson's and my grandma has diabetes." Somehow neither caught COVID. When everyone in her family recovered, Linda, an aspiring photographer, took out her camera and explored the neighborhood. She shot Corona Plaza, where long lines formed outside the pharmacy and the check cashing service, hungry men begged for handouts, and outdoor vendors sold toilet paper and disinfectant for a premium price. To find out what was happening in the neighborhood, she went to the place where everyone goes for gossip: the bodega. "There's always people there talking," Linda explained. "The one on my street is owned by a Dominican family. They're always around, listening to Spanish music, watching games on TV. Usually there's, like, five to ten people around. Some people hang out by the deli, have a little conversation, see what's going on. Some people sit outside, smoking weed or waiting for people. Everybody talks here. We don't all know each other, but we know each other's faces." In the dark days of March and April, people talked about who was in the hospital, who was sick at home, who had died. But then Linda's brother told her that someone at the bodega caught COVID. "I stopped going," she said. "And I didn't really need to, because my father had all this food from the restaurant." Of course, most people around her didn't have that luxury. Shopping in the neighborhood was their only way to survive.

Private homes and the public hospital are not the only severely crowded places in Corona. Commercial venues—bodegas, bakeries, grocery stores, check cashing services, and the like—are small but exceptionally busy, serving not only as sites for shopping but also as crucial gathering places that absorb social life that spills outside the domestic sphere. By the summer of 2020, it seemed clear that residential congestion and doing essential work during the pandemic had made people in neighborhoods like Corona particularly susceptible to contracting COVID, and that lacking health insurance or access to quality medical care compounded the risk of death. Epidemiologists would soon confirm these facts.[12] But as low-income, Black and brown neighborhoods in cities throughout the United States experienced spikes in COVID deaths akin to what happened in Corona, a group of social scientists and big data analysts led by Jure Leskovec at Stanford University began to wonder if there were other factors driving up the number of cases and deaths in poor communities. What if, they asked, spending time in crowded shopping centers was not just an inconvenience, but also an important way of catching or transmitting the disease?

To answer this question, Leskovec's team, which included the sociologists David Grusky and Beth Redbird as well as scientists from Northwestern, Stanford, and Microsoft Research, drew on a remarkable dataset. SafeGraph, a private firm that aggregates anonymous location information from mobile devices, released fine-grained data tracking the hourly movements of roughly 98 million people in ten of the largest American metropolitan areas between March 1 and May 2, 2020. The data allow researchers to observe mobility across census block groups (CBGs), geo-graphical areas that typically have between six hundred and three thousand people, and measure the time people spend in specific nonresidential points of interest (POIs), such as grocery stores, restaurants, and churches, where they are likely to have social contact. They also provide information about the characteristics of these places, including the square footage of each facility, the number of other people present in a given hour, and the median duration of a visit.[13] To this unusually precise location data, the researchers added the confirmed COVID case counts published by *The New York Times*. These numbers understate the likely number of COVID cases in each metropolitan area, but they remain the best measures available.

The results of their analysis, published in *Nature*, are as extraordinary as the data. Predictably, mobility declined precipitously across all ten cities in the study during March and April 2020. In Chicago, for instance, overall visits to points of interest dropped 55 percent between the first week of March, before the first major coronavirus outbreak, and the first week of April, when cases were surging. The reductions in mobility were not evenly distributed. People who lived in high-income census block groups were far more likely to stay home, protecting themselves by establishing physical distance from potential agents of contagion, whereas people who lived in low-income areas maintained circulation patterns much closer to their norms. More intriguingly, simulated models that track the spread of the virus alongside visits to POIs showed that "a minority of POIs account for the majority of predicted infections"; in Chicago, the simulations suggested, about 85 percent of predicted infections came from just 10 percent of the POIs. The implication of this is straightforward: some places fostered super-spreading interactions, while others generated little risk of contagion. Naturally, the researchers wanted to know which sites were especially dangerous, and why.

Here their research is revelatory. When they scrutinized the data, Leskovec's group discovered that the points of interest that low-income urban residents visited were dramatically different from those other people used during the pandemic, as were the amounts of time they spent in each place. Consider grocery stores, which, despite home delivery services, were hard for most people to avoid. "In eight of the ten metro areas," the scientists found, "visitors from lower-income CBGs encountered higher predicted transmission rates at grocery stores than visitors from higher-income CBGs." The difference was not trivial, either; in poor areas, shoppers had twice the risk of catching COVID each time they shopped for food. What accounts for that disparity? The mobility data culled from smartphones show that "the average grocery store visited by individuals from lower-income CBGs had 59% more hourly visitors per square foot, and their visitors stayed 17% longer on average."[14] In other words, people who live in poor neighborhoods tend to shop in substantially more crowded places, and to stay there considerably longer, than people who live in more affluent areas. Some of this lingering may stem from the fact that congested stores often have longer lines. But spend a little time around bodegas in neighborhoods like Corona and it's clear that people stick around longer because they are social spaces, not just sites for instrumental exchange. Ordinarily, they deliver benefits; but in the pandemic, they exacted a terrible price.

Flushing, another densely populated Queens neighborhood with a large immigrant population, is a straight two-mile walk from Corona Plaza, up Roosevelt Avenue, past the National Tennis Center and Citi Field, and across the Flushing Meadows Corona Park. When you get there, you cannot help but notice some important differences from Corona, particularly in its ethnic makeup. Of Flushing's 81,000 residents, 72 percent are Asian (mainly Chinese and Korean), 16 percent are Latino, 8 percent are white, and 2 percent are Black.[15] The median age, forty-four, is higher than most New York City neighborhoods, including Corona, as are the poverty rate, 22 percent, and the proportion of immigrants, 70 percent.[16] The physical environment is also distinctive, with the feel of an Asian city (some call Flushing the "Chinese Manhattan"). It features a Chinatown that's dense with people, commercial establishments, and colorful signage; large shopping malls with high-end restaurants and national chain stores; a smattering of high-rise apartment buildings; a cluster of nursing homes and housing for the elderly; and, like other neighborhoods in central Queens, small residential streets packed with low-rise apartment complexes and family houses.

Flushing may feel busy and congested, but its residential units are nowhere near as crowded as the dwellings in Corona.[17] Single-family homes with just one nuclear family are far more common, and apartments where new immigrants take shifts in a bed or cram several people into each room are relatively rare. Although its households are older and, on average, poorer than those in Corona, it's also gentrifying more quickly. There is a growing supply of newly constructed buildings, some marketed as "luxury housing" even though they're adjacent to corridors with concentrated poverty; a spike in shops and restaurants catering to young professionals; and an emerging group of more affluent residents raising eyebrows with their entrepreneurial designs.[18] The transformation is visible, but it was another change—one less perceptible to outsiders but seen by everyone in the local Asian community—that decisively shaped Flushing's experience with the coronavirus: weeks before their neighbors in Corona, Flushing's social networks were buzzing with news about the deadly new disease.

Yang Zhen doesn't live in Flushing, but she has spent fifteen years working in the Queens Public Library system, and in 2017 she became director of its branch in Flushing, one of the largest and most heavily used neighborhood libraries in the city. In Flushing, the responsibilities of a library director involve learning everything you can about the patrons, the community, and the many cultural and political issues that organize daily life there, not reading or recommending books. In her first years on the job, Zhen had become something like a neighborhood anthropologist, charting relationships and deciphering social patterns so she could make the library work better for local residents. When 2020 started, she could tell that something was off.

"I remember Lunar New Year's Day. January 25, 2020. That was the first time I felt something changing," Zhen told me. "The Lunar New Year is always one of our busiest days. There's a parade right outside, and since it's always in January or February, it's very cold! People come into the library to warm up or use the bathroom. We do a daily gate count, and in 2019, we had more than six thousand people on Lunar New Year. Much higher than usual." Zhen and her staff prepared for something similar in 2020, but when the parade got going, the crowd seemed smaller and more subdued than she anticipated. "I can't remember the exact number," she said, "but it was around three thousand, much smaller. [Later, she tracked down the statistics: the gate count on Lunar New Year dropped 44 percent from 2019.] The president of the library was here. He was a VIP marshal for the parade. We were talking about why there weren't many people here. We couldn't figure it out."

Zhen has friends and family in China, and she was well aware of how worried people were about the coronavirus outbreak there. But it wasn't until the New Year's parade that she registered the level of concern among Chinese Americans in Flushing. "We knew what was happening in Wuhan. The whole city was locked down," she said. "But we didn't know how fast this virus would spread." By February, the gate count was dropping daily (according to Zhen's numbers, attendance that month was down 16 percent from 2020), and people started calling the library to cancel or postpone their programs. "We have one we do every year with the Chinese American Parents Association, on the fifteenth day of the new year. They wanted to reschedule, because some of the parents were too worried to come to the library." Requests like this kept coming through the month, even from groups that had already signed contracts and paid to reserve space. "People just weren't comfortable doing things here," Zhen recalled. "Then I started seeing people around Flushing wearing masks. That didn't happen in other communities in the city at that time, just the Asian ones."

By late March, people all over New York City would be taking precautions like this; what was remarkable about Flushing, Zhen explained, was that residents began hunkering down and masking up in January and February, when their friends and family in China and Korea sounded the alarm. Their reaction, the sociologist Gil Eyal has argued, was not based solely on what they were learning about COVID. Chinese Americans and Korean Americans in New York City had paid close attention to the lessons of the SARS crisis that hit Asian countries so severely in 2003. Unlike most other New Yorkers, they were aware that corona-viruses can spread through aerosols, not just droplets on con-taminated surfaces, and that wearing masks or avoiding crowded indoor areas can reduce the spread of disease.[19] They weren't just avoiding libraries. Parents were pulling their children out of neighborhood schools and child care centers. Small business owners were closing their shops. So many grocers shuttered their doors that, in March, someone started a Reddit thread, "NYC Chinese Supermarket Closure," where people could track which places were still selling food.[20]

Ann Choi is a journalist for *The City*, a daily newspaper cov-ering local New York City issues, and when the outbreak started in Asia she and her husband were living a few miles away from Flushing, in Jackson Heights. "My parents are in Korea," she told me. "They got really worried about COVID in January. They started calling me, telling me to be careful, that this was com-ing, and I listened. I went out and ordered masks. I had a cloth mask, but my husband and I also ordered N95s on Amazon. In January—and no one else was really doing it, so it was easy, and cheap. We just paid regular price. I remember going into the office in January or February with a mask on and people were teasing me about it. It just seemed weird to them."

Jackson Heights was one of the city's hardest hit neighbor-hoods, and she could tell that her part of Queens was plum-meting into catastrophe. "I am a data reporter," she explained. "Most of what I do is numbers. And that's what most of us rely on—numbers of this, numbers of that. It's how we know things. But living here in Jackson Heights during March and April, it wasn't the numbers. It was the sirens. They just kept coming, every few minutes, all through the day and night. I was pregnant. I was home, not going anywhere. But I couldn't get away from the sirens. It was scary, I have to be honest. I was sitting here, so scared, because I knew every siren meant someone in the neigh-borhood was going to die."

It didn't take long for the numbers to confirm what her senses perceived directly. Her part of Queens was one of the deadliest places in the world in March and April. But Flushing, she learned, when she started to report on its condition, was surprisingly stable, and she couldn't help but think the difference was the extent to which residents and business owners there were connected to people in Asia who warned them about the virus, and the extensive measures they took to stay safe. On May 3, Choi published a story about the stark disparities in COVID cases across Queens. Corona, she wrote, is an "early epicenter of the outbreak in New York City and shows no sign of slowing down." This proved to be an understatement. Between the weeks ending March 21, 2020, and May 30, 2020, Corona would record 480 deaths from COVID, for a mortality rate of 428 per 100,000, among the highest in the city. "Meanwhile," Choi explained, "the rate of test-confirmed positive cases of the virus among Flushing residents has remained among the lowest in the five boroughs."[21]

Choi was right about the divergent fate of the two neighboring neighborhoods: Corona would remain one of the deadliest places in New York City, while Flushing, despite its older and more impoverished population, fared remarkably well. But the vital information that Asian residents got from their friends and relatives was not enough to protect everyone in the area. Flushing's nursing homes were devastated, for the same reasons that nursing homes across the United States were so vulnerable to COVID: residents were cramped together in crowded environments. Workers circulated from one facility to another, while living in low-income, immigrant neighborhoods that were similarly congested.

The consequences were brutal. According to data from the New York City Department of Health, 189 residents of Flushing died of COVID between the week ending March 21, 2020, and the week ending May 30, 2020, for an overall COVID mortality rate of 233 per 100,000 residents. At least sixty of the decedents, or roughly one third of the total, died in Flushing's nursing homes; one facility, the New Franklin Center for Rehabilitation and Nursing, had forty-four COVID deaths by mid-April.[22] Subtract these cases from the neighborhood's toll and the mortality rate drops to 159 per 100,000, on par with places where residents were considerably younger and wealthier. Flushing's social

networks, and local knowledge transmitted from a geographically distant but culturally close continent, made the difference
between life and death.

Flushing was just one of countless neighborhoods, across the
country and around the world, where locally based but globally
connected social networks were galvanized by the pandemic,
inspiring people who hardly knew their neighbors before 2020 to
spend hours each week protecting them from hunger, isolation,
or disease. Some helped out casually and informally, calling to
check up on an old neighbor, picking up groceries for a family
that lost their income, sending money to a friend in need. But
thousands of Americans made a deeper commitment. Like Nuala
O'Doherty, they created, joined, and became regular participants
in mutual aid groups that operated primarily at the neighborhood
level, doing collaborative work that benefited everyone, the giv-
ers as well as the recipients of services and goods. In so doing,
they helped revive an ancient institution that human societies
rarely acknowledge but often turn to in times of distress or
upheaval, particularly when their governments fail to meet people's basic needs.[23]

 This is not a trend that featured prominently in media coverage of America's response to COVID. By the summer of 2020,
divisions among Americans who disagreed about how to handle

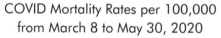

COVID Mortality Rates per 100,000
from March 8 to May 30, 2020

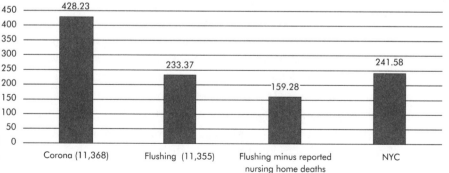

the new virus—masks or no masks, remote school or return to the classroom, restrict social gatherings or "open it up"—gave rise to complaints about a crisis in civil society, or, potentially, its imminent demise. The pandemic, pundits proclaimed, was bringing out the nation's worst tendencies: Conflict, not solidarity. Polarization, not common cause. It's hard to argue with this diagnosis. Democratic and Republican leaders were accusing each other of undermining America's most sacred values: democracy, freedom, the pursuit of health and prosperity. Ordinary citizens were fighting over masks on airplanes and distance requirements in grocery stores. But at the local level, at least, another picture emerges, as do possibilities for cooperation that are otherwise difficult to see.

Alice, thirty-seven, was a new mother living in Jackson Heights with her husband and ten-month-old daughter when the pandemic started. She had occasionally volunteered for neighborhood projects, helping friends with their campaigns for local office or supporting community organizations. Nothing too demanding, not with a full-time job and an infant at home. Like many working women raising a family, Alice had become active in a few online forums for parents. The Facebook groups Jackson Heights Parents and MOMally Astoria, and a Google Group called JHFamilies. "We also have a Buy Nothing group in Jackson Heights," she told me. "It's great. People share everything from a $2 lightbulb to a home printer or a bicycle, something they bought and don't need." She's not a fan of social media, but she appreciated how much it helped her make connections with people in her situation. Critics always complain that the internet keeps people on their screens, estranging them from friends and neighbors. Alice recognized that problem, but she also had the opposite experience. In Jackson Heights, social media helped her connect.

Alice wound up on her screen more than ever in March 2020, when work went remote, the governor urged New Yorkers to shelter in place, and her apartment turned into an office, child care center, and home. It was a stressful, unsettling moment. Like everyone in Jackson Heights, she heard ambulance sirens every few hours, and at night bright red and white flashes from the emergency vehicles lit up her block. To ward off anxiety, Alice started cleaning out her cabinets, a task she had put off for months.

"I found all these old samples of baby formula," she recalled. "I'd received box after box from all the big manufacturers. Enfamil. Carnation. I had plans to breastfeed my child, but I held on to them because a mother friend of mine had told me that if it's the middle of the night and breastfeeding isn't working out, it's good to have it around. Well, I was kind of horrified because I had like five full-size canisters of formula. I had completely forgotten they were there!" Immediately, Alice realized that someone else in the neighborhood could use them, and she offered them on one of her social media groups. "When I went back online, I had seventeen requests from mothers who needed the formula. It was, like, whoa!"

Sharing the formula was not just a good way to clear space in the cabinet. When mothers came by to pick up the canisters, Alice felt a surge of energy course through her body, a sensation she had forgotten since the outbreak started and the city locked down. She also had a revelation: What if, instead of cowering in her small apartment, she found a way to scale up the simple act of sharing? Everyone, herself included, would be better off.

"One of my cousins had seen what I was doing. I'm not sure who she works with, but she had gotten all kinds of donations—baby things, food, you name it." Her cousin lived in a middle-class suburb where most people had their basic needs covered, and local support networks were less active. "So, she said, 'There's probably people in your community who could use this stuff. Could I bring it to you?'" A few days later, she arrived in Jackson Heights with what Alice described as "bags and bags and bags of formula and diapers and canned food." Fortuitously, Nuala, who had organized the COVID Care Neighbor Network, was Alice's neighbor. She had set up a drop-off site and was trying to build a distribution network, and already they could tell that formula, diapers, and baby wipes were among the community's greatest necessities. Alice delivered her bounty, but now she and the organizers had another problem: finding a regular source of supplies for the parents who would need more to feed and change their babies the next week.

"Being a newish mom, I thought, let me tap into these networks. I'm online in a couple of due date groups, some sleep safe groups, moms and dads and caregivers just giving advice and being a village, you know, a community. So I put up a call to these parenting groups, saying, listen, if you're local to Queens or anywhere in New York City, I have a car. I'll, you know, I'll load up the Subaru. Let me know what you've got." Alice wasn't asking people to buy things. She hoped that parents would clean out their cupboards and turn up things just like she had. "That canister of formula, it's, like, $30 at the pharmacy. I told people, I'm a parent in the community, you've probably got some of these cans laying around your house, too." She quickly learned that the cabinets of middle-class new parents in New York City are lined with unused formula and diapers that no longer fit. "People would message me and say, like, 'I only have two cans, will you really pick it up?' Yes, I've got a Subaru. I will!"

By April, Alice's family had a new ritual. "My poor kid. She was ten, eleven months at the time, and every Friday night we'd strap her in the car seat, my husband would drive, and I would get on Google Maps with my phone and figure out where we're going to go. We'd start in Middle Village, then go to Elmhurst, maybe make four stops in Astoria before winding up back in Jackson Heights. I'd mask up, glove up, go in and do the pickups. We did that for weeks. And from the due date groups, I got women from as far away as Utah sending me packages. Then my friends—high school friends, college friends, neighborhood friends—they saw what we were doing and they started buying stuff, sending it here. My house was just getting, like, an influx of packages." Alice juggled as much as she could through May and June. At times the work felt overwhelming, since she was still responsible for her regular job and, of course, trying to see her daughter, her husband, and herself through the pandemic. On June 27, her father died, suddenly and unexpectedly, of a heart attack, and she left New York to be with family. First, though, she reached out to all the people who had been mailing packages of baby supplies to mothers in her neighborhood. "I asked them to send everything directly to COVID Care."

Debi, a mother, small business owner, and—until she lost the gig in the pandemic—part-time personal assistant who lives near Alice, helped Nuala when she started COVID Care. During the initial outbreak, she had posted notes on her neighbors' doors asking people if they needed anything. The response was unambiguously yes. "Within weeks, people were getting desperate," she told me. "What surprised me was not how much people needed, but how many people wanted to help. A lot of people didn't know what to do when the pandemic started. They were home. They were scared. But they wanted to do something. They wanted to help their neighbors, even total strangers!" The mutual aid society made it easier for people like Alice to plug into a collective project, whether they wanted to give, receive, or, as was often the case, do a little of both.

Hunger was a major problem. It's common for immigrant workers in Queens to live paycheck to paycheck, without savings or even a bank account. Suddenly, thousands of them—restaurant workers, domestic cleaners, taxi drivers, hairstylists, and the like—had no job, no income, no way to pay for their next meal. Job numbers analyzed by *The New York Times* indicated that, between February 2020 and June 2020, the unemployment rate in central Queens went from between 2 and 5 percent (depending on the neighborhood) to more than 17 percent in every neighborhood. In the area around Jackson Heights, Corona, and Elmhurst, the unemployment rate hovered around 25 percent.[24] For mutual aid societies across the borough, securing and delivering food was the most urgent task. Debi and her collaborators developed strong ties to local food providers. They found wholesalers who agreed to donate staple items, like milk, eggs, produce, and rice. They recruited unemployed restaurant workers who volunteered to cook hot meals most days of the week. They partnered with mosques and churches that wanted to build out food pantries.

COVID Care was just one of many local groups that helped La Jornada, the food pantry, scale up their operations to a level that would have been unimaginable before the pandemic. They went from providing meals to a few dozen new clients each week to hundreds, and eventually thousands. In the neighborhoods they serve, including Jackson Heights, Corona, and Elmhurst, lines for food stretched for blocks. By the end of the year, amid the enduring unemployment crisis for low-wage workers in the borough, La Jornada had established partnerships with community organizations throughout Queens, and was feeding more than ten thousand families on a regular basis. Food pantries popped up all over the borough during 2020, and in most other parts of the city as well.

"It's incredible to see what people are doing here," Debi told me. But she was incensed about the fact that so much voluntary labor was necessary to provide the most basic human needs to people in the city. "I've been surprised by how alone we really are. Why don't we have pandemic food stamps? It's not just a federal failure. Why isn't New York City doing this? Why are we not doing more for undocumented immigrants? I mean, we're supplying the food, we're supplying the diapers. Where is our government, to this day?"

No government—not the city, the state, or a federal agency—ever did meet the needs of New York City's most precarious people, and as the pandemic wore on, mutual aid societies throughout the area expanded their projects. "The food was always just a Band-Aid," Debi offered. "We also wanted to give people a deeper level of help." Groups that began by offering food and cleaning supplies wound up offering new services. Mental health care. Legal advice about rent obligations and eviction notices. Determining eligibility for public benefits and programs. Providing access to vaccinations. Counsel for small business owners facing bankruptcy or trying to revive operations. Veterinary care.[25] In December, Debi and her friends realized that, without a community effort, scores of families in the neighborhood would have nothing for the holidays. "So, we started getting Christmas trees and toys for children. And thank God we're all doing it, because if we didn't, who would?"

CHAPTER 11

"COVID Was Not
My Primary Concern"

BRANDON ENGLISH

In September 2019, the Atlanta-based photographer Brandon English got a call from a friend in Sunset Park, Brooklyn. There would soon be an open bedroom in their apartment and they wanted to know if he was interested. The place was well located. It wasn't too expensive, at least not for New York City. There was only one issue: it was directly upstairs from a funeral home.

English, who was thirty at the time, wasn't bothered. In fact, it seemed appropriate. Fated, even. "I was coming off a time when several family and friends had passed away," he told me. "Atlanta felt like a shell of its former self. Physically, personally, I needed to move on." Living above a funeral home might not have been an ideal arrangement, but English believed that it could only make things more interesting. "I know it's too grim for certain people. They wouldn't want to live in a place like this. But it is work that is being done whether you see it or not." And after all that he had been through, he said, "there was an aspect to it that was almost fated."

The point of moving to New York was to live more intensely, take risks, do things he wouldn't do anywhere else. For English, there's a high bar for all that. He had been working as a photojournalist for the better part of a decade. Since 2016, when Americans elected Donald Trump, an outspoken nativist and unapologetic bigot, as president, English began seeing things differently—especially the images he produced on the job. He had been shooting political demonstrations by extreme-right-wing organizations, including the Ku Klux Klan. As a six-foot-five Black man, his presence at these events never failed to stir up everyone's emotions. Journalism, he felt, didn't have room for all the things he wanted to say and show about America. "I was disenchanted," he explained. "It felt like it had reached its natural end." It was time to let himself embrace a life as a visual artist, and New York would help him achieve that.

Initially, though, English just had to pay the rent. He found a job in the mail room and handling art at a gallery in Chelsea. Anything to be close to the creative world. "I had a bit of pensiveness about my own art. I was in a new place, and I didn't really have a voice yet, or even the statements that I wanted to make," he explained. "I spent the first months trying to understand the city." He took long walks and late-night bike rides, tried plugging into local groups working on racial justice issues. One day, a friend messaged him about a demonstration against the New York Police Department, which had been accused of "brutalizing some kids" on the subway. "She just texted me: 'Tomorrow. Union Square,' with the time," English said. "The next day, I was there." The protest felt just like the ones against police violence in Atlanta. In so many ways, New York was different from Georgia. But on some matters, things looked pretty much the same.

Soon, however, everything in New York City got upended. "I wasn't here very long before the lockdown started," English recalled. In March, the media reported a spike in coronavirus cases. The numbers seemed low at first. A case in the suburbs. Where's New Rochelle? Another from a woman who had just returned from Iran. But then they were everywhere, and COVID was all anyone wanted to discuss. Inevitably, the gallery closed. So did the other cultural institutions that had drawn him out of Atlanta, the music halls, the theaters, the clubs. Suddenly, English had endless blocks of time to take photographs and develop his art. But it felt like the world had been shuttered, and he couldn't help feeling estranged. "I had developed this routine of waking up and hearing the people downstairs working," he recalled. "And on that first day, when things started, I woke up and it was just quiet. The quietest my neighborhood, the quietest the funeral home has ever been. And I woke up with goosebumps. Literally. I was like, 'Okay, something is different. Something has just changed.'"

It took twenty-four hours to find out exactly what happened. When he first looked out the window the next morning, English could hardly believe the scene. "Bodies were coming in, like multiple, multiple bodies, every hour. The street was lined with hearses. There were four or five, blocking the street, taking every parking space available. And I could hear the workers trying to handle all the people coming in. At times they were screaming at each other, with expletives used in ways that I've never heard." The stress was palpable, English recalled, and it persisted far longer than he anticipated. "There was that one day of unsettling quiet, and then they were processing bodies for the next, well, I kind of even lost track, but it felt like it didn't stop for the remainder of that year."

It didn't take long for English to hear about people clearing out of New York City. "There were a lot of communities, privileged communities, where people were able to leave," he told me. "But that wasn't happening much in my neighborhood. There are a lot of undocumented people here. Asian Americans. Latinos. People who had to keep on working. They had barriers. They stayed." English had some options. His mother, who lives on her own in the rural area outside Atlanta where English grew up, got anxious about his situation. In early March, she sent him a package with gas masks and Clorox, which were hard to find in New York City. When people started dying, she offered to pay for his ticket home. "That was a very emotional conflict for me," he confessed. "I was worried about her. I didn't want her to be alone. But knowing myself, and the kind of person I am, I couldn't just leave here. How do I move to this neighborhood for the cheap rent, then leave when things get kind of tough and come back, like, 'Hey, yeah, I'm an artist!' I was like, 'No, if I'm going to be a part of this community, then I gotta be an actual part of the community. Good and bad. I'm gonna be here.'"

Every morning, English would wake up to the sounds of hearses delivering corpses and funeral home workers grunting, shouting, arguing about where to put the next body. One day, he walked outside and tripped over a stack of coffins that they had left close to his building's entrance. "I didn't take many pictures of the funeral home," he told me. "It just didn't seem respectful. But I definitely took a picture of those coffins. I didn't want to forget that." It was surreal, English said, being inundated with the material reality of so much death while skeptics, including the president, were all over TV and social media saying that the virus wasn't all that dangerous, that soon it would just disappear. From his vantage, all the signs were ominous. The plague may have been invisible to people who escaped the city or lived in healthier places. Where he was, though, you couldn't help but see.

How did people see the pandemic in those first weeks of the outbreak? What was happening? To whom? And where? English may not have been taking many photographs of the daily death parade around his building, but his mind had frozen the images, and he couldn't stop flipping through them. What more was there to see? "I started seeking out more information," he told me. "I love to be out there, taking images. But when the world is shut down, how I do explore and examine it? I was biking around the city at night taking photos, but it wasn't really what I was seeking. I wanted more." English paused for a beat and considered how much he wanted to tell me; then he continued. "I feel like I can say this, and hopefully I don't get into trouble. But I found a way to get access to CCTV feeds in countries all across the world." He was particularly interested in seeing what was happening in countries where the virus had begun spreading before it hit New York City. He figured out how to find them.

"I began using these cameras to continue my practice of photography in a new way. I screen-recorded the feeds. And these experiences became sort of an oracle for me, because, you know, I started seeing articles that were about Italy being maybe two weeks ahead of New York. So I would check the cameras in various cities in Italy and I would see, you know, the hospitals. I would see the funeral homes. I would see the grocery stores. And when I began to see lines around the block for the grocery stores in Italy, I would say, like, 'I'm gonna go to the grocery store today and pick up some things.' Not that many people there. I was like, 'I'm gonna mark this date and go back in two weeks and see what it looks like here.' And in two weeks, the line is wrapped around the building at the grocery store. And I'm like, 'Okay, this is becoming an eerie method of telling the future.'"

English kept one eye on the global situation, the other on New York City. He got curious about the stories behind the bodies that kept arriving at the funeral home downstairs from his apartment. Who were the people? Where did they come from? What, other than the virus, was making the crisis so dire?

He could tell that things were not going well in his part of Brooklyn. Ambulances were everywhere, their sirens announcing each new neighbor who had fallen gravely ill. "I saw the fallout in my neighborhood," English said. "I don't want to quote any statistics, but for a time we were one of the most heavily impacted neighborhoods in New York City. And we're also one of the most economically downtrodden neighborhoods. So it made sense to me, why these things were happening. There's a context. Causality."

It wasn't just a matter of economics, English told me. Race mattered, as it always does in America. He could see it when he biked around Brooklyn. He could see it in the case numbers and death figures that the media reported, in New York and across the U.S. By April, it was already clear that Black people were dying more than white people. On television, medical experts talked about the risk of having "pre-existing conditions," like hypertension, heart disease, diabetes, and obesity. English knew that all of these health problems affect Black people disproportionately, because living with racism means being sick more often, feeling stressed more often, and, too often, not getting good care. He also knew that Black people were more likely than others to be working through the pandemic, exposing themselves to the virus to make ends meet. And really, with so little wealth despite such a long history of hard labor to build the country, what choice did they have?

"It wasn't surprising to me," English said. "Disappointing, you know? But I've never not been disappointed in how this country responds to issues of race, or racial issues of injustice."

There was, however, something that did surprise English. It infuriated him, and everyone else he knew, too. Beginning in late March, New York City police officers began stopping and, in some cases, arresting people for social distancing violations. The arrests, people complained, seemed unfair and suspicious. Some questioned whether they were racially motivated. Were police using masking and social distancing rules to crack down on Blacks and Latinos, while giving white people a pass? "You would hear stories about police cracking down on Black people who weren't wearing masks but not doing the same thing with white people," English said. "Like, in Midtown, police were asking people if they wanted masks. But in the Bronx or in Brownsville and the Black parts of Brooklyn, police were stopping people, arresting people, fining them, ticketing." It was as if the police had discovered a new form of criminal activity: living in a pandemic while Black.

At first, English said, these were just stories people told, things you would hear from a friend or read on social media. Who knew if the police were really discriminating that way? But in May 2020, journalists dug up the actual numbers, and things were worse than English had suspected. In Brooklyn, *The New York Times* reported, police arrested forty people for social distancing violations between March 17 and May 4. "Of those arrested, 35 people were black, four were Hispanic and one was white." What's more, the police appeared to be targeting Black neighborhoods. "More than a third of the arrests were made in the predominantly black neighborhood of Brownsville," the *Times* found. "No arrests were made in the more white Brooklyn neighborhood of Park Slope."[1]

The pattern of discrimination wasn't limited to Brooklyn. Across New York City, "officers made at least 120 arrests and issued nearly 500 summonses for social-distancing violations between March 16 and May 5," the *Times* reported. "Citywide, black people make up 68 percent of those arrested on charges of violating social-distancing rules, while Hispanic people make up 24 percent."[2] The proportion of those arrested who were white was far lower, just 7 percent.

. . .

English couldn't recall exactly where he learned about these numbers. But he did remember how upset he and his friends were in May 2020 when the patterns of racial inequality that shaped the nation's pandemic experience began coming into view more fully. The crowded hospitals. The funeral homes. The bread lines. The arrest sheets. The prisons where COVID ran rampant. All were packed with Black and brown people. "This virus, this, like, invisible thing that is affecting and killing all people around the world without prejudice," English said. In America, "it winds up being about race."

As the injustice of the situation became more visible, English felt compelled to do something about it. At first, most of his options were local. He joined a mutual aid network and began making food deliveries to old people who didn't feel safe going shopping. He helped post signs with public health advice and instructions on how to get help in Spanish, Cantonese, and Mandarin. He volunteered in a community garden that grew vegetables for low-income families. He made banners to memorialize neighbors who had died of COVID. It had been months since the art gallery in Chelsea had closed, and it felt good to work on these projects. He was contributing something meaningful. He was also developing new relationships. A community, even. "It was a lot of people my age, late twenties and early thirties, who were out there doing it. Our elders couldn't really be present because of COVID. So it was our job to do," English said.

At first, the group bonded over shared fears about the pandemic. "At the garden," English recalled, "we were just getting ready for whatever was going to happen. I mean, for a while there was a pretty apocalyptic mindset, like, is this the end? How far is this going to go?" As the weather warmed and conditions stabilized, the conversations turned more political. The election was coming. Joe Biden had clinched the Democratic nomination and Bernie Sanders, the socialist from Vermont who had been running on a platform of radical transformation, had suspended his campaign. The outcome disappointed young progressives, but the people English had been working with in Brooklyn were even more concerned about the prospect of a second Trump administration. Soon, the president would be holding MAGA rallies across the country, attracting white Christian nationalists and anti-immigrant groups with divisive ambitions. The threat of them holding on to power was palpable. English thought back on the violence he had observed covering extreme-right demonstrations. He felt himself on edge.

Memorial Day, May 25, was supposed to be a respite. It was true that, during the lockdown, holidays didn't feel quite as special. The office was closed, as were most gathering places. Not many people were traveling or visiting relatives. Parades were canceled. Restaurants and bars were still shuttered. It would be weeks until they could begin serving outdoors. Somehow, though, the day seemed different. The weather was mild and pleasant. The parks were busy. People lined up, at a distance, to buy ice cream on Coney Island. You could feel summer coming and, with it, the possibility of better times ahead.

Instead, on Memorial Day, America turned in a different direction. That night, shortly after 8 p.m., police in Minneapolis responded to a call from a store clerk at Cup Foods who reported that a customer had just paid for cigarettes with a counterfeit $20 bill. Four officers, Thomas Lane, Tou Thao, J. Alexander Kueng, and Derek Chauvin, approached a vehicle where the suspect, a forty-six-year-old Black man named George Floyd, was sitting in the driver's seat. Officer Lane tapped on the window with his flashlight and asked Floyd to show his hands. He repeated the demand several times, until Floyd opened the door and apologized. Six seconds later, Lane drew his gun and pointed it at Floyd. "Put your fucking hands up right now!" Lane shouted, and then yanked Floyd out of his seat without explaining why.[3]

Officers Lane and Kueng put Floyd in handcuffs and walked him to their car. When they forced him into the backseat, Floyd resisted and complained, saying that he was claustrophobic and refusing to be locked in the vehicle. Instead of sitting, Floyd pushed his way out of the opposite door and said he was going to lie down on the ground. Three of the officers, Chauvin, Kueng, and Lane, rushed to pin him, facedown. Lane held Floyd's legs.

Kueng knelt on his upper legs and held his wrist. Chauvin knelt directly on his neck, and held his position.

Floyd gasped for air. "I can't breathe," he told the officers, repeatedly.

Chauvin kept his knee in position, pressing it into Mr. Floyd's neck. He continued, despite Floyd's pleas, for more than eight minutes.

"I need some water or something, please, please," Floyd asked.

"They're going to kill me, man," he cried.

"Mama!" Floyd called out.

"I'm through."

The other three officers did nothing to stop Chauvin. Lane and Kueng maintained their hold on Floyd's limbs. At one point, six minutes after they had pinned him down, and with bystanders shouting for someone to help, Kueng checked for Floyd's pulse. He told his partners that he could not find it. The officers continued holding him down for another two minutes, until medics arrived, loaded Floyd into an ambulance, and drove him to a hospital nearby.

That night, the police announced Floyd's death. "Man Dies After Medical Incident During Police Interaction," read the department's initial news release, published on the website insideMPD.com.[4]

The statement said that Floyd "appeared to be under the influence." It said, "He physically resisted officers." It said, "Officers were able to get the suspect into handcuffs and noted he appeared to be suffering medical distress." It said, "Officers called for an ambulance." It said, "At no time were weapons of any type used by anyone involved in this incident." It said, "No officers were injured in the incident."[5]

A few hours later, at 1:46 a.m. on May 26, a seventeen-year-old girl named Darnella Frazier logged onto Facebook and posted a video of the incident that she had taken with her phone, along with the caption, "They killed him right in front of cup foods over south on 38th and Chicago!! No type of sympathy </3 </3 #POLICEBRUTALITY." At 3:10 a.m., after learning how the Minneapolis Police Department had characterized Floyd's kill-

ing, she added an update. "Medical incident??? Watch outtt they killed him and the proof is clearlyyyy there!!"[6]

By afternoon, it seemed like everyone in America had seen the video of the police killing Floyd on television or heard about it on social media. That day, the Minneapolis Police Department fired all four officers involved in the incident. No long review. No suspension with pay. Fired. "Separated from employment" is how the police spokesman put it.[7] The Minneapolis mayor endorsed the decision. "Justice must be served for this man and his family, justice must be served for our community, and justice must be served for our country," Amy Klobuchar, U.S. senator from Minnesota, tweeted.[8] The FBI announced that it was opening an investigation.

None of these statements satisfied Black residents of Minneapolis, or anyone, regardless of race, who was outraged by the pattern of police violence against Black people in the U.S. On the night of May 26, hundreds of protesters arrived at the scene of Floyd's murder. Some held signs saying, "I can't breathe." Many wore face masks. The pandemic was still raging, and convening in public was a risk. Another group of demonstrators gathered outside the 3rd Police Precinct, where the four officers had been assigned, chanting and calling for change. People were angry. Someone smashed a glass window on the façade of the station. Others vandalized police vehicles with graffiti.[9] Officers tried to calm and disperse the crowd. But the protests were only beginning.

"I didn't watch the video," English said. "I didn't want to subject myself to that. I've seen these videos because I've grown up Black in America, I know the realities of that video, and I honestly didn't need to see a lynching again to know what was about to happen."

There was nothing surprising about the fact that the Minneapolis police killed an unarmed Black man, English told me. It was predictable. Expected. Since English turned twenty, he had seen the police kill Black people over and over again, across the U.S. There was Eric Garner (July 17, 2014), who died in a choke hold after saying, "I can't breathe" to New York City officers eleven times. Michael Brown (August 9, 2014), shot dead by police on the streets of Ferguson, Missouri. Laquan McDonald (October 20, 2014), a seventeen-year-old shot sixteen times by Chicago police while attempting to walk away. Tamir Rice (November 22, 2014), a twelve-year-old child killed by the Cleveland police for holding a toy gun. Freddie Gray (April 19, 2015), who died of spine injuries after Baltimore police handcuffed him and left him in the back of a wagon on a rough ride through the city. Stephon Clark (March 18, 2018), shot multiple times by Sacramento police while in his grandmother's backyard holding a mobile phone. And, just before the lockdown, Breonna Taylor (March 13, 2020), shot eight times by Louisville police who raided her apartment without identifying themselves.[10] These are just a few of the cases that made headlines. There were others before; there would surely be more later. It was only a question of where and when.

Still, English was infuriated. "The rage that I felt wasn't new," he explained. But the pandemic changed the context. As long as he could remember, police violence had always been both an immediate threat to Black people and a symbolic reminder of their place in America's political order. Floyd's murder took place while he and so many people in his community were stewing in anger over racial injustice related to the pandemic. The high Black death rate from COVID was a product of the same social system that gave rise to police brutality and, too often, legitimated it as well. Firing the officers who killed George Floyd wouldn't do anything to fix the systemic problems that made Black people so unsafe in America. For that, people would have to go into the streets.

In some ways, the conditions for protests were ideal. Rarely had so many people had so much unstructured time. Most of those with jobs were working remotely, without the fixed schedule or direct oversight they got in the office. Millions were unemployed because their companies had scaled back operations or closed. With work life diminished, people also had more mental space to focus on public issues. COVID. Trump. And now George Floyd's murder and the pattern of police violence.

There's a concept sociologists use to describe how a person's life situation affects their likelihood to join a social movement or participate in demonstrations: "Biographical availability." In ordinary times, for instance, mothers with full-time jobs have trouble finding time for regular protests. Students are more available than people who clock into work daily, so it's easier for them to get involved. Waiters, bartenders, and artists often control their daytime hours. Teachers are free in summer. The lockdown disrupted these patterns—so much so, in fact, that it's hard to imagine a moment when people would be more available than they were in May 2020. The only impediment was the fear of contracting a lethal illness from all the others who wanted to join the protests. And that was a risk that people were willing to take.

English didn't hesitate. The moment he found out about the first demonstration in New York City, he knew he would be there. Was he worried about catching COVID? "Not any more than I was about being murdered by the police," he said. "That was the way I thought about it. Like, yes, COVID was something on a global scale. It was frightening to a lot of people. But this sort of invisible threat that's looming, that you don't know when it's gonna happen, when it's gonna attack, when it's gonna find you. As a Black person in America, I've lived with that my entire life. And so the virus didn't change things for me. The fear that I had going to the grocery store during COVID is the same fear that I had when I was walking down a country road as a child and didn't know whether a pickup truck full of white men was gonna pull up like they did with Ahmaud Arbery and, you know, pull out a shotgun, or do something else. What I told myself while I was out there in the streets is that COVID is just another in the long run of invisible assailants, potential assailants, against my body, that at least I could wear a mask for COVID. There's not a mask that I can wear so racial injustice doesn't find me, at least in this country. So no. COVID wasn't. . . . It wasn't a primary concern."

Still, English took precautions. He wore a mask to the protest—not just any mask, he told me. "It's the one with dual chambers, a respirator. It's like, for carpentry, or if you're in a metalworking shop or something like that. People would come up to me and be like, 'Yo! You're the dude with the gas mask!'" Other protesters, English said, stood out for a different reason. "There was a rage in people who I had not seen angry in this way before. White people! There were white people who were visibly angry, willing to fight the police, willing to put their bodies in front of Black and brown people so they didn't get arrested or attacked by the police." English had been to countless racial justice demonstrations, in the South and the North. He had never seen anything like the ones after George Floyd's murder. "It was palpable, the energy that was there. The frustrations. The anger. That first day, we went all the way to Wall Street. All around Manhattan. I just knew that this was a different movement. It was going to be sustained."

It's exhilarating to be part of a surging crowd that's marching for social justice. This, English said, was another level. Maybe it was the release it provided, after so many months of lockdown anxiety and isolation. The "collective effervescence," as the French sociologist Émile Durkheim called it, from taking part in such a vibrant shared experience, fueled by passion and moral fervor.[11] Maybe it was the urgency of the moment, or the sense that, in 2020, anything was possible. The economy. The government. The social order. The criminal justice system. Nothing felt rock solid any longer. Radical transformation was usually just a fantasy. Now it seemed possible. Look what was happening in America. Beyond America, too. The world had been shattered. How could things stay the same?

English threw himself into the movement. He brought his activist friends, his artist friends, his partners in the mutual aid network, the community gardeners, too. "I couldn't be inside," he told me. "If somebody broke my legs, I would have crawled out to be out there. There was no other place I could be." The protests—organized around the theme Black Lives Matter!—were spreading. Brooklyn. Queens. The Bronx. Staten Island. *Staten Island!*[12] And that was just New York City. There were protests in suburban Westchester, in New Jersey, Pennsylvania, and Connecticut. There were protests in every state, including the red ones, and across the planet, too.

Although most of the demonstrations were peaceful, many were enraged by the situation and intent on leaving their mark. In some places, including New York City, the protests turned violent, with packs of marchers hanging back behind the masses and looting shops along the route.[13] In previous uprisings, including those that followed the assassination of Martin Luther King Jr., rioters lashed out at businesses and institutions in Black neighborhoods, leaving communities that were already suffering from racial segregation and hatred in even more abject conditions. In 2020, however, the targets changed. On May 31 in lower Manhattan, for instance, vandals peeled off from the crowds and ransacked stores with abandon. They robbed opulent boutiques, high-end fashion shops, expensive department stores, and chain pharmacies. Chanel and CVS. Bloomingdale's and Wells Fargo. To *The New York Times*, the pattern of destruction seemed "widespread and indiscriminate."[14] To others, it marked an attack on the emblems of economic inequality and runaway global capitalism.

Black Lives Matter protesters, including English, saw the looters as criminal opportunists, saboteurs rather than allies in their cause. There were, to be sure, people who showed up to condemn police violence and wound up inflicting violence. But there were also strange cases of right-wing extremists who engaged in vandalism during social justice demonstrations to discredit the larger project, and, more commonly, outsiders who arrived on the scene to rob or cause trouble.[15] In Minneapolis, for instance, observers were dumbfounded by the video recordings of "Umbrella Man," a tall man, dressed in black clothes, wearing a black gas mask, and carrying a black umbrella, who smashed storefront windows with a sledgehammer as activists called for social change. Eventually, police issued an affidavit for a white supremacist who belonged to the Hells Angels and a prison gang in Minnesota and Kentucky called the Aryan Cowboys.[16] In Detroit, at least thirty of the forty people police arrested for vandalism or attacks against officers during demonstrations on May 28 did not live in the city.[17] They clearly had reasons for driving in to the protests, but many doubted that Black Lives Matter was among them.

It was hard to tell exactly who was doing the looting in New York City, but each night brought a new set of broken windows and burglaries. Businesses began boarding up their storefronts, and each new demonstration felt more tense than the last. Police wore riot gear, deployed blockades along the sidewalks, and carried lethal weapons. "The cops were scared," English said. "I saw that fear in their eyes." Police didn't know what the crowds would do, or where things were heading. They felt the crowd's anger, and knew how much of it was directed at them.

The battle gear was not the only thing that concerned activists. In defiance of city and state rules, most officers at the protests refused to wear face masks, even among thousands of civilians who were taking precautions to ward off the virus. "The policy is police officers are supposed to wear face coverings in public, period," Mayor Bill de Blasio insisted. "Police officers should be wearing masks," Governor Andrew Cuomo confirmed.[18] To English, their refusal to mask up felt like an act of aggression. At best, they placed themselves at risk and disregarded the health and wellbeing of the people they were supposed to be protecting. At worst, they disdained them. Either way, activists interpreted the gesture as another way the NYPD said "fuck you" to the residents of New York City, especially those who cared about social justice. Officers would follow the law if and when it pleased them, no matter the consequences. And that, protesters noted, was the very reason that so many of them were out there, demanding change.

The hostility from police caused real problems for racial justice activists. So did the looting and vandalism. Black Lives Matter organizers feared that they would lead to more police violence, if not martial law. On June 1, President Trump threatened, "If a city or a state refuses to take the actions that are necessary to defend the life and property of their residents, then I will deploy the United States military and quickly solve the problem for them."[19] That same day, New York City implemented an 8 p.m. curfew and announced that patrols would keep people off the streets. Inevitably, English believed, Black people would wind up getting hurt.

June 4 was the day they would find out. "There was a march happening in Mott Haven, in the Bronx," English told me. "You could write a whole book about what happened in the Bronx during COVID. Things were bad." The Bronx is the poorest New York City borough. It also has the highest Black and brown population; about 85 percent identify as African American or Hispanic.[20] In ordinary times, the relationship between the Bronx's Black communities and the NYPD are strained and contentious.

After George Floyd's murder, tensions were high, and the June 4 demonstration threatened to elevate them further. The rally was organized by an alliance of grassroots activists and led by Black and Latina women from a Bronx-based group called FTP Formation; and while FTP can stand for different things, like Free the People or Feed the People, for most it simply means Fuck the Police.[21]

English and some friends from Brooklyn made the long trip to the Bronx that afternoon. It was warm and sunny, and the energy was positive, he recalled. About three hundred people showed up at the intersection of 149th Street and 3rd Avenue in Mott Haven, a place known as the Hub. They marched peacefully, clapping, drumming, singing. One demonstrator, Andom Ghebreghiorgis, recalled the optimistic tone of the protest. The march wove through the neighborhood and passed by the Patterson Houses, a hot spot of COVID deaths during March and April, a place where poverty and suffering are rampant even in stable times. Residents leaned out their windows, banging pots and pans and shouting out support for the activists. Some left home to join the march, raising everyone's spirits as they made their next turn.

The 8 p.m. curfew was approaching, but the activists had more than enough time to continue their protest. When they reached Willis Avenue, however, more than fifty police officers were blocking the street. The demonstrators reversed course and walked down 136th Street. It was 7:50 p.m. At this point, according to a report by Human Rights Watch (HRW), which obtained video recordings and eighty-one eyewitness accounts of the event, "scores of police officers surrounded and trapped the protesters—a tactic known as 'kettling.'" Participants caught between the officers had no way to escape. "We were being packed and packed like sardines," one remembered. Some chanted, "Let us go!"[22]

When 8 p.m. arrived, HRW found, "the police, unprovoked and without warning, moved in on the protesters, wielding batons, beating people from car tops, shoving them to the ground, and firing pepper spray into their faces before rounding up more than 250 people for arrest." The human rights organi-

zation documented "at least 61 cases of protesters, legal observers, and bystanders who sustained injuries during the crackdown,
including lacerations, a broken nose, lost tooth, sprained shoulder, broken finger, black eyes, and potential nerve damage due to
overly tight zip ties."[23] The next day, at a news conference, New
York police commissioner Dermot Shea defended the officers'
conduct. "We had a plan which was executed nearly flawlessly in
the Bronx," he said.[24]

At least 263 people were arrested that night, considerably
more than at protests in the city after George Floyd's murder.
Some were released from custody that night, but others were
detained until the next afternoon, and one was detained for a
week. The Bronx district attorney issued summonses or desk
appearance tickets and court dates for those arrested. In September, however, the DA's office filed to dismiss the summonses and
the tickets. The protesters were free.[25]

But not exactly, English told me. "That event was planned
to suppress the Bronx," he insisted. "To tell that borough, this
is what happens if you come out into the streets. When we were
marching, we had people in the projects stick their heads out of
the windows and call out their support. They were ready to come
and join us. I think the NYPD decided that this was their moment
to suppress it. And they did it successfully. [Though not without
a cost. In March 2024, New York City agreed to pay $21,500 to
each of the hundreds of people who were kettled and then either
charged at or assaulted by the police.[26]] From then on, people
didn't want to go to the Bronx for actions."

Still, the protests continued. The demonstrations lasted far longer than anyone anticipated, and spread far wider, too. "As a historian of social movements in the U.S., I am hard pressed to think
of any time in the past when we have had two straight weeks of
large-scale protests in hundreds of places, from suburbs to big
cities," Tom Sugrue, the historian of civil rights, tweeted. "The
breadth and scale of #Floyd protests is staggering. We have had
some huge one-day demonstrations, e.g. March on Washington
for Jobs and Freedom (1963); antinuclear march in NYC (1982),

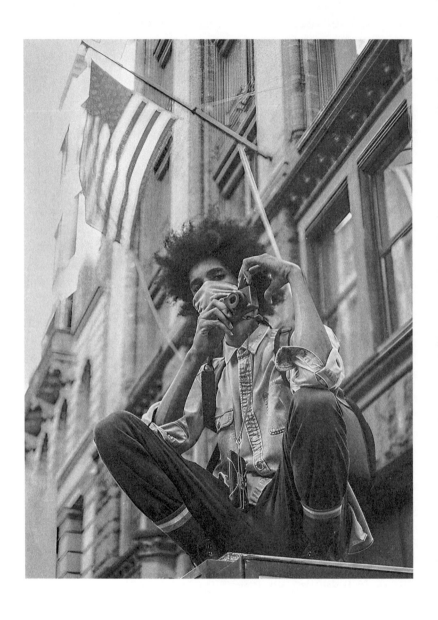

and Women's March (2017). We have widespread, simultaneous protests, such as in the days following MLK Jr.'s assassination (1968). But the two together—very unusual."[27] Polls suggest that somewhere between 15 and 26 million Americans participated in racial justice demonstrations in the two weeks following Floyd's murder alone. "These figures would make the recent protests the largest movement in the country's history," *The New York Times* reported.[28]

English felt compelled to be part of it, and the movement was becoming a part of him. He was bringing his camera. Taking photographs. Shooting videos. English wanted to go to everything now, and not just in New York City. He traveled to Minneapolis to protest. He returned to Atlanta, saw his mother, and protested there, too.

Now there was no pretense of journalistic detachment and neutrality. Nor was there a fantasy about creating a typical art object, something he'd show in a gallery like the one in Chelsea where he was working when the pandemic began. "I think what I was making was an archive for myself, a vast, very personal archive of what happened and what is happening right now. Because I don't understand the moment. None of us do," he explained. "The medium isn't necessarily photography. The images aren't meant for newspapers or for Instagram. It isn't necessarily video, either. It's the lived experience. That is the medium." He hasn't decided whether, or when, he will share them. It depends on what comes next.

CHAPTER 12

Race

Every global crisis produces the same fantasy: humanity, suddenly confronted with its shared vulnerability, bonds together to ward off a universal threat.

Climate change. Nuclear annihilation. An earthbound asteroid. Plague. In the fantasy, each peril induces fear across nations and societies that might otherwise oppose one another. Ultimately, political leaders and ordinary people realize that, as the clichés go, the looming catastrophe is "the great equalizer," or "we're all in it together," or "we're all in the same boat."

These sentiments were ubiquitous during the first year of the pandemic. "Together we will beat this," British prime minister Boris Johnson tweeted, after being diagnosed with the disease.[1] "Coronavirus: We're in This Together," *USA Today* announced in April 2020 when it launched the "In This Together" series, a recurring feature of "powerful, human stories [that] offer some good news: our families, friends and neighbors are moving forward amid coronavirus."[2] In June, the United Nations Department of Global Communications pushed this idea to the international level. "We're all in it together," it proclaimed.[3]

By then, however, it was already clear that the coronavirus had not put everyone "in the same boat." Same storm, perhaps; but people would ride through it on different ships, and their course would be shaped by the very same factors that shaped the course of their daily lives.

Class mattered, as it always does, since wealth and education allowed the most privileged to keep distanced, avoid the virus, and access the best available health care. Politics mattered, too, since some nations had robust public health systems and effective infectious disease policies, while others had neither. Soon after the initial outbreak, however, it was clear that another factor would play a key role in the social life of the pandemic, dividing rather than uniting, amplifying inequality, and inducing violence across the planet: racism, in both structural and more rudimentary, interpersonal forms.

Spikes in racial prejudice, discrimination, and violence have become typical features of modern infectious disease outbreaks. AIDS. Ebola. SARS. Monkeypox. Major media, political officials, and humanitarian groups consistently use loaded rhetoric and imagery to mobilize emotional (or affective) responses to health scares in ways that, as the anthropologist Adia Benton has illustrated, foreground race as the central mediator of risk.[4] To address this problem, in 2015, the World Health Organization issued a statement on "best practices in naming new human infectious diseases to minimize unnecessary negative effects on nations, economies, and people." Names such as "swine flu" (a disease tracked to Mexican pig farms) and "Middle East respiratory syndrome" (MERS) stigmatized the regions or racial groups associated with the novel illness. WHO called for officials to avoid labeling new diseases with geographic locations, people's names, species of animal or food, cultural, population, industry, or occupational references, or terms that incite undue fear.[5]

When the World Health Organization first learned about the new coronavirus in China during December 2019, it anticipated trouble. The agency, intent on preventing another wave of ethnonational or racial hostility, explicitly urged journalists and officials to avoid associating the new disease with China or Chinese people. "Viruses know no borders and they don't care about your ethnicity, the color of your skin or how much money you have in the bank," said Mike Ryan, executive director of WHO's Health Emergencies Programme. "This is a time for solidarity, this is a time for facts, this is a time to move forward together, to fight this virus together."[6]

The statement was entirely admirable. It was also utterly ineffective. The virus might not have cared about borders and skin color and money in the bank, but people throughout the world did. Some, including the president of the world's most powerful nation, could not have cared less about WHO's advice on naming or visual imagery. They were hell-bent on lashing out.

As we have seen, "the Chinese virus" was Donald Trump's preferred way of labeling the new coronavirus, though sometimes he called it "the China virus" instead. "It's not racist at all," he insisted, when critics denounced him for stoking racial antagonism and violence. "Because it comes from China, that's why."[7] Key members of the Trump administration used similar language. Secretary of State Mike Pompeo called it the "Wuhan Virus," and defended the phrase as a tool for combating "Chinese misinformation" about the disease.[8] Trump even called it "Kung Flu."[9]

Anti-Asian hate crimes in the United States soared after Republican officials and right-wing media outlets invoked this terminology. They were racially targeted, against people of Asian descent generally, and not just people from China.[10] In early March 2020, the National Public Radio program *Code Switch*, which focuses on race, encouraged listeners to send in stories about their experiences with xenophobia as Americans grew concerned about the coronavirus. "Judging by the volume of emails, comments and tweets we got in response," one editor wrote, "the harassment has been intense for Asian Americans across the country—regardless of ethnicity, location or age."[11]

One key theme that emerged involved harassment in public spaces, particularly public transit. A woman from Brooklyn reported "that when visiting D.C., she saw a man making faces at her on the Metro train. She tried to move away from him, but he wouldn't stop. After a while, she said, he confronted her outright, saying: 'Get out of here. Go back to China. I don't want none of your swine flu here.'" The next week, when she was riding a Muni train in San Francisco, "another man yelled the same thing to her—'Go back to China'—and even threatened to shoot her." A listener from Boston had a similar story: "A man on a bus muttered about 'diseased Chinese people' when she sneezed into her sleeve. When she confronted him, he told her: 'Cover your fucking mouth.'" A man from Seattle recounted that "a Costco food sample vendor told his Korean wife and mixed-race son to 'get away' from the samples, questioning whether they had come from China."[12] None of these incidents resulted in a formal police report, so it's hard to know precisely how much harassment of this type increased in 2020. But sociological research, including a series of studies by the organization Stop AAPI Hate, suggests that public harassment against people of Asian descent became far more common in 2020 than it was before.[13]

There are better data about more serious crimes against Asians and Asian Americans. According to the Federal Bureau of Investigation, reported hate crimes against people of Asian descent increased some 73 percent from 2019 to 2020, while hate crimes in general rose a more modest 13 percent.[14] In cities, the attacks escalated even more sharply. Researchers at the Center for the Study of Hate and Extremism at California State University, San Bernardino, found that anti-Asian hate crimes—including intimidation, simple assault, destruction of property, and aggravated assault—increased 145 percent from 2019 to 2020 in America's largest urban areas, with the first major spike taking place precisely when Trump and his allies framed the pandemic in xenophobic terms.[15] The majority of these cases occurred on public streets and sidewalks, particularly in neighborhoods that had long served as safe spaces for Asians and Asian Americans.

Before the pandemic, anti-Asian hate crimes had become rare events in most of America; after March 2020, Asian Americans came to expect them.[16] According to a survey conducted by the Pew Research Center in April 2021, 81 percent of Asian Americans said that violence against them was increasing (compared to 56 percent of all American adults); 32 percent said they feared someone might threaten or physically attack them (a higher proportion than any other racial or ethnic group); and 45 percent said they have experienced at least one of five specific offensive incidents—fearing attack; seeing people acting as if they are uncomfortable around them; being subject to racial slurs or jokes; being told they should go back to their home country; or being told they are responsible for the pandemic—since the initial coronavirus outbreak.[17]

There's no doubt that right-wing rhetoric linking China and Chinese people with the coronavirus contributed to the climate of racial hostility in America during 2020. But it's impossible to know exactly how much anti-Asian crime and violence that year is attributable to Republican scare-mongering—in part because American conservatives were not the only organized political actors framing the virus in racial or ethnonational language (recall the Black woman who complained "they're everywhere" when she saw May Lee at a magazine store in Chinatown, inciting the principal's ire); and in part because anti-Asian hate crimes spiked outside of the United States as well.

By May 2020, reports of racial discrimination and attacks on people of Asian descent were so widespread that Human Rights Watch published a report on the "worldwide" spread of xenophobia, and called on governments to "take urgent steps to prevent racist and xenophobic violence and discrimination linked to the COVID-19 pandemic." The organization turned up evidence of political officials stirring up ethnonational and racial discord to rally support for their larger agendas. "Government leaders and senior officials in some instances have directly or indirectly encouraged hate crimes, racism, or xenophobia by using anti-Chinese rhetoric," the report explained. "Several political parties and groups, including in the United States, United Kingdom, Italy, Spain, Greece, France, and Germany have also latched onto the COVID-19 crisis to advance anti-immigrant, white supremacist, ultra-nationalist, antisemitic, and xenophobic conspiracy theories that demonize refugees, foreigners, prominent individuals, and political leaders."[18]

The violence was directed mainly at Asians, however, and it began early in 2020, as political leaders, pundits, and ordinary people around the world drew on a deep well of racial resentment and fears of the "Yellow Peril," the myth that Asians threaten national security and public health. In February 2020, the governor of the Veneto region of Italy proclaimed that the coronavirus would be less deadly there than in China because of Italians' "culturally strong attention to hygiene, washing hands, taking showers, whereas we have all seen the Chinese eating mice alive." Beginning that month, the Italian civil society group Lunaria reported, the nation experienced a spate of "assaults, verbal harassment, bullying, and discrimination against people of Asian descent."[19] Human Rights Watch documented a similar trend across Europe. The violence was particularly bad in the U.K., where a series of physical assaults on Asian people sent a clear message about who would be blamed for the outbreak. But nearly every country on the continent saw a wave of vicious beatings and public harassment. The veneer of civility was gone.

The climate of hatred extended beyond Europe. In Brazil, the education minister tweeted that the coronavirus was a weapon for advancing the Chinese government's "plan for world domination."[20] Harassment and "shunning" of Asian people followed. Australia's Human Rights Commission reported a wave of anti-Asian hate crimes, including vandalism and physical assaults. In Sydney, someone spraypainted "Death to Dog Eaters" in front of one Asian family's home; near Melbourne, the home of a Chinese Australian family was attacked and vandalized, once with a rock thrown through a window and twice with racist graffiti— "COVID-19 China Die" and "Leave and Die"—in just one week. In Kuwait and Bahrain, migrant workers from Asia complained that they were being quarantined without cause and demeaned by managers for being dirty and diseased.[21] "In Africa," Human Rights Watch found, "there have been reports of discrimination and attacks on Asian people accused of carrying coronavirus," with notable cases in Kenya, Ethiopia, and South Africa.[22] The pattern was predictable, the sociologist Yoon Jung Park explained, because "across the continent there have been periodic kinds of outbursts of what looks to be anti-Chinese sentiment" even before the pandemic. "Sometimes the Chinese are a scapegoat," she added. "There's a tremendous amount of fear about the unknown, and this unknown disease is now attached to Chinese bodies."[23]

·   ·   ·

While visible forms of racial discrimination and interpersonal violence disproportionately targeted Asian bodies, the more insidious types of racial violence—being segregated, exposure to dangerous conditions, lacking access to good health care, and other kinds of what sociologists call "structural racism"—proved most dangerous for Black and brown people, particularly in the United States.[24] The pattern was as predictable as the spike in hate crimes against Asians.

Among the many forms of race-based inequality in America, the gap in health and life expectancy is especially glaring. In the year before the pandemic started, for instance, the overall life expectancy for white Americans was 78.9, compared to 75.3 for Black Americans, and Blacks had higher rates of obesity, diabetes, and heart disease, as well.[25] How, exactly, race shapes these patterns is a matter of considerable debate. Historically, scientists and political officials attributed the short life span of Black people to biology and culture, but in the twentieth century scholars debunked these views. Race, as the historian of public health Merlin Chowkwanyun puts it, became more of a "social myth" than a "biological fact." In 1972, he recounts, the population geneticist Richard Lewontin showed that 85 percent of genetic variation occurred within so-called racial groups, not across them. "By extension," as Chowkwanyun puts it, "health disparities . . . could not be explained away by them."[26]

Americans, however, have held fast to biological explanations, and they have hardly disappeared from popular culture or politics. The same is true for behavioral accounts. American individualism has long supported the view that each person's conduct ultimately determines their fate, and when it comes to Black health problems, the media encourages this view. In a study of U.S. news coverage, for example, a team of public health scholars led by Annice Kim found that Blacks' health issues are more likely to be framed as symptoms of behavioral deficiencies than the health problems of whites.[27] Identifying this inconsistency did little to change things. In public health and public policy, the behavior of Black people remains an object of scrutiny, and Black people get blamed for suffering that is usually structurally imposed.

In recent decades, scholars have established the relationship between health disparities and place-based inequalities (such as segregation), stress from discrimination, and public policies that shape access to education and medical care. Researchers have grown particularly interested in cases where racial disparities cannot be explained by class alone—cases, for instance, where Black and white communities with similar levels of income and education have unequal health outcomes, or where Black and white mortality diverges despite similar incidence of disease. Consider low birthweight, which is related to infant mortality as well as a host of developmental problems. "The black-white disparity in the prevalence of this condition actually increases with higher levels of educational attainment," reports a team led by the Harvard epidemiologist Ichiro Kawachi. Since it's hard to believe that the biology of more educated Black women explains this outcome, social factors, such as stress related to racial discrimination or inequities in health care, are more likely to be the cause. The same is true for deaths from cancer. Blacks and whites do not have significantly different rates of cancer incidence. In fact, as the Kaiser Family Foundation reports, "As of 2019, Black people had similar or lower rates of cancer incidence compared to White people for cancer overall and most of the leading types of cancer examined."[28] Compared to whites, however, Blacks are significantly more likely to die from cancer. Among the likely reasons: less access to health care, which means later diagnoses; less access to the most advanced medical treatments, which are often offered in the prestigious private hospitals located far from Black neighborhoods; less support for long-term care in the health system; and more "comorbidities," also known as "pre-existing conditions."

During 2020, both exposure and "pre-existing conditions" emerged as key explanations for the fact that, in the U.S., Native Americans, Blacks, and Latinos had both a higher incidence of COVID and higher pandemic mortality rates than whites and Asians.[29] Their exposure was rooted in social conditions, from concentration in "essential jobs" and dangerous low-wage work to residential crowding and segregation. So, too, were their pre-existing conditions. One of the most powerful explanations for the prevalence of underlying medical conditions in racial and ethnic minority groups comes from the public health scholar Arline Geronimus, who claims that Blacks and Latinos experience physical *weathering*—"early health deterioration as a consequence of the cumulative impact of repeated experience with social or economic adversity and political marginalization."[30] According to the theory of weathering, Black Americans' relatively low life expectancy and high levels of vulnerability after they become ill are due not to genetic factors or behavioral deficiencies, neither of which have been systematically established. Instead, they are due to routine conditions in a society where prejudice, discrimination, and segregation are commonplace, and Black people are disproportionately exposed. Weathering is not necessarily a racial phenomenon. Poverty, as the sociologist Matthew Desmond writes, takes its own toll on the body, and makes poor whites, for instance, more likely to have chronic illnesses and disease.[31] But in America, race compounds the risk of physical suffering, which is why structural racism helps explain why Blacks faced elevated risks of contracting and dying from COVID-19 during the first pandemic year, too.

This risk was not widely acknowledged by American political officials and scientific leaders when the initial outbreak hit. The Trump administration was notably silent about the dire public health threat to both Blacks and Latinos, but so, too, were more liberal voices. "This virus is the great equalizer," New York governor Andrew Cuomo tweeted in late March 2020 after his brother, Chris, was diagnosed with COVID-19. By then, however, inequalities around escape, exposure, and access to good health care had already emerged across the state, and his brother, self-quarantined in the basement of his beach house in the Hamptons, could have been Exhibit A.[32]

Soon, though, evidence of racial health disparities in COVID-19 cases and mortality appeared in even more dramatic fashion. In New York City, for instance, there was the constant song of ambulance sirens and the overcrowded hospitals in Black and brown neighborhoods. There were grim reports of devastating COVID clusters in the city's most racially segregated areas, including parts of the Bronx and outer Brooklyn. During the first few weeks of the outbreak, it was hard to get reliable demographic information on local COVD infection rates; tests were scarce, even for people with high fevers and difficulty breathing, and neither asymptomatic carriers nor people with mild illness could find out if they had the disease. Still, clear patterns emerged. COVID deaths, while by no means easy to count with precision, were more apparent, and on April 8, the city released data showing that, after adjusting for the size and age of the population, Blacks and Latinos were dying at twice the rate of whites and Asian Americans. Media outlets began publishing color-coded maps that illustrated precisely which places were "hot spots" and which were relatively safe. "The virus map of New York boroughs turns redder along precisely the same lines as it would if the relative shade of crimson counted not infection and death but income brackets and middle-school ratings," the writer Zadie Smith observed. "Untimely death has rarely been random in these United States. It has usually had a precise physiognomy, location and bottom line."[33]

Consider the Bronx. The poorest and, in proportional terms, most Black borough in New York City, the Bronx was also, as *The New York Times* reported in May 2020, the place where COVID "inflicted the worst toll" on residents, with "the highest rates of coronavirus cases, hospitalizations, and deaths in the city, while the most well-off borough, Manhattan, has the lowest rates."[34] Neither virology nor genetics can explain these disparities, but sociology can. People in the Bronx tended to work in "essential jobs" that could not be done remotely, and personal protective equipment was in short supply. They tended to live in crowded apartments, where everyone, working or locked down, faced higher odds of contracting the disease. They endured high levels of air pollution, which made them more likely to develop asthma and other respiratory problems.[35] They faced relatively high levels of crime and violence, which made them more likely to experience stress-related illnesses, too.[36] They had less access to primary care than their neighbors in Manhattan, less than half as many hospital beds per capita, and, inevitably, lower quality facilities.[37] In ordinary times, those differences make residents of the Bronx far more likely to suffer from illness and early mortality. During the pandemic, they were even more consequential.[38]

High levels of racial segregation placed Black people in other parts of New York in similarly dangerous conditions, and their fate reflected this fundamental inequality. According to the COVID Tracking Project, a volunteer organization supported by *The Atlantic* that was dedicated to collecting and sharing reliable data about the pandemic, during the first year of the outbreak, the rate of hospitalization for COVID-19 was 848 per 100,000 among Blacks in New York, compared to 766 among Latinos, 501 among Asian/Pacific Islanders, and 199 among whites. Blacks, in other words, were more than four times more likely than whites to be hospitalized with the disease. The rate of reported deaths from COVID-19 followed a similar pattern: 352 per 100,000 among Blacks in New York, compared to 268 among Latinos, 184 among Asian/Pacific Islanders, and 156 among whites.[39]

New York City was by no means alone. A study published in the *Annals of Internal Medicine* showed that Blacks and Latinos in New York City, Chicago, and Philadelphia experienced similar levels of vulnerability during the first six months of the pandemic, an expression of what they call "spatial inequities." In Chicago, the authors note, Blacks represent 30 percent of population but accounted for 50 percent of COVID-19 deaths between March and the beginning of October 2020. In Philadelphia, "age-specific incidence, hospitalization, and mortality rates are 2 to 3 times higher for Black persons and Hispanic persons than for non-Hispanic White persons." Most strikingly, the researchers found that higher levels of social vulnerability in racially segregated neighborhoods were associated with dramatically higher rates of COVID cases and deaths. "Notably, Chicago, Philadelphia, and New York are among the 10 most segregated cities in the United States," they conclude, calling attention to the plight of "areas of concentrated poverty and with a history of extreme racial segregation, including West and North Philadelphia, the West Side of Chicago, and the Bronx in New York."[40] In these cities, and others, the past has an enduring impact. As stacks of urban research show, patterns of racial segregation that were established in the twentieth century shape American residential life to this day, with communities "stuck in place," and Blacks subjected to the harshest conditions.[41]

Racial inequities in COVID mortality during 2020 showed up at the national level. When a team of health scholars from New York University examined COVID deaths in ten major cities across the U.S., they found that Blacks and Latinos had substantially higher rates of infection and death than whites, even when they lived in counties with comparable class status. "Among both more-poverty and less-poverty counties," they report, "those with substantially non-White or more diverse populations had higher expected cumulative COVID-19 incident infections compared with counties with substantially White or less-diverse populations (e.g., more diverse counties with less poverty). . . . Similar associations were observed for deaths."[42] In the *Annals of Internal Medicine*, an article that reviewed more than fifty studies of race and ethnic disparities during the first six months of the pandemic found that Blacks and Latinos faced significantly higher risks of getting infected, being hospitalized, and dying of COVID than whites. "Analysis of data from the CDC's National Center for Health Statistics shows that African American/Black populations experience approximately 15% excess deaths (defined as the percentage of COVID-19 deaths for a racial/ethnic group compared with the percentage of that racial/ethnic group in the population), and data from APM Research Lab show that African American/ Black populations have 3.2 times the risk for mortality compared with White populations," the authors report. Latinos, they write, "have approximately 21% excess deaths, and . . . 3.2 times the mortality risk compared with non-Hispanic White persons."[43]

What explains these disparities? There was a widespread impulse, from prominent conservatives as well as from some medical experts, to ascribe them to the cultural tendencies or biological traits of different groups. Such narratives were ubiquitous throughout the first year of the pandemic: in hospitals, where medical staff tried to understand why so many of the people coming in with severe symptoms of COVID were Black or Latino, but focused on behavioral and physiological problems rather than social conditions; and in the media—and not just conservative cable news channels and talk radio stations—where journalists, pundits, and officials did the same.

On April 7, for instance, National Public Radio invited Bill

Cassidy, a medical doctor who's also a Republican U.S. senator from Louisiana, onto its popular program *Morning Edition*. "Can you tell me what is being done to help the black community in your state right now, which clearly is being disproportionately hit by this disease?" asked David Greene, the host. Cassidy began by explaining that hospitals had brought in "a surge of ventilators," but he quickly pivoted, adding that, "if you're going to look at the fundamental reason, African Americans are 60% more likely to have diabetes. The virus likes to hit what is called an ACE receptor. Now, if you have diabetes, obesity, hypertension, then African Americans are going to have more of those receptors inherent in their having the diabetes, the hypertension, the obesity. So there's a physiologic reason which is explaining this. Now, as a physician, I would say we need to address the obesity epidemic, which disproportionately affects African Americans. That would lower the prevalence of diabetes, of hypertension. And that's what would bring benefit."[44]

Greene pushed back, quoting an earlier interview with Cedric Richmond, who at the time was a Democratic member of the House of Representatives from Louisiana. "I mean, we heard Congressman Cedric Richmond say, as well, that this is rooted in years of systemic racism. Aren't there other forces at work here?" Cassidy immediately shot down the idea. "Well, you know, that's rhetoric, and it may be. But as a physician, I'm looking at science."[45]

The authors of the *Annals of Internal Medicine* study on racial disparities in COVID mortality drew different conclusions from the data. Overall, they report, "exposure" and "health care access" appear to underlie racial inequality in COVID rates. This means that pre-existing social conditions likely mattered more than pre-existing medical conditions (which they call "susceptibility" or "comorbidity").[46] In other words, the source of America's pandemic inequalities is not merely in the body, but in the body politic as well.

It's striking how little this insight informed America's policy response to COVID. Instead, as the sociologist Eduardo Bonilla-Silva argues in an article about "color-blind racism" in the pandemic, health officials such as Anthony Fauci emphasized the dangers of "their underlying medical conditions—the diabetes, hypertension, the obesity, the asthma," without linking them to the pre-existing condition of racial inequality. Fauci is a medical doctor, and his expertise involves explaining the physiological conditions that elevate the risk of severe disease or death. But as Bonilla-Silva sees it, Fauci's statement about the individual-level medical risk factors "reifies the deficiency narrative and opens the door for racist 'culture of poverty' discourses."[47] Vulnerability, this story goes, was rooted in the behavior of Black and brown people, who had failed to take care of themselves.

Scholars of race and racism refused this perspective. "Without question, African Americans suffer disproportionately from chronic diseases such as hypertension, cardiovascular disease, diabetes, lung disease, obesity, and asthma, which make it harder for them to survive COVID-19," wrote the prominent historian Ibram X. Kendi. "But if [Senator Bill] Cassidy were looking at science, then he'd also be asking: *Why are African Americans suffering more from these chronic diseases? Why are African Americans more likely to be obese than Latinos and whites?*"[48]

The truth is, we know the answers to these questions, too.[49]

By April 2020, progressive voices in American politics were making the connections that Senator Cassidy was so adamantly denying, insisting that the pandemic toll was both a product and an expression of racial inequality, and demanding a response. Death and disease, which Black and brown people experienced so much more than whites and Asian Americans, were only part of the problem. The lockdowns also had a disproportionate economic effect on Black people, who—due to the legacy of structural racism—have far less wealth than white people and were significantly more likely to report that they had been financially hurt by the pandemic.[50] The lockdowns of schools hurt Black students more than white students, too.

Police crackdowns on people who were not wearing masks in outdoor public spaces also had an outsized impact on Blacks, who—in the pandemic as in ordinary times—were prosecuted for offenses that white people could commit with far less risk of arrest. In fact, as six U.S. senators, including Kamala Harris and Cory Booker, noted in a letter to the Department of Justice and the Federal Bureau of Investigation, Black men were being persecuted no matter what they did. Sometimes they were charged for not wearing a mask, and sometimes (in Illinois, two men wearing surgical masks in a Walmart were followed by an officer gripping his gun and told that masks were prohibited) they were profiled for wearing one.[51]

It was an intolerable situation. Although Black Americans are always disproportionately exposed to public health threats and targeted by the police, the problems felt especially acute during the first months of the pandemic. What's more, the reduction of other activities—office life, social gatherings, travel, church, eating out—meant that most people were home, following news about the pandemic, stewing in their frustrations and anxieties about the state of the world. In Black communities, conversations often turned to the ways that racism—prejudice, discrimination, segregation, and police violence—was shaping the crisis, putting Black people in danger. It wasn't exactly that the pandemic "revealed" things about racial inequality in America; most Blacks knew just how unjust things were. But it did put a spotlight on the problem of racial justice, making it harder to tolerate, impossible to ignore. As the virus spread across the country, a growing number of people felt the urge to push back and do something. But the public realm was closed and gated, the ordinary options for action blocked.

That changed on May 25, 2020. When Minneapolis police murdered George Floyd. Within hours, video of the homicide began circulating online and on major media outlets, domestic and international. Protesters, undeterred by restrictions on public gatherings or the risk of contracting COVID, began demonstrating in Minneapolis on May 26. Soon, people like Brandon English and Enuma Menkiti were taking to the streets in cities around the world.[52]

The United States, after all, was not the only nation where glaring racial inequalities during the pandemic had primed people for protest that summer. In the U.K., for instance, the Office of National Statistics analyzed racial and ethnic disparities in

COVID-19 deaths in England and Wales during the first wave of cases, from March 2 to May 15, 2020. "After taking into account size and age structure of the population," the agency reports, "the mortality rate for deaths involving COVID-19 was highest among males of Black ethnic background at 255.7 deaths per 100,000 population and lowest among males of White ethnic background at 87.0 deaths per 100,000." Black men, in other words, were roughly three times more likely than white men to die in the first few months of the pandemic. "For females," they found, "the pattern was similar with the highest rates among those of Black ethnic background (119.8) and lowest among those of White ethnic background (52.0)." Strikingly, the British statisticians claim that socioeconomic factors explain only a fraction of these disparities. After controlling for class and geographical location, they found that Black men were twice as likely to die of COVID than white men, and Black women were one and a half times more at risk. In the U.K., as in the U.S., structural racism and racial inequality get under people's skin.

Race also mattered in Canada, though it took some time to establish that, because the national and provincial governments initially did not track COVID mortality by race or ethnicity. Civic groups, concerned that failing to collect group-level health data would render important risk factors invisible, pushed for change. Once Canadian provinces began counting, it was impossible to ignore just how much race and ethnicity determined who lived and who died in the initial outbreak. In Ontario, for instance, the infection rate for what the state calls nonwhite "racialized" groups was up to seven times higher than for the white population, with Latino, Middle Eastern, and South Asian communities being hardest hit.[53] A team of sociologists from the University of Western Ontario pushed further, making creative use of publicly available records to examine whether localities with high proportions of Blacks, immigrants, and low-income residents were experiencing higher incidence of COVID-19. "Similar to the U.S. and U.K.," they found, "urban regions in Canada with higher shares of Black residents have been disproportionately impacted by COVID-19. This may help explain why places like Toronto and Montreal, with relatively large numbers of Black Canadians and Black immigrants, have emerged as epicenters of the pandemic." As in the U.K., the authors report that "socioeconomic disadvantage" does not explain the heightened level of Black cases. In Canada, too, racial health disparities were not driven solely by class.

"These results may be surprising to those who believe that racial discrimination against Black communities is less severe, and as such, Blacks are not as disadvantaged in Canada as they are elsewhere like the U.S.," the authors write. In fact, they conclude, when it comes to race-based disparities, "we may be underestimating the severity."[54] At the end of 2020, Canada's national statistics agency, Statistics Canada, confirmed this when it reported on COVID-19 mortality. In regions where 25 percent or more of the residents identified as "visible minorities" (the government's term for nonwhite and non-Indigenous people), the mortality rate was more than twice the level of regions where less than one percent of residents were classified as minorities. "The data," the Canadian Broadcasting Corporation explained, "affirms what some Canadians have reported anecdotally for months: Black people in particular have been far more likely to succumb to the virus than members of other groups."[55]

Perversely, however, news about the heightened risks for Black people did not have the effect that advocates for racial justice imagined. When psychologists at the University of Georgia surveyed Americans about their attitudes toward COVID, they found that white people who were more aware of racial disparities reported feeling less afraid of the disease and less supportive of public health measures designed to reduce spread of the virus. When given additional information about the specific dangers for Black people, whites became less empathic toward COVID victims. "These findings," they conclude, "suggest that publicizing racial health disparities has the potential to create a vicious cycle wherein raising awareness reduces support for the very policies that could most protect public health and reduce disparities."[56]

As Black people in North America and Europe called attention to the ways that the virus was threatening their communities, white people on the political right expressed a different concern. Some claimed that the new coronavirus had been manufactured by the Chinese or "globalist elites," mainly Jews such as George Soros or the Rothschild family, as a biological weapon and deployed to assert control over the "white race."[57] Immigrants, others said, were responsible for transmitting the virus. "Wake up people," one post implored. "The Jews own COVID just like all of Hollywood."[58] The Voice of Europe, an antimigrant media outlet, claimed that " 'asylum seekers' are rioting against quarantine and flying ISIS flags."[59] No matter the trends on racial disparities in COVID mortality, on Telegram, 4Chan, and platforms popular among right-wing extremists, there were rumors that COVID-19 was designed to be most harmful to white people, that Black people were immune from the disease, and that the virus was part of a plot to achieve "white genocide."[60] These narratives circulated quickly and widely, in some cases outpacing the official recommendations from health officials.

In March, when governments in Europe and North America began implementing COVID-19 restrictions, activity on far-right internet platforms soared to its highest levels, the Institute for Strategic Dialogue (ISD), a research organization that conducted extensive studies of pandemic disinformation, reported. According to "The Conspiracy Consortium," the ISD's analysis of 239 Telegram channels and nearly 500,000 messages in 2020 and early 2021, there was "consistent crossover in topic relevancy between white supremacist and conspiracy communities on Telegram when discussing COVID-19."[61] Infowars.com, the website developed by the prominent conspiracy theorist Alex Jones, was the most cited source of information in posts about COVID-19 shared on explicitly white supremacist and conspiracy channels. The second most popular source of information was Twitter, and the third was Zero Hedge, a conservative financial and political website that U.S. intelligence agencies have accused of amplifying Russian propaganda.[62]

The economic insecurity, physical isolation, and generalized anxiety created by the pandemic left people feeling powerless, in search of new sources of meaning and order. Right-wing extremists, including neo-Nazis and emergent white nationalist groups, exploited these fears as opportunities for recruitment, adding links to join or follow their organizations into the conspiratorial COVID-19 articles they posted. "White supremacist channels that engage in COVID-19 conspiracy content and gain considerable subscribers as a result can and do regularly revert to more explicit white supremacist and extremist material," the ISD explained. "Such activity has the effect of exposing audiences and people who were initially interested in perhaps lighter conspiracy content to more explicit material, which can foster radicalization and recruitment risks."[63] The right, said Ciarán O'Connor, author of the ISD report on Telegram messaging, called the pandemic "a catalyst for radicalization. It allows conspiracy theorists or extremists to create simple narratives, framing it as us versus them, good versus evil."[64]

The Proud Boys, a right-wing men's group of self-proclaimed "Western chauvinists" that has endorsed and committed acts of violence, were among the many extremist organizations that catalyzed participants with narratives framing white people as victims of a globalist pandemic plot. In April 2020, Proud Boys members helped rally people against public health policies that restricted social and economic activities in several states.[65] In spring 2020, an investigation by the Center on Terrorism, Extremism, and Counterterrorism (CTEC) found that Proud Boys members promoted the idea that the "New World Order" or "Zionist Occupied Government" was responsible for the pandemic and that the health crisis was part of an orchestrated Plandemic. "They have used coronavirus policies as excuses to further advocate for civil unrest and violence," the CTEC researchers conclude. "Their use of the pandemic to accelerate calls for a new civil war with liberals indicates a significant and notable escalation of their ideology."[66]

Ideology, for this extremist group, was only prelude. In May, Proud Boys members claimed responsibility for taking down a memorial in Spokane made up of wooden white crosses for each person who died of COVID-19 in Spokane County, Washington. A video posted on a Proud Boys social media page shows an image of the crosses piled up beside Spokane's City Hall, with the message: "Antifa made a fear propaganda cemetery. We cleaned it up. We dont stand for Communist Fear!" If you look closely, you can also see a man's hand making the OK symbol, which right-wing groups have adopted as a sign of white supremacy.[67]

In September 2020, the moderator of the first presidential debate asked Donald Trump whether he would condemn white supremacists and military groups. The president pushed back. "Give me a name," he demanded. "The Proud Boys," his opponent, Joe Biden, interjected. "The Proud Boys," Trump said, before sending out what sounded like a call to arms for an imminent conflict. "Stand back and stand by."[68]

CHAPTER 13

"Travels Far"

THANKACHAN MATHAI

"We were very blessed," Mathews Thankachan told me in March 2022, near the second anniversary of his father Thankachan Mathai's death from COVID. I respected his gratitude, and could not help feeling humbled by the sentiment. When I heard his family's story, the blessings were not what stood out.

Mathai was born on a rubber farm in Kerala, India, in 1963. He loved school, especially math and physics, but didn't have much time to study because his family needed him in the fields. "His life as a young person was very busy," Mathews told me. "The farms there are not like the ones in America. They didn't have all of our machines. To extract the rubber, you had to open a scab in the tree. That allows the rubber to drip out, bit by bit. For each tree, you had to manually open the scab. Our family's farm had two hundred, maybe four hundred rubber trees on it. He had two younger brothers who helped out. They'd do that in the morning, and then they had to walk, like, an hour to get to school." As a teenager, Mathai took a factory job after school to supplement his family's income. He kept the job through high school and college, filling his waking hours with farming, the factory, math, and physics. "He didn't see his parents very much," Mathews explained. "He didn't have much time for playing games or sports." What's more, Mathews added, was that none of the work he did was going to take him anywhere in Kerala. Mathai had family in America, however, and they promised things would be better if he joined them. That's exactly what he did.

Naturally, Mathai found his way to Queens. The physics degree from Kerala didn't do much for him in the New York City job market, but since he no longer had to split his time between the farm and the factory, it was somehow easier to see family and friends. Dating was more complicated. But one year, on a trip home to India, he met a nursing student named Sheeba and they clicked. They got married—even though Sheeba didn't have a visa to come to the U.S., and they could only see each other on holidays. She got pregnant and gave birth to Mathews in 1997. The next year, they both moved to New York City, where she found work as a nurse. In 1999, Sheeba gave birth to a second son, Cyril. "Around that time, my father got hired by the MTA," the Metropolitan Transit Authority, Mathews told me. "He was a custodian, mostly working nights. It was a hard job, but it was steady work. They had a union. Good health insurance. Dental. Vision. It was a job where he could support our family. He liked doing it. He liked the people he worked with, too."

Mathai worked the night shift for most of Mathews's child-hood. He'd get assigned a station to clean and stay there for a few years before rotating to another one. In each location, he'd get to know the station managers, the fare collectors, the operators, the security staff. People moved around a lot, but they usually spent their careers in the system, and they couldn't help but develop relationships—some loose, some tight and meaningful—because they spent so much time together underground. Occasionally, Mathai complained. People made messes in subway stations— big messes, as bad as you can imagine. Passengers could be rude, obnoxious, or violent. Sometimes a colleague acted out of turn. But mostly he took pride in his work, and in the community of coworkers who made the job all the more worthwhile. New York City relied on public transit, and neither would work without public servants. Mathai, ever the mathematician, understood how it all added up.

"My father really did love the subway system," Mathews remembered. "He was always trying to get us to learn how to use it. He'd make us stop and look at the maps so we could figure out how to get around. When we went into a station that was getting renovated, he'd always explain what they were doing, what they were trying to improve. I don't think I appreciated it that much when I was growing up, but later I'd meet people from here who hadn't traveled around the city a lot. We'd been everywhere. I think my brother and I went to the Empire State Building like, ten times!" Mathai also loved to take the family outside the city, and his job left time for that. His mother and two brothers had moved to America, and his favorite cousin was just outside of Philadelphia. "We'd travel every few weeks," Mathews told me. "That would be so exciting for us. It was my favorite place. We'd get in the car. See the bridge. I was always so happy to get outside of the city. We were immigrants. We didn't have much money. My parents saved so they could take us to India every few years. So those driving trips to see family, they were always really important to my father. They were the best things we did."

When they were home in Queens and, eventually, Long Island, where they found a house they could afford, Mathai spent afternoons with Mathews and Cyril while Sheeba worked at the hospital. "He liked to teach us math the way they taught it in India," Mathews told me. "They learned multiplication differently. That was the best. I remember being in third grade. I came home and told him about this cross box method we were using, and he was just so happy. Like, as if his team had just won the Super Bowl! He was very excited and interested, and he decided to teach me multiplication tables with this older, Indian method. He knew it would be useful for us, so we'd practice it." For Mathews, it became something like a secret superpower, one he rarely deployed. "But once the teachers started teaching tables, I just knew them already. I'd absorbed it. And they couldn't figure out what was going on. It was amazing." Another time, in fifth grade, the math teacher gave the class a challenge that they had a year to complete. "He explained it to me. We did a little practicing, a little theoretical explanation. And I did it right away! The first time." Mathai delighted in his son's successes. "Those are very good memories," Mathews said. "Very good."

Mathai swelled with pride when Mathews finished high

school and enrolled at the State University of New York at Stony Brook, a prestigious school whose campus was close enough for a commute from home. Mathews was there in January 2020 when the coronavirus outbreak reached New York City. "My father was nervous about the situation," he recounted. "It was confusing. We couldn't get much information about it at first. We didn't know much about the disease. But my mother was working in the hospital and my father was in the subway station. They were both on the front line, exposed to everyone. And the MTA didn't have masks for workers. It seemed inevitable that they would get it, and my father was mostly worried about bringing it home to us."

Staying home was not an option. The family still depended on Mathai's income. The transit system still depended on his labor. Custodians don't get to be remote. "My father felt a deep sense of responsibility to his job," Mathews said. "He was a little scared of the unknown, but he had a very strong immune system. He didn't even get colds. I can only remember him using sick days so that he could take care of us."

Among all the unknowns that the family was dealing with at that moment, the question of whether Mathai and Sheeba needed to wear face masks was especially confusing. In the hospital, administrators were doing everything they could to get high-quality masks for all staff members. Nurses were advised to wear them at all times. The MTA issued the opposite advice. On March 6, 2020, the agency sent a memo, "RE Frequently Asked Questions Regarding COVID-19" to all employees. One section read: "Should I wear a mask to work? No. At this time, masks are not being recommended by the relevant medical governmental authorities." The following section pressed the point. "I understand that masks are not recommended, but can I wear a mask if I want to? Current medical guidance indicates that respiratory masks do not protect healthy people—they are designed to keep infected people from spreading the virus to others. . . . [I]t is currently understood that the virus is transmitted through droplets, not through the air. This means you cannot randomly breathe it in and that the standard surgical masks you see people wearing will not help." Following this, the MTA specifically prohibited masks, deeming them a violation of employee dress codes.

"Since masks are not medically necessary as a protection against COVID-19, and not part of the authorized uniform, they should not be worn by employees during work hours."[1] The message was unequivocal: Mathai did not have a choice.

It did not take long for MTA workers to begin getting infected. On March 20, Peter Petrassi, a forty-nine-year-old conductor who had worked in the system for twenty years, checked into a hospital with respiratory problems. On March 26, he became the first known MTA worker to die from COVID-19.[2] Reports of MTA employees getting sick circulated widely. Bus drivers. Mechanics. Operators. Custodians. The transit workers union demanded better protection. The MTA rescinded the mask ban, but otherwise they got little traction. Mathai and his colleagues grew increasingly anxious. No one knew how to avoid the disease.

"My father got sick on March 31," Mathews told me. "He was tired and he had shortness of breath. He called an ambulance, and that night they put him on a ventilator at the hospital. The first day we had hope. The doctor told us he was doing tremendous. But the second day the doctor said he was not looking good. My brother, who's the youngest in the family, was the most attached to dad. He told the doctor, 'Please, try everything you can. Try to get him back to us.' The doctor promised to do that. 'We're trying our best,' he said. 'But we know so little. Sometimes we're just as confused as you are.'"

Mathai didn't get better, and while he was isolated in the hospital, struggling to breathe, Sheeba, Cyril, and Mathews came down with COVID, too. None had severe symptoms, but there was no way for them to visit Mathai, nor even to speak with him because of the ventilator. The two-way confinement was excruciating, a slow torture unlike anything they had experienced or could have imagined. So much closeness, obliterated by an impossible virus.

On the morning of April 4, the hospital called to inform the family that Mathai would not last much longer. They scheduled a short phone call, enough time for everyone to say a distant goodbye. "A few hours later they called to tell us that he'd passed away," Mathews told me. "It was so tough. At first there was this intense rush of emotions. Time stood still. Days passed, but everything felt frozen. People from our church called to offer their condolences. Ordinarily, they'd come and visit. But of course, we had COVID and we couldn't welcome them in. My dad had younger brothers, cousins. At a different time, we would have been surrounded by our family and friends. Having people around, their presence helps you. They bring food, and you don't feel like eating but you do because they're there. But we didn't have anyone. It was just my mother, my brother, and me."

The pandemic forced people to give up nearly all sacred rituals, and none felt more necessary—and impossible—than grieving together. "The MTA is a community, and if somebody here dies, everybody shows up," said Sandra Bloodworth as we sat in the living room of her towering apartment building on the Queens side of the East River, watching trains, buses, ships, and ferries course through the city below. "Whether it's a wake, a visitation, a funeral home, whatever the culture, we just surround that family. They're bonded. Over the years, I've probably been to thirty-five, forty of these gatherings. We're different people, different groups. We come from far-away places, speak different languages. But we have something bigger in common. And when there's a death, yeah, we come together for a big embrace."

Bloodworth, who grew up in Mississippi and never lost her accent, moved to New York City in 1980 to pursue a career as a painter. Many artists support themselves by waiting tables, others teach. Bloodworth had a different idea. In 1988, she took a job in the MTA's Arts & Design department, overseeing art installations and live performances in stations and public spaces throughout the city. Some of her group's projects are grand and highly publicized, with majestic works by world-famous artists in storied locations. Some are more modest, designed to bring something beautiful into the day of passengers in an outer-borough station. Bloodworth became director in 1996, and when the coronavirus outbreak hit New York City in March 2020, she feared that the transit system would turn dark and grisly, the specter of death and disease rendering every mosaic, sculpture, or painting irrelevant. When cases spiked, her division went remote. Bloodworth knew she had to be careful. But back home, perched high above the city, she also knew that most of her colleagues were still underground, invisible, and stuck in harm's way. She couldn't help feeling like the city had failed them, that there was a substantial moral debt to pay back.

"We're in March, April, and my husband and I are sitting here at home, watching TV news every day," Bloodworth told me. "MTA workers were starting to die, and one of the reporters touched on the fact that they couldn't come together and support each other. I knew what that meant for that community. I knew what was gone. And I remember standing right here and looking out and going, 'Oh God, I wish we could do a painting for every one of those workers who died.' Of course, I knew we couldn't, but I also thought, maybe there's a way."

It was not the first time that Bloodworth had thought about how to honor people who died doing their jobs in New York City. After September 11, 2001, she was part of the MTA's efforts to design new memorials to victims of the attacks on the World Trade Center, from a pair of monumental murals and an accompanying soundtrack in Grand Central Terminal to a mosaic with text from the Declaration of Independence and the United Nations Universal Declaration of Human Rights at the Cortlandt Street subway stop, set beneath the fallen towers.[3] Working on those projects had been soulful and fulfilling, Bloodworth told me. It felt important for New York City, and personally significant as well. COVID would hit her even more directly. Her colleagues, after all, were playing the role that firefighters played on 9/11, making it their duty to work in the danger zone, and paying the steepest price. People throughout the MTA were already talking about paying homage to the workers who had died. The question was how.

April 2020 was too early to work on memorials. The MTA, like most other public agencies in New York City, was focused on how to prevent the disease from spreading. They weren't particularly successful. Bloodworth kept getting emails with data on new cases among her colleagues, and occasionally she'd see one of their faces on television after they died. By April 8, at least forty-one

MTA workers had died of COVID, around 1,500 had tested positive, and more than 5,600 had called in sick or self-quarantined.[4] It was, *The New York Times* reported, a "staggering toll."[5]

That month, New York governor Andrew Cuomo took the extraordinary step of shutting down the twenty-four-hour subway system during early morning hours, during which the MTA sent in special crews—full-time employees as well as thousands of contractors, primarily Latin American immigrants—to clean and disinfect the seats, handrails, floors, and platforms, every surface that, officials feared, could get contaminated and spread the disease.[6] The work was challenging. Although ridership had plummeted, essential workers in other industries continued to use the system, as did the growing ranks of people without homes. Dealing with their waste—food, trash, excrement, even—made the job difficult and dangerous, as did their inevitable confrontations with passengers who refused to leave or follow the rules. The fact that the work was largely invisible, and that it paid around minimum wage, made it particularly unsavory. But the city needed laborers, and laborers needed work.

No one knows the exact number of MTA employees and contractors who caught COVID during the initial surge, because it was so hard to get tested in the early stage of the pandemic. One study shows that between March and August 2020, roughly one quarter of all MTA workers had been infected, and at least 125 had died.[7] By fall, when the death rate had slowed, Bloodworth and her team decided that they couldn't wait any longer to pay tribute. They wanted everyone to see just how much transit workers had given to keep the city going, to give the families of those who perished the embrace they deserved.

Abstract art, which had been so effective for memorializing September 11 and its terrifying imagery, seemed inappropriate for commemorating the MTA's fallen workers. They needed to be made visible, rendered fully human. For that, Bloodworth knew, portraits would work best. "I went through all the newspapers and found photographs of some of the people who died early on," she explained. The first one was Peter Petrassi, who, at forty-nine, was a difficult subject. He just looked so healthy, and far too young to die. "I had my husband's iPad, and I copied some images, put them in a design program, and made them black-and-white. I had this idea of taking out the background so I had just the person, and then filling the area around them with color. I could see them looking almost like stained glass windows, with the colors running across images." She made a few mockups, showed her husband and sent them to her deputy. But the truth, she confided, is that she didn't need their confirmation. "Immediately, I knew it would work."

In late September, Bloodworth presented the idea to a group of MTA deputies and designers who had been thinking about a memorial project since July. They responded the way she thought they would. She had a green light. "Now we needed to get the families engaged," Bloodworth said. "We needed their permission, of course. And we wanted them to choose the photograph, the color. I mean, this was about celebrating their loved one. This was for them." The MTA set up a team of liaisons who would work with each family, explaining the concept, helping them find the right image, making sure they felt comfortable with the public project. "It wound up being a little complicated," Bloodworth told me. "Some families didn't want to do it. Some didn't have a good photograph. You'd be amazed at how many families don't have a great image of a person they lose." She asked Gary Jenkins, a graphic designer at the MTA, to rework the images, improve the resolution, and remove other people and objects from view so that the subject came into relief. Bloodworth's team selected a color palette, drawing from the ones used in the transit system, and laid out the images, first one by one and then in groups of three. "They all became individuals," she explained. "You could see who they were."[8]

Because they were digital, you could also see them anywhere. Instead of installing the memorial in one central location, the MTA decided to display the images on triptych screens in 107 transit stations throughout the city, as well as in Penn Station and online. Calling the piece "Travels Far," the Arts & Design group produced a nine-minute video, with an original score by the composer Christopher Thompson, and an introductory poem by U.S. Poet Laureate Tracy K. Smith.

Travels Far
What you gave—
brief tokens of regard,
soft words uttered
barely heard,
the smile glimpsed
from a passing car.
Through stations
and years, through
the veined chambers
of a stranger's heart—
what you gave
travels far.[9]

The memorial project went live in January 2021, at a jittery moment for the city and the U.S. The first COVID vaccine was becoming available. President Trump, who was wildly unpopular in New York City, was on his way out of office, and a new administration, promising to shore up the nation's public health system, was on its way in. But the transition was rocky, violent, even. On January 6, when Congress convened to count votes from the Electoral College and declare Joe Biden the next president, Trump and his allies led a rally on the Mall in Washington, challenging the legitimacy of the election. When they finished, hundreds of people, many armed, stormed the Capitol, disrupting the official ballot count, looting congressional offices, and threatening to kill or capture Vice President Mike Pence or House Speaker Nancy Pelosi, who refused to go along with their plans. The attempted insurrection failed, but there was a dark, foreboding mood throughout the country. The virus contributed to the generalized sense of insecurity. It was surging again, and New York City was on edge.

On January 25, 2021, the MTA opened the memorial to the public—first in transit stations, and then in a small, physically distanced press conference at the new Moynihan Train Hall in Penn Station. Originally, Bloodworth had considered holding a ceremony for the families, a gathering for those who had mourned in isolation and fear. The surge made that impossible. But relatives of the MTA workers made their own way to the memorial, each at their own pace. Those who went to Penn Station found the space transformed by the installation. The bold colors cast a spectral light on the cavernous, empty train hall; the musical score, measured and solemn, slowed the pace. Instead of a commuter hub, it felt like a modern cathedral. "You can't imagine the feeling of walking into that space," Bloodworth said. "It was breathtaking. You could see the images so clearly, each one of them. And the colors. Oh my God."

On January 26, local and national news outlets featured the memorial in stories about the fate of public service workers, in New York City and beyond. "Here's an example of the incredible risks and burdens that our essential workers have been facing," former president Barack Obama tweeted, with a link to a triptych of three MTA employees who had died of COVID.[10] *This American Life* did a long radio segment on the installation, "Goodbye Mr. Facey," featuring a testament to the decency and dedication of Clarence Facey, a fifty-eight-year-old superintendent who had perished, just eight months before his planned retirement, and a

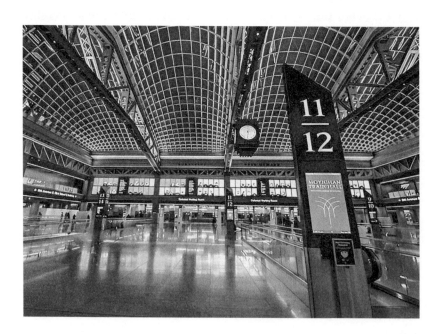

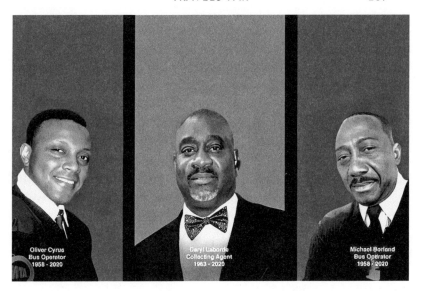

Oliver Cyrus
Bus Operator
1958 - 2020

Daryl Laborde
Collecting Agent
1963 - 2020

Michael Borland
Bus Operator
1958 - 2020

station agent who said the memorial was so important that it belonged in the Metropolitan Museum of Art. "The important thing was the attention that went to the families and the way that the workers reacted," Bloodworth told me. "Someone sent me a picture of a worker standing and looking at the screen in a subway station." Some of them, *This American Life* reported, wanted to watch the video over and over again.[11]

The portraits of 111 MTA workers who died from COVID were included in the Travels Far memorial. It was, Bloodworth told me, a tremendous collective effort. It was also, she acknowledged, completely inadequate for recognizing the pandemic's toll on New York City's essential workers, let alone on the city and country writ large. More than 350,000 Americans died from COVID during 2020, and in the spring of 2022 the mortality figure topped one million. If, in the early days of the pandemic, each COVID death sent shivers through the nation, as months passed Americans grew accustomed to the carnage. Mass casualties from the virus became normal and acceptable, as if the body politic had become numbed.

In her small world, at least, Bloodworth refused to let this happen. She could not force a national reckoning. She could not honor every essential worker who lost their life so that the rest of us could move along. But she could do something to help others understand what people gave so that the trains could keep running. She could make each MTA family's tragedy process a little less lonely, a little less invisible, a little less muted. She could help her city feel what they had been through.

"It was an acknowledgment of the losses in our community. The workers and the families. It was a way for them to pay tribute to those they lost," she told me. "I don't think many people know what art does for us, because it's so embedded into our lives. The memorial showed people the power that art has. It gets short shrift on funding, but it carries so much water. People needed it in this pandemic. That's why they were drawn to these portraits. The art helps us heal."

Mathews Thankachan only saw the installation once, at Grand Central Terminal in Manhattan. "It was a difficult experience," he told me. "I saw Dad, but I also saw a lot of his coworkers at the MTA. I know that they went through the same thing that Mom, Cyril, and I went through. I started thinking: if there's three of us, and there were a hundred other workers at the MTA who died, that's like, at least three hundred people who experienced this. Probably a lot more. And even if they had just one person—it's more of an intense emotion, because that one person carries all of that alone."

There was a journalist at Grand Central when Mathews visited, and she recorded a few moments of him watching the images before interviewing him about how it felt to be there. "Seeing this video helped me know that I'm not alone," Mathews told her. "My dad was always very grateful for this job, and this memorial, it's like the MTA is grateful for him."[12]

The experience helped Mathews and his family reach a turning point in their grieving. A few months later, at the one-year anniversary of Mathai's death, they invited friends and relatives to join them in a service. "We're Catholic," he said, "and our priest is from the same part of India where my parents are from. He did a ceremony for us, said the traditional prayer for the dead. We did it first in the church and then went to the gravesite. It was a very sunny day, and my close friends were there. We went the day before and put some nice flowers there. It was very beautiful, very good to do."

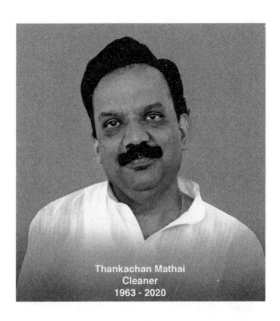

Thankachan Mathai
Cleaner
1963 - 2020

CHAPTER 14

Home Alone

There's no such thing as a good time for an infectious disease outbreak, but a pandemic that takes place during what pundits and policymakers call an "epidemic of loneliness" is especially unfortunate. In most of the world, the advice to socially distance hit at a moment replete with anxiety over the perception of fraying social bonds in general, and the atomization wrought by social media in particular. When, in March 2020, governments began to issue instructions for people to stay at home and avoid face-to-face interaction, they triggered fears of what journalist Ezra Klein called a disastrous "social recession," marked by a spike in loneliness and distress.[1]

Although everyone faced challenges related to lockdowns and distancing, one demographic group seemed particularly likely to suffer from the emergency public health measures: people who live alone. In ordinary times, those who are "going solo" are surprisingly social. They are more likely to visit with friends and neighbors than those who live with others, and also more likely to spend time in public gathering places such as bars, restaurants, cultural performances, and gyms.[2] During the pandemic, however, many public spaces that support collective life were shuttered, and people who were living alone by choice one day found themselves without the option of physical companionship the next.

Despite widespread concern for the wellbeing of people living alone, it was unclear whether it would be an advantage or
disadvantage for getting through the initial outbreak of COVID.
After all, going solo during a pandemic means not worrying about
whether a romantic partner, child, or roommate comes home
with the disease, or whether you will infect one of them. Perhaps
being alone offered some peace of mind? But within weeks of the
outbreak, psychologists were warning about a "double pandemic"
of social isolation and COVID-19. The Brigham Young University professor Julianne Holt-Lunstad reported a 20–30 percent
rise in overall loneliness and a tripling of emotional distress during the first month of the lockdown. The pattern, she suggested,
indicated that "the pre-existing public health crisis of social isolation and loneliness may be far more widespread than previously
estimated."[3]

International surveys designed to track levels of loneliness and
isolation during the first year of the pandemic failed to confirm
these patterns. Instead of a spike in perceived disconnection, they
showed, in aggregate, a series of squiggly lines. In some places,
the lines were basically flat. Consider, for instance, the results
of a weekly survey of 38,217 adults from the United Kingdom
during the seven-week, "strict lockdown" period between March
and May, 2020, conducted by a team from the University College
London COVID-19 Social Study. They found that people who
self-reported high levels of loneliness before the pandemic experienced a "slight increase" in loneliness during the lockdown, but
also that those who reported low levels of loneliness in ordinary
times felt even less lonely when they had to stay at home. People with more moderate levels of loneliness before the outbreak,
however, reported hardly any changes, leading to the surprising
conclusion that, in the U.K., at least: "Perceived levels of loneliness under strict lockdown measures due to COVID-19 were
relatively stable."[4]

Researchers in the U.S. observed something similar. Psychologists who surveyed a nationally representative sample of
1,545 Americans in late January/early February 2020 (before the
outbreak), in late March (during the federal government's initial
"15 Days to Slow the Spread" campaign), and in late April (when

most states implemented "stay-at-home" policies), reported no significant changes in overall loneliness levels across these three assessment periods. Improbably, they found, "respondents perceived increased support from others over the follow-up period." Their conclusion: when it came to managing loneliness, at least, Americans exhibited "remarkable resilience in response to COVID-19."[5]

The United States was not unique. In Norway, a group of health scholars compared self-reported loneliness among 10,740 adults, drawing on surveys conducted before the pandemic and again in June 2020. In a paper published by the *Scandinavian Journal of Public Health*, they reported "slightly increased loneliness" during the lockdown period among single people and older women. "Overall," however, they found that "loneliness was stable or falling during the lockdown." In fact, they continued, "individuals with low social support and high levels of psychological distress and loneliness before the pandemic experienced decreasing loneliness during the pandemic." The reasons for this unexpected decline in disconnection are unclear, but the authors speculated that it had to do with an "enhanced sense of togetherness" rooted in shared values and experiences in a moment where Norwegians felt a sense of linked fate.[6] Researchers in Germany observed this same phenomenon. A study published in the *International Journal of Psychology* reports that during the lockdown, Germans experienced stable levels of "emotional loneliness," the perceived lack of emotional connections with others, and "social loneliness," the perceived lack of a broader social network. What increased, though, were reports of "physical loneliness," due to the sudden impossibility of getting close to people who lived outside one's own domestic space.[7]

These surveys on loneliness are helpful for establishing patterns of connection that are noticeably different from what pundits feared, and journalists reported, when they raised concerns about the "social recession" in the pandemic. What they cannot do, however, is help us understand how people who were forced to make such immediate and dramatic cutbacks in their social interactions experienced the transformation, or why most people were able to fend off the feeling of being on their own. To answer those questions, I designed a study based on interviews with an ethnically and geographically diverse group of fifty-five adults (ages twenty to eighty-six) who lived alone in New York City between March and July 2020, when the coronavirus initially surged. (I use pseudonyms to identify them here.) Jennifer Leigh, a graduate student in sociology at NYU, conducted the interviews, and together we assessed what people said.[8]

One clear takeaway from these conversations is that living alone during the first COVID outbreak, even in the epicenter of the pandemic, did not induce the kind of emotional disconnection or social isolation that so many people feared. Too often, public debates about loneliness frame it as static and corrosive, as if it leads only to lasting suffering and pain. It's true that for some people loneliness is chronic and dire; they lack the capacity to form the relationships they long for, or the resources to break through their psychological impasse. Usually, though, people who feel lonely respond by searching for better connections. Often, they find them, and their sense of loneliness diminishes. The experiences of people who lived alone during the most restrictive phase of the pandemic illustrate this social fact. The knowledge is relevant not only in crises, but in ordinary times, too.

Although most people we interviewed reported experiencing loneliness at some point during the pandemic, hardly anyone described it as a personal crisis. Loneliness, after all, need not be debilitating, and usually is not. In small doses, loneliness is the body's way of signaling that it needs stronger and more meaningful connections, and, as the late psychologist John Cacioppo explained, most people respond to it by seeking out those very things.[9] When the initial COVID outbreak hit New York City, people who lived alone made special efforts to contact their friends and relatives. Those we interviewed consistently described themselves as being quite strongly tied to friends and family, and did not perceive themselves to be isolated so much as physically distant from the people who mattered to them. Physical distance, not social distance, was paramount, whereas chronic, existential loneliness was rare.

That said, being physically alone was confusing and distressing. The people we met struggled with the loss of everyday social interactions with neighbors and familiar strangers who, while neither friends nor confidants, provided regular companionship in gathering places such as coffee shops, bodegas, public transit, and sidewalks. They told us that despite the social and emotional challenges of living alone, "structural isolation"—feeling abandoned by government or marginalized by society at large—was a greater emotional burden than they had anticipated, greater, even, than being confined to a place of their own.

People living alone do not have the support of another person in their immediate home environment. However, the vast majority of the people interviewed said that during the first wave of the pandemic lockdowns, they were able to connect with their loved ones easily via phone, Zoom, FaceTime, or social media. Even those who previously had not particularly enjoyed using social media or communication platforms such as Zoom described pushing themselves to connect with others by making accounts or attempting to use technology that they had never used before.

Not only were most people able to virtually connect with their loved ones, nearly all were in touch with distant friends or family even more often than they ordinarily would have been. Jennifer, a woman in her fifties, described a sharp increase in her communication during the pandemic, saying, "There are some people I could have gone a month or two without talking to, but we all felt the need to talk to each other." She didn't think that the frequent contact would last forever, but she wondered, as did most people, whether some of her relationships would wind up closer on the other side.

Others found that they were able to enjoy conversations with friends and family in a way that they were not able to in the past. James, a health care worker in his forties living in Queens, said that using the phone brought him back to his childhood experiences, when he was able to call his friends after school and talk for hours. Home, alone, in the shuttered city, James rediscovered the pleasures of slow media in unstructured time. "I don't think this current society affords that type of connection as much anymore, like a long phone call," he explained. "'Cause everybody's so busy, everybody's so into all these other things."

Remote conversations were not always satisfying, however; in some cases seeing a close friend or family member on a video call wound up reminding solo dwellers of how far they were from the people they loved. Deborah, a woman in her fifties who described immense difficulty being alone during the peak of the pandemic, said that Zoom could be a source of both connection and isolation, and often did both at the same time. "I feel like there was support there," she said. "Like, there was 101 Zoom calls every week for birthday parties and drinks or class." But there was a dark side to the interactions online. "I found Zoom to be extremely exhausting pretty early on. And I felt like a freakin' wreck, so I didn't want to be on Zoom. I had to drop off of some family calls when it was really in the thick of it, because I just started crying when I saw people on the screen."

When it comes to social media, less is more. Using it too often left people longing for more intimate connection, something more solid and real. "We're all made of energy, and it's not the same over video," Diane said. "I think it's just that lack of human interaction and like, being able to hug them when you greet them and then to, you know, to touch them, to say goodbye . . . I think that makes a difference." Darren, who's in his thirties, reinforced this distinction: "Because I've had to socialize with people online, nothing really seems real, or people don't really seem real. Like, I'm talking to my friends online, and I see them on a screen, but there's no connect." The dissatisfying aspects of such interactions suggest aspects of loneliness that don't come across in surveys where people rate their level of social bonding on a numerical scale. It's the quality, not the quantity of interactions, that most directly affects people's feelings of connection, and in general, conversations through screens proved less fulfilling than our informants wanted them to be.

Although solo dwellers are quite social during ordinary times, the pandemic created serious obstacles. The problem was not simply that the usual meeting places were closed and inaccessible, but also that norms around communication were shifting, in ways that people living alone found hard to track. The New Yorkers we interviewed said it was hard to know exactly how and when to reach out to others, especially when they needed support. Robert, who's in his thirties, told us that he had an easier time attending to strangers than providing for his own needs. "I'm trying to think about like, reaching out to people. I'm very loath to reach out and ask for help and say, 'Hey, I'm not in a good place right now.'" No one wants to be a burden. Helping others, however, was a compelling way to connect. For Robert, getting involved in mutual aid projects around the neighborhood became a vital source of social integration. It served a dual purpose; caring for others turned out to be an essential way to take care of himself.

That care proved important, since the restrictions on social life lasted longer than most people anticipated when the coronavirus first arrived in New York, and social relations remained distorted for months. The initial surge of video calls eventually receded. "Zoom fatigue" became a widespread phenomenon, and some solo dwellers wound up feeling left out. Sandra, who's in her thirties, had been living alone after her roommate moved out in the initial outbreak, and she said group conversations online became a lifeline. "I honestly think everyone got tired of it, and we stopped doing it," she recounted. "And then I got kind of upset at them, 'cause I was like, you all live with four roommates or your partners or all of this stuff, and I'm totally alone." She didn't feel desperate to change her living situation, but when she started to feel lonely she decided to remind her friends who lived with others that she needed extra attention. "I felt kind of, you know, abandoned in that sense by them. . . . Even if it's just a text saying, 'Hey, what's up, how are you doing?' I'd appreciate it, just 'cause I feel like it's easy to forget about me because I don't have all these other people around me who sort of have to check on me." It takes genuine self-knowledge to make those calls, and strong social skills, too. Of course, not everyone has those capabilities. For those who lacked them in the pandemic, the emotional toll was real.

·   ·   ·

The more common emotional pain that solo dwellers felt came not from typical feelings of social disconnection, but from the difficulty of being physically alone through the extended suspension of collective life. Nothing had prepared them for that experience, and nothing they could do remotely could compensate for the loss of intimate, tactile, or face-to-face interactions with other human beings.

The people we interviewed were careful to distinguish between the state of being alone and the condition of feeling lonely. One may lead to the other. Then again, it may not. When asked whether he had felt lonely during the pandemic, Dean, a man in his twenties, responded: "Yes, but lonely, isolated . . . I mean, these are all kind of words that don't necessarily have to be associated with feeling bad about yourself. I think you can feel really, really lonely and go to parties every weekend." Indeed, some mentioned that their friends who lived with family, roommates, or spouses felt as lonely as they did, if not more so, despite not being physically alone. But the struggle with physical loneliness was far more difficult for those going solo. When discussing his own experiences of loneliness, Peter, an Asian American physician in his forties who had moved out of his home to protect his wife and children, said: "I mean, it's hard to say; I think everybody has their different meaning of what loneliness means to them. It's kind of a strong word, loneliness, 'cause that sounds like you're alone, emotionally, physically. But that's kind of how . . . I guess physically, I'm lonely. Emotionally, to cope with it, I would call folks, family, friends . . . just to kind of get by."

Sam, a man in his sixties whose partner of more than thirty years died of COVID early in the pandemic, also insisted on the difference between feeling lonely and being alone. "People ask me if I'm lonely," he said. "And I don't feel lonely, I feel alone." Sam identified mundane moments, such as eating dinner or watching TV, as times when he felt most alone. "If I'm watching a program, there's nobody to like, say, 'This is crap,' or 'This is good,' or 'Did you see that?' Although I get to the point sometimes where I talk to the dog and I say, 'Did you see that?'" he said. "But there's no human being to do that, so I just look at it as a feeling of being alone, not being lonely." Sam was just one of the many people who told us that highly touted coping mechanisms for dealing with the quarantine—cooking, baking, organizing one's home, making cocktails, even—didn't work as well for solo dwellers. Elena, who's in her thirties, described her frustration with the suggestions for how to spend time at home that she saw on social media. "I'll never be someone to make a big fancy dish just for myself, just 'cause I'm like, who else is gonna appreciate this?" she explained. "I would've been fine with making mac 'n' cheese. So a lot of the things that were being encouraged, and were helping a lot of other people cope, were not really necessarily options that made sense for me." Vicki, who's in her fifties, said that although social media had been an important source of connection for her, seeing others cooking with their loved ones when she could not compounded her emotional stress. "When you're alone—who the fuck are you cooking for?" she exclaimed, laughing. She had lived alone for years and took pride in being an independent person, but as the pandemic dragged on she began to wish for domestic companions: "I got more depressed, like oh, if I had a family, if I had someone, then at least . . ." she sighed. The distress of being alone ultimately motivated her to move in with her romantic partner, and they decided to get married that summer.

Cooking alone was connected to larger problems in the phenomenology of being alone in the pandemic. Solo dwellers specifically identified the lack of physical touch as a unique challenge of living alone when gathering places were shuttered. Even those who identified themselves as generally not affectionate reported that they longed for physical connections. "I'm not like, super clingy or touchy," said Maria, who's in her twenties. "Now it's like, I crave that, I want that." With few options available to her, Maria found that immersing herself in a bath was the closest way to feel "embraced by something." But warm water was no substitute for human touch. Similarly, Dep, a Vietnamese woman in her fifties, was shocked to find herself "really kind of hell-bent on trying to find a lover, like, just to have somebody to kind of have an interaction with," a response that she emphasized was extremely out of character.

Others developed psychological strategies for minimizing the pain of isolation. Some explained that they could manage loneliness by reminding themselves that it is usually a passing feeling, and that the extreme situation they were stuck in would eventually end. Katie, who's in her forties, recounted, "My therapist was like: 'What do you do when you're lonely?' And I was like, 'I cry, 'cause I'm sad. And then it's over!' That's sort of how it is, I'm sad sometimes, and sometimes it's just sad to be alone. I'm like, that's fine. You don't have to always distract yourself, sometimes you can just be sad and alone." Katie had contracted COVID-19 early in the initial outbreak, and when her roommate moved out, she found herself sick, scared, and alone. But fighting off the disease and the anxiety related to her new situation gave her a renewed sense of self, and a belief in her own resilience. If some solo dwellers responded to the crisis by seeking out a spouse or permanent companion, Katie had the opposition reaction. If it was affordable, Katie said, she would prefer to keep living alone.

In summer, when the first wave of cases receded and New York relaxed its distancing guidelines, people who had been living alone were eager to reconnect with friends and family in person. Some seemed downright euphoric, with impromptu dance parties breaking out on city streets and people of all ages expressing pure joy and relief. Most of the solo dwellers we interviewed reported some anxiety about the return of more ordinary social life. Face-to-face interactions that had always been routine were suddenly shot through with risk. But no one questioned their value. Universally, solo dwellers said that having physical contact lifted their spirits and improved their mental health. Terri, who's in her thirties, described the thought process behind her decision to go on picnics with friends she had not seen since the outbreak. She couldn't help but feel guilty, even though she knew it was the right thing to do. "Beforehand, it's this whole, 'Oh my God. Are we being horrible people if we're gonna do this?'" she said. "I have sort of made the decision that at some point my mental health needs it. I have to make a risk calculation." For Terri, and everyone else we interviewed, the ultimate choice was clear.

·   ·   ·

It was striking, how many people who had been living alone before the pandemic said that they still liked doing so, despite the challenges of isolation. As they explained things, everyone was struggling with the new restrictions on social life and public gatherings. There were, no doubt, specific problems related to going solo, but people with spouses, children, or roommates were hardly free of challenges. They knew, from conversations with friends and family, that living alone meant not worrying about someone else bringing COVID into the apartment, not being asked to do day care for a toddler or manage remote school for an adolescent, not finding oneself with a mountain of domestic labor that no one else was willing to share. The kinds of comparisons people make when they assess a situation shapes their own emotional wellbeing. Too often, we heard, those who live with others assume that people on their own are suffering from extreme levels of loneliness and isolation. They don't necessarily recognize how being confined with other people can make their own lives difficult, too.

No matter how much people valued having a place of their own in the pandemic, most had a hard time dealing with the loss of their option to not be alone. The inability to visit friends and family was only one part of the problem; the other was how difficult it was to forgo spontaneous interactions with the neighbors and strangers who once populated their daily lives. These social exchanges, a staple of urban living, have particular value for those going solo. Jack, who's in his forties, said that normally, when one feels alone, spending time in public spaces yields casual conversations, shared smiles, elementary forms of human connection that alleviate the loneliness so many people feel. In ordinary times, he explained, "at least you can go on walks or like, just randomly strike up a conversation with someone who's sitting outside your porch. Like, random interactions if you can't have very specific ones. That has become exponentially more difficult now than it was before." These sorts of anonymous interactions—a wave to a neighbor, a nod from the commuter who's always on the same morning train, a conversation about the weather with the barista—are fundamental features of everyday social life, and not only in cities, but they were lost in the distance that COVID imposed.

Many had not been aware of how important these interactions were to the structure of their life before the pandemic. Leon, who's in his fifties, reflected on missing the "bite-sized interactions" that he had grown accustomed to, unconsciously. "I have someone I can be intimate with and affectionate with, but just that giving someone a fist-bump or sharing a joke with a stranger about some ridiculous part of life, that kind of all disappeared. Those casual interactions that sometimes lead to new friendships and sometimes don't lead anywhere, but greatly spice up your day, have all disappeared." Although Leon decided to keep visiting his girlfriend during the outbreak, their relationship did not provide the same structure that he got from anonymous interactions. "You find that they are part of the fabric of your daily life that you had not noticed before," he remarked.

Some of the people we interviewed told us that, when the pandemic started, they actively sought out spontaneous interactions in public, even if they were discouraged, because they knew how much these occasions buoyed their spirits. Doing the laundry in the building's common area. Lingering on the front steps or in the hallway. Planting oneself on a park bench and hoping someone else stopped to do the same. Kira, who's in her fifties, and has a long history in her neighborhood, explained, "I realized how important that is for me, that I get this kind of social support, my need for connection and just to talk to people spontaneously. I can walk out and have that." For Kira, the interactions need not be with close friends; familiar strangers made her feel connected, and at home, too. "These are people that literally I've known for twenty years. Often enough, they may not know my name—and that's by choice, we don't know each other's name—but they're people I've been saying hi/bye to, and it's like a very real conversation," she said. Mary, a nurse in her fifties, reported that "I'd go to the grocery store, sometimes just to get conversation on your day off. People didn't understand that, that you'd be going to Stop N' Shop—not to buy anything, just to talk."

Not everyone had equal access to shared public spaces that

fostered these important interactions. The social infrastructure of New York's neighborhoods varies dramatically, with some places, like Park Slope in Brooklyn or the Upper East Side of Manhattan, offering an abundance of open parkland, with ample green space and paths for walking or biking, and others, such as Jackson Heights in Queens or East Tremont in the Bronx, saturated in asphalt and concrete. Those differences always shape the quality of social life in New York City. But in the pandemic, their impact was profound.

The people we interviewed conveyed a deep appreciation for their local social infrastructure, particularly the public parks and community gardens that allowed them to spend time around other people outdoors. Not every city condoned this kind of activity. In Chicago, for instance, Mayor Lori Lightfoot made the controversial decision to close the city's most popular public parks as well as the busy lakefront walking and biking paths, due to concerns that the social life they attracted would exacerbate the public health crisis.[10] San Francisco and Seattle established similar temporary restrictions.[11] New York City closed its playgrounds, public swimming pools, and beaches, but it kept parks open.[12] Sandra, who's in her thirties, appreciated that decision. "One of the great things about parks is it's one of the few things you can do that's always free, right? So they're free, and we didn't close," she explained. "The mayor very intentionally did not close the parks, even though lots of people were calling for them to." Lou, who's in his seventies, spent hours walking through the park every day of the pandemic, and he insisted that it was the key to his physical and mental health. He did other things to protect himself, too. After seeing how many people did not respect the recommended six feet of space for physical distancing, Lou made a sign that said, "In case you aren't sure, this is six feet," and carried it around on a curtain rod. Though not everyone responded positively to his message, he recounted the reactions of people around him with some amusement: "It was very interesting, because I got, you know, a lot of thumbs-up and a lot of smiles, but also a lot of people were angry that I was carrying it. Which I found interesting." Lou was good-natured about both responses. Whether positive or negative, they were social experiences that alleviated his isolation, and he was grateful that the park made them so easy to produce.

Isolation, as sociologists generally define it, refers to the level of people's social ties and contacts. When people report having few confidants to speak with, or infrequent visits with friends and family, we call them socially isolated. Whether or not they feel lonely, social isolation can be harmful. It means not having support when you need it, not knowing where to turn when something goes wrong. Isolation is especially dangerous in an emergency. During heat waves and hurricanes, people who lack social ties face greater risks of death and desertion. They have more trouble recovering, too. Isolation during an infectious disease outbreak is a more complicated matter. On the one hand, strong social ties are important for anyone who needs assistance with food, medication, physical or mental health. On the other, being isolated means being less exposed to the virus. Temporarily, at least, a condition that's bad for the body can help keep someone alive.

It was not social isolation, but structural isolation, a sense of being marginalized or neglected from the broader society, that proved particularly challenging to the solo dwellers we interviewed. When we asked what kind of support would have been most helpful for coping with the challenges of living alone during the pandemic, people were far more likely to identify material support—lost income, rent relief, access to PPE and health care—than social or emotional attention. Marta, who's in her twenties and had lost her job at the start of the pandemic, reported, "I don't really feel like I lack support in any area at this time; I've got family, friends . . . just not work!" Terence, who's in his forties and had lost his job prior to the outbreak, said unemployment was his main problem. "It's not necessarily emotional, but obviously, my biggest challenge is finding employment, by far. Like, I'd say that prospects have obviously gotten smaller, and especially with COVID, the supply and demand curve has only gotten more extreme."

People who live alone tend to feel more economically precarious than people living with others, because there's no one else to provide income if they suddenly lose their job. In the first months of the pandemic, unemployed Americans had no idea whether, or for how long, the government would provide financial assistance, nor did they know how much support they would receive. No one knew what would happen if they couldn't pay their rent or mortgage, how far they were from being out on the street. "The fact that even now, they're sort of waiting until the last minute to let us know if they're gonna pay us next month, like, that's not pleasant," said Michael, an actor and bartender in his thirties who had lost both sources of his employment. He was considering moving in with a roommate to ease the financial burden. He felt unseen or forgotten by the political officials whose decisions would determine his fate. It wasn't clear that anyone noticed how treacherous it had become for people in his situation.

Some embraced their invisibility by decamping from the urban environment and venturing into what soon became known as "van life," a nomadic existence organized around adventure and novelty, and a lifestyle now compatible with remote work. Once countries lifted the first set of pandemic travel restrictions, a wave of younger and more affluent professionals left the country altogether, renting apartments in places like Lisbon and Mexico City and logging into the virtual office when necessary, their location a secret, or no longer relevant to their firm. Among financially secure young adults who lived alone or did not have children, there was hushed talk of the virtues of the pandemic. They were living well, and in new if not exotic places, saving money, streaming films and TV shows, enjoying the calm.

Most people didn't have this luxury. Several solo dwellers reflected on how their socioeconomic status and material needs influenced their sense of loss during the pandemic. Pamela, a Thai woman in her seventies, expressed gratitude for the city's COVID-19 Emergency Home Food Delivery program and the Zoom classes offered by her local community center. In some ways, the special public services gave her a greater sense of stability during the crisis than she had during ordinary times. "I told them I'm happier because I have food delivered to me. I don't have to cook, and I can exercise. I can do anything!" she recounted. But other old people around her had different emotional experiences. Despite having greater financial security than she did, her more affluent classmates at the senior center felt that they had lost more during the pandemic. "I think they're retired with a lot of money, so they lost their freedom to eat out, to see friends, to go to theater, everything," she reported. "They lost more than me."

Again, the kinds of comparisons that people made—upward, against those who seemed to be flourishing despite the virus and the social restrictions, or downward, against those who appeared to be coming undone—shaped their experiences. Steve, a Black man in his forties, told us that his white, wealthier friends seemed to be reaching out for support more than his Black friends. "They're probably less used to coping with extremely adverse situations. And I'd say that my minority group is . . . How do I put this? They're used to—not used to, but maybe conditioned to—having to hunker down, if you will." Steve didn't think that his more privileged friends were actually worse off during the pandemic, but they acted as if they had lost more.

No one could solve the problem of structural isolation single-handedly. What they could do, however, was re-engage and make things better. A number of solo dwellers we spoke with did exactly that during the pandemic. Volunteering in mutual aid networks. Working in food pantries. Demonstrating for racial justice. Participating in civic action was a powerful antidote to structural isolation, and to the problem of physical loneliness, too. It gave people a sense of agency and camaraderie. It brought them out of their solitary domestic environments, and back up-close to people they had been told to avoid. Julius, who's in his thirties, said that he joined the Black Lives Matter protests in part because "I'm personally longing for physical interaction." He was furious about the murder of George Floyd, and the pattern of racial violence that preceded it. But moral outrage was not the only thing that brought him into the streets in the summer of 2020. "Ignoring the reason I'm there, I feel alive being around people," he explained. The social movement helped him return to himself, and also offered a release.

For others, basic community work provided similar benefits. After becoming more concerned about economic inequality during the pandemic, Jeff, a white man in his thirties, got deeply involved in mutual aid efforts. Though he had never before felt tied to his neighbors, the pandemic gave him a newfound sense of empathy and linked fate. Collective projects, from organizing grocery deliveries to planting public gardens and cleaning streets, brought him closer to people he'd never paused to consider, creating bonds where before there was distance, and opening avenues for support. He called attention to "that switch, where they put out into the world, 'Hey, I really just want to help anyone who needs help.' It makes it so much easier to ask for help, and it adds so much safety to the community." It added just as much to his own local life.

Teresa, who's in her forties, had a similar experience. She lived in one of the neighborhoods in Queens that was hit hardest by COVID, with a crisis in hunger as dire as the disease. "It was really hard to see so much need and desperation," she explained. "I live in an area where like, people were blocks and blocks just on line to get food, Pampers, things for babies, like, baby necessities. It's just like, we've gone through a lot here." She was distraught about the situation, and even though there was nothing safer than being home, alone, doing that felt useless and wrong. "I gotta tell you, it felt really good to like, buy groceries for a family. It felt good to like, show up at their door or meet them at the supermarket. To me, it was probably one of the most satisfying feelings that I've had in my life."

Teresa's words are a reminder that feelings of deep satisfaction can come directly out of isolation or emotional distress, as long as the person enduring them has opportunities to change the situation. They also point to a fact about loneliness that's easy to miss if we approach it as a problem of individual psychology rather than collective action: shared social experiences, and the sense of being part of something greater than the solitary self, cut against the feeling of radical disconnection. What's more, these experiences are possible even in the most extreme and isolating situations. That's why this case study is so instructive: The city that's hit hardest by COVID. The people who are most at risk of being alone.

The way we understand the social and emotional pain that people experienced during the pandemic is hardly an academic matter. Focusing on loneliness and isolation as the most worrisome symptoms of life in a locked-down, distanced, remote world leads to a certain set of prescriptions: Call your friends and family. Reduce your time on social media. Seek out companions wherever you can. There's nothing wrong with calling for these social remedies, but if, as the evidence suggests, loneliness did not spike dramatically during the pandemic, and most of those who felt its sharp edge found ways to blunt its impact, they may not offer much help.

More worrisome, though, is that public attention on individual and relatively apolitical problems like loneliness and isolation may distract attention from larger structural problems. Stress from social and economic insecurity. Anxiety about viral or material threats. Existential concerns about the world we have created, and the catastrophes that may come next. In 2020, not many people were free of these fears, and the sources were not merely psychological. Social conditions—where we work and live, where we learn and play, where we get care and support, and how we're treated by the powerful institutions that determine our fate—are the root causes of distress for those going solo, just as they are for most everyone else. An individual may well get help in the therapist's office, but the best remedies require collective action, and a change in the system that makes so many people feel abandoned, if not alone.

CHAPTER 15

Growing Up

In January 2020, Luis was twenty-one and beginning the second semester of his junior year at a public college in New York City. He had just changed his major from biology to political science, and stepped up his participation in a political group that advocated for Puerto Rican causes. Luis lived with family in Queens, and everyone pitched in to make ends meet. His father was retired. His mother collected disability insurance. His older sister, with whom he shared a bedroom, was a veterinary technician. Luis worked at a law firm in Manhattan. The apartment was crowded, loud, and sometimes crazy. But in New York City, what isn't? Luis was usually out in the world, anyway. School was in Harlem. Friends were in Brooklyn, Queens, and the Bronx. Work was everywhere, because his main job was serving legal papers, and the law had tentacles everywhere. Luis was going places. He just didn't know where.

That month, Luis started hearing about a potentially lethal new coronavirus that was spreading around Asia and possibly heading to America. At first COVID-19 seemed like a distant threat. There was always talk of potential crises; he and his family had more pressing concerns. By March, however, there were confirmed cases in New York City. His professors told him to prepare for remote classes. He went shopping at a store in his neighborhood and suddenly, Luis remembers, "everything was gone. People were just hoarding. There was nothing." One day, Luis's sister came home with news that her veterinary clinic had closed and terminated her position. Soon after, Luis lost his job, too. "Then I actually caught it," he recounted. "I'd never gotten the flu. I didn't know what it was. I had fever, coughing. I lost my [sense of] smell." Luis went online, looked up the symptoms for COVID, and found a pretty good description for what he was feeling. "They're saying, 'Oh, you've had symptoms, we don't recommend you get tested because you really have to just stay inside.'" He stayed home, as did his parents and sister. Before long they all had the virus. It was scary, because by then they knew that Queens was a COVID-19 hot spot. Ambulance sirens blared around the clock. Local hospitals were filled to capacity, with so many dead bodies that they needed refrigerated trucks to store the remains. But no one in Luis's family got a severe case of the illness. Luis still couldn't smell anything. Otherwise, they were safe.

Among medical scientists, Long COVID refers to the condition in which patients experience sustained physiological symptoms of the disease for months after the typical duration of the illness. For Luis, and millions of other people whose lives have been shaken up by the coronavirus pandemic, Long COVID could also refer to the enduring social and economic effects of the crisis, from lost educational opportunities to chronic unemployment, mental illness to fractured friendships and strained family ties. It could refer to the long-term changes in political values and civic participation as well.

By summer of 2020, Luis had fully recovered his sense of smell and taste. "But I lost everything," he reported. His family, once stable, was now impoverished. They relied on food pantries, which helped with the basics but satisfied no one. "It was just repetitive, the basic food you get. Eating crackers and cheese every day is not gonna help anything." Luis looked for government programs that could help them with rent, food, jobs, dignity. There wasn't much on offer. "So I ended up just going into stores to shoplift. I used to do it when I was younger, because I had no source of income. I was kind of going back to those days." Luis lied to his parents, making up stories about odd jobs or gift cards he'd picked up. "It was harrowing," he recalled, and not great for his pride or dignity, either. "But I didn't get caught."

As the year dragged on, Luis found himself feeling trapped by the pandemic and its many burdens. The apartment was confining. The food insecurity, the problem of paying rent, the joblessness, the small businesses closing, the desperation that was suddenly visible across the city, the anxiety that lingered everywhere—all of it weighed on Luis and his family. There were also bright spots. In the absence of reliable public assistance, New Yorkers started mutual aid networks and neighbors helped each other like they had never done before. He got a job as a contact tracer, though that also involved getting bombarded with sad stories from people who'd gotten sick and were afraid of what would happen next. After a police officer killed George Floyd, Luis joined thousands of New Yorkers in protests that lasted through the summer. "It was connected to the pandemic," Luis said. "It was boiling over at that point, this kind of mistreatment. And the reason I went was because it kind of showed that yeah, we've lost our jobs, we lost all our money. People are gonna do what they need to survive."

Some things, though, got lost or put on hold. Luis had been planning to apply to graduate school in 2021. "But then I thought, why am I rushing back into education? I'll be in Zoom calls for probably the first year of the PhD program. Why go into that?" His social life was still nonexistent. "Being social has been one of the hardest things to give up," he explained. "I worry about my family and not getting really sick, so I have really distanced myself from hanging out this year, haven't really socialized at all." When the vaccine arrived, Luis found himself looking forward to the world reopening. "I'm thinking of putting one continent on every side of a dice and just rolling it and just seeing where it lands," he told us, before pausing a beat and sharing his new, albeit more modest ambition: "Breathe."

It will take decades to assess the full impact of the pandemic on Luis and other young adults who experienced the crisis at a pivotal moment in their development, to understand whether they will undergo social and personal changes on par with what the sociologist Glen Elder Jr. called the "children of the Great Depression," in his classic study of that formative event.[1] Already, though, people in their twenties worry that nearly everything important to them—education, career, relationships, health—may be shaped by what they endured, or escaped, as the historic plague spread across their families, neighborhoods, schools, and workplaces. So, too, do scholars studying the consequences of being infected or affected by COVID-19. Some, despite the surprisingly resilient labor market, have suggested that young adults who were entering postsecondary schools or launching new careers when the pandemic hit are at risk of becoming a "lost generation," their immediate security shattered, their future economic prospects bleak.[2] Others have reported a dramatic spike in anxiety, depression, and suicidal ideation among young adults during the first year of the pandemic, warning that the long-term effects of mental illness could be as consequential as the acute distress.[3]

Of course, young adults are a large and diverse demographic, unified in age but differentiated in just about every other way: social class, race, ethnicity, religion, gender, geography, nationality, and the like. For that reason, sociologists are generally skeptical about the usefulness of the concept "generation." It clearly works as a marketing tool, but for analysis, it doesn't get you very far. I was interested in learning more about what challenges young adults were experiencing in the first year of the pandemic, but I knew I'd have to focus on a specific set of questions and a particular segment of the group. I designed an interview-based study of people aged eighteen to twenty-eight who were either college students or recent college graduates. Along with Isabelle Caraluzzi, a student of mine at New York University and the main research assistant for this book, we interviewed thirty-three people from three institutions in the New York metropolitan area: a public college known for its racial and ethnic diversity and accessibility; an affordable Jesuit college where roughly two thirds of the students are Latino or Black; and a highly selective, expensive, private university where undergraduate students identify as roughly 20 percent white, 20 percent Asian/Pacific Islander, 15 percent Latino, 10 percent Black, 25 percent international, and 10 percent "other."[4]

I make no claim that this sample represents the general population of young American adults, and of course it does not represent the entire generation at the global level. But it does allow us to learn about the experiences of college-educated young people in dramatically different situations, including those from poor families who relied on public assistance and those from wealthy families who faced no financial hardships; those with jobs and those who were unemployed; immigrants; Black, white, Latino, and Asian American people; residents of cities and suburbs; those who provided for their parents, those whose parents supported them, and those who are parents themselves.

The interviews were designed to elicit young adults' own accounts of their experiences in the pandemic, and to examine how they dealt with a series of challenges that were imposed or amplified by the crisis: Economic insecurity. Educational disruption. Managing social networks. Caring for others. Caring for the self. Coping with uncertainty. Dealing with stress and anxiety. Each interview began with an open-ended question about whether there was anything important that we should know about what happened to them, their family, and their core friend group. We then asked about whether they experienced changes or stresses in their living situation, family, school, work, social life, romantic life, and personal health. We asked about whether the pandemic had altered their views about careers, education, relationships, and politics. We asked whether and how they had altered their daily routines and practices to protect themselves, their family members, and people in their social circle from COVID-19 and related dangers. We ended by asking if there was anything important that we missed.

In our interviews, we learned that the COVID-19 pandemic disrupted some important developmental processes for highly educated young adults, delaying transitions to graduate school, cutting them off from important work experiences, forcing returns to the parental home. But we also discovered that the pandemic sped up their march toward adulthood. The people we spoke with told us that, during the pandemic, they sacrificed their social lives and pruned their social networks to protect their older relatives, felt added pressure to put food on the table or rent money in the bank account, decided to stand up for their values and beliefs, learned who they are and what they want to become. Although it's unclear whether the changes they made during the plague year will hasten, stall, or reverse their track to conventional benchmarks of adulthood such as marriage or a career, the young adults we interviewed consistently reported that they had aged and matured in 2020. In fact, a recurring theme in our conversations was that, as Luis put it, "I grew up like ten years in the pandemic." So much happened while no one did anything and time stood still. Inevitably, young adults came out in a different place.

Some were laid off. Some felt the cushion of parental support ripped out from under them suddenly, and quickly took on the responsibility of supporting their parents instead. Some who began 2020 without any dire financial pressures found themselves wondering how they would pay for rent and food. Jobs disappeared. The specter of student debt loomed larger than ever. Protests felt necessary and urgent. Career paths that looked open seemed unreachable. For most of the young adults we interviewed, the pandemic induced a deep sense of economic and personal anxiety, consistent with what young adults have felt in previous recessions.[5] The feeling was well founded: according to the Pew Research Center, at the beginning of 2020, roughly 12 percent of Americans aged sixteen to twenty-four reported being "disconnected"—neither enrolled in school or employed— about the same rate as in previous years. By April, the number had spiked to 20 percent, and by June it was 28 percent, translating to more than 10 million "disconnected" Americans between ages sixteen and twenty-four.[6] Disconnected or not, for nearly everyone, the pandemic sparked a reckoning about the things they wanted and needed, and a rethinking of the kind of future they would have.

Angelica, a twenty-one-year-old Latina student, had a job as a paralegal before the pandemic hit, and she used her income to pay for things like clothes and nights out at restaurants and bars. She lost her position, and the promise of a full-time job in the firm after graduation, soon after the economy contracted in March of 2020. It was painful and challenging, as was her decision, a few weeks later, to file for unemployment. Going on welfare just didn't seem like the kind of thing she would ever do. The experience made Angelica realize how important financial stability was to her sense of identity. As an economics major, she felt some shame at not being "economically independent." By summer, Angelica had found a new job, but she told us that she no longer feels entitled to "the luxury" of spending money on things like drinking with friends. The shock of insecurity she experienced led her to invest in her future. She paid down her maxed-out credit card, chipped away at her student loans, and made sure she sent in her rent check on time. "My name is on this lease," she explained, "and I have to pay my bills." She also got fixated on improving her credit score, using the number as a marker of her accomplishment, a sign and symbol that she was back on her feet. "It's so funny, being a finance and economics major and finally understanding the value of a dollar in my last year because of a personal experience through COVID," she remarked. She viewed the crisis as a hard but important life lesson, one that would ultimately take her to a better place.

Not everyone retained that confidence. Keisha, a twenty-four-year-old Black woman who lives with her mother, stepfather, and younger sister in Brooklyn, was studying for an associate's degree and working full-time as a sales representative for a fashionable athletic company before the pandemic hit. "I've always wanted a job," she told us. "My mom told me to just focus on school, but from the time I was seventeen, I wanted to start working and get my own actual money." Partly, Keisha said, she felt compelled to help her mother, who was also enrolled in college while working full-time and raising a family. "But I was young at the time," Keisha recalled. "I kind of took advantage of it. I wanted to buy shoes and clothes." The job, which required her to work on the floor of a well-known shoe store, came with lots of perks and benefits. Free outfits. New shoes every few months. Trips to the corporate headquarters. Advanced knowledge of what was coming in a high-status industry, one she and her friends dreamed about. The sense that she was making it. Being part of a team. After a few years, Keisha began to share a little more of her income with her mother, covering part of the rent and the occasional food bill. "That's a pretty good feeling," she explained. "Yeah, I started feeling really good. And I was like: Yes, this is what I want to be doing. This is what I want to do."

In January 2020, Keisha lost her job in a wave of corporate lay-offs. Stores everywhere were struggling to compete with internet vendors. She'd heard rumors of cutbacks, but she wasn't expecting it to come for her. At first, Keisha didn't worry much about her situation. She felt confident about her work experience and her prospects in the labor market. Also, she had been thinking about different ways to work in the industry. What if, instead of selling shoes, she became a journalist and covered the industry? She had already been writing for websites, and she knew there were col-lege journalism programs nearby. In February, Keisha registered with a job search site and started submitting applications.

Around that time, the coronavirus arrived in America—first far away, then in New York City. Initially, political officials encouraged everyone to go about their business. The mayor called for residents and tourists to eat out in restaurants, see shows on Broadway, support their local bar. By mid-March, it was clear that the strategy had backfired. The virus was spreading exponentially. Local leaders reversed course, closing schools and all nonessential businesses. Keisha found herself among hundreds of thousands of New Yorkers who had lost a job in the retail and service industries and were looking for new positions. The econ-omy was in free fall. Suddenly, Keisha was, too.

Unemployment was not her only problem. Keisha's grand-parents, who had fled New York to be closer to their parents in South Carolina, had unknowingly contracted COVID-19. Instead of escaping the virus, they wound up carrying it with them. Soon Keisha's great-grandmother had it. Days later, she was dead. The family was traumatized and guilt-ridden, and there was no funeral, no convening, no songs or prayers to salve their wounds. Instead, everyone was cooped up indoors, listening to the ambulance sirens, wondering when and how the dying would end. In April, Keisha's stepfather, a firefighter who had continued working, came down with COVID. Fortunately, his symptoms were mild. Then Keisha caught it. "I was sick for like, three or four days," she recalled. "Oh my God. I couldn't move, like, I just felt weird. And then the next couple days I couldn't smell and taste anything." After she recovered, her mother's turn came. She was fatigued, feverish, and bedridden. Keisha, like so many women during the pandemic, had no choice but to take on more domestic work.[7]

We interviewed Keisha in early 2021, and she still had not found a full-time job. Sales jobs in the athletic shoe business remained scarce. Jobs in media were even more competitive, and the college journalism program she wanted to take rejected her application for a scholarship. Instead, Keisha took a part-time position at a shoe shop in Times Square, and an internship at a website covering the industry. "I feel like now I have to work my way up versus I was already kind of up there," she explained. "I'm moving way slower. It's a different pace for me." If, in some ways, the losses were painful, in other ways Keisha found them productive. "Now that I lost my job, I've started looking at the bigger picture. I want to go back to school. I want to apply to jobs, start my career. I want to fast-track it." The question was whether, or when, the opportunities would come back.

The coronavirus arrived in New York City just as local universities were beginning the winter semester; by March, most schools had shut down their campuses, temporarily suspended classes, and switched to remote education. For college students, the disruption was both sharp and long-lasting, and the consequences included mental health problems, food and housing insecurity, and problems keeping up with schoolwork.[8] At first, the shift required adjusting to a new way of learning: distanced, digital, impersonal, and individual. There were no more office hours with professors, no more study sessions in libraries or dorms; no impromptu get-togethers after class discussions or debates at cafeterias and coffee shops. Some students had to leave the city and move in with their parents. Some never made the transition to remote education; they stopped "attending" or missed assignments and wound up failing classes they otherwise would have aced. Others simply lost interest and motivation. Subjects that had always fascinated them seemed irrelevant as the pandemic set in and their social worlds collapsed. Their performance slipped. When the semester concluded, a second set of problems emerged, and these had more durable significance. Was college really worth it? Should they drop out and help support their family instead? Did they really need to go to graduate school? Should they change their course of study? Do something to increase their odds of financial success?

It's not surprising to learn that the pandemic disrupted, altered, and, in some cases, prematurely terminated the educational paths of young adults.[9] Crises, including economic recessions, climate disasters, and infectious disease outbreaks, typically inflict damage on young adults and students, with more impoverished people suffering disproportionally. "The COVID-19 pandemic created the largest disruption of education systems in human history, affecting nearly 1.6 billion learners in more than 200 countries," write Sumitra Pokhrel and Roshan Chhetri.[10] Young adults in the U.S. higher education system faced a specific set of challenges, including the steep cost of tuition, the burden of substantial student debt, and the expectation of graduating into a tight labor market without a strong safety net.[11] According to U.S. Census surveys, between 7.7 million and 10 million Americans "canceled plans to take post-secondary classes last fall because of financial constraints related to the pandemic," while another survey reported that the number of high school graduates who went immediately to college dropped 7 percent.[12]

Antonio, a twenty-one-year-old psychology student at the expensive private university, lived with his family in Corona, Queens, one of the first hot spots for COVID-19 cases and deaths. Being there was traumatic, Antonio told us. Ambulances were everywhere, and their sirens blared around the clock, each shrill sound giving notice that a neighbor would soon be dead. He worried about his parents, albeit for different reasons. "My mother worked as a house cleaner," he explained. "But she was laid off because her patron didn't want to risk transmitting the virus." Her unemployment was a cause for concern, as was his father's job. "My dad works as a butcher and he never stopped working. I was nervous because he's immunocompromised and he's old. There was always anxiety that something would happen."

As cases mounted, Antonio experienced a loss of control. He stayed at home as much as possible, only going out to walk the dog. He felt lucky for being able to keep his job as a research assistant in a university laboratory, but paralyzing guilt for not being able to meet deadlines or fulfill his required hours. He went to his online classes, but failed to meet his own high standards. "I was feeling really unmotivated," Antonio recalled. Before the pandemic, he was gearing up for graduate school applications, feeling passionate about a career doing academic research. In late 2020, he told us that "I actually don't remember what classes I took last semester. Everything is a blur." He had put off registering for the next semester, too. With everything virtual, he worried that "I won't be able to try my best, that I won't be able to retain a lot of the information. I'm scared."

Antonio still gets nervous when he talks about his education. He spoke quickly, almost frenetically, when our interview touched upon school issues. His anxiety was palpable, as was his disappointment at opportunities lost. He had planned to study abroad, which is one of the perks of his university. COVID killed the option. He had hoped to develop close relationships with professors in the laboratory, relationships that could help him get into graduate school. That possibility was disappearing, too. The coronavirus hadn't gotten to him, but Antonio knew that his mental health was a problem. "The pandemic has made me really burned out," he acknowledged. "I just want to take a really long nap all the time. I feel that I'm doing something wrong, like I'm not doing my best in a way."

As a psychology major, Antonio has his own theories of why he's suffering. "I didn't have an outlet for all of the trauma that I went through. I internalized everything. So everything that I should have been feeling, I just felt inside and I felt like shit." But his self-diagnosis has not yet produced a remedy. Once a careful curator of his academic experience, he remains too unsettled to plan his next semester. Once assured enough to lead the student psychology club, he's now worried that he doesn't know enough to go to graduate school. Once eager to travel, he's now afraid that if he leaves home, he will forget what he has learned in college. In our interview, Antonio shared the way his anxiety spirals: "I wish I could take a gap year! But I have a scholarship. So even if I wanted to take a gap year, I'm scared that I would lose my financial assistance. My entire family is low-income. Losing that scholarship would mean that I lose my ability to attend [college]. That might have just been anxiety talking, but it was always there. I have to go to school and at least push through, because if not I lose the scholarship and I lose all of the finances, and I guess I lose my degree. I can't really do that. So even if I wanted to, I can't."

Fear, disorientation, and self-doubt were common themes in our conversations about young adults' educational ambitions. Shanice, a twenty-five-year-old public university graduate, told us that she had lost her sense of direction in the pandemic. "I don't know what I want to do anymore," she acknowledged. "I met with a career adviser and they asked what I was interested in. I went blank. I told my therapist, she asked me what I was interested in, I went blank. Before this whole pandemic happened, I had an answer for that. I don't even know anymore, I really don't know. Because everything looks so uncertain now, we don't even know how things are going to be by next year, or even the next few months. . . . I feel like I'm just wandering."

Craig, a twenty-three-year-old private university graduate, told us that he had elaborate plans and aspirations before the pandemic started. "I'm, like, a theater dude. I like to be in plays and make them, and that's just been wiped off the face of the earth for the foreseeable future." He got a job at "one of those Instagram museums" so that he could make ends meet. "I've basically given up on any kind of planning for the future," he acknowledged. "I'm, like, what's the point? Ambitions are just dangerous right now. I don't even know that the world's going to be here!" What Craig would really like to do, he says, is to take things a little less seriously and have some fun. Getting a van, traveling around, and busking for money. "That's the dream!"

Some of the young adults we interviewed had the opposite reaction to the pandemic. Instead of losing focus, they sharpened their vision for the future and committed to a new project. Diane, a twenty-two-year-old, had planned to take a year off from school after graduation. She had always wanted to move to the Great Barrier Reef, work in ecotourism, and indulge her interest in marine life. Now she is determined to get a job and apply to graduate school as soon as possible. Cindy, who's twenty-five, made the same decision. She took advantage of the lockdown to cram for the LSAT and did better than she had hoped or expected. When we interviewed her, Cindy told us that she will soon move to Chicago, where she got a generous scholarship to law school. Cindy was done with insecurity, and eager to establish stronger footing. If that meant locking into something a bit earlier than she had anticipated, so be it. The important thing was to take care of herself.

Many young adults got politicized. Some grew furious about the Trump administration's bungled response to COVID; others became enraged about school closures, lockdowns, and threats to their liberty. They joined mutual aid networks, like Nuala's, to help support neighbors. They rallied outside of small businesses, like Daniel Presti's bar, Mac's, calling for the government to reopen everything and let them live free, again. They poured into the streets to protest against police violence and racial inequality. They raised their voices in the workplace and the university, condemning bosses, colleagues, teachers—everyone who tolerated and upheld unjust and discriminatory systems. They lost faith in leaders, and searched for something else to believe in, another way to live.

Through all of this, they learned—about the forces that had shaped the world they inherited, about the reasons their country worked the way it did. "There's so much that they don't teach in schools," said Justine, who joined her first protest for racial justice during the summer of 2020. "And there's so much that I learned this past year. Like, I never would have known about these movements if the pandemic hadn't occurred. I'm grateful for that." After participating in BLM demonstrations, Luis told us that he had grown more aware of "systemic issues" around urban inequality, policing, and criminal justice that he had not recognized before the COVID crisis. "I don't want to toot my horn, but I feel like I've gotten smarter. Now, I'm kind of viewing a situation and actually understanding why this occurred, the origins of it." The challenge, he said, was figuring out how to effect change.

Active, dynamic, and, occasionally, experimental or boundary-crossing social relationships are key features of what social scientists call the "extended adolescence" stage of character development. During ordinary times, most young American adults enjoy an open, freewheeling, permissive cultural environment, one that encourages and rewards the formation of social ties. The psychologist Jeffrey Arnett emphasizes the optimism and emergent sense of possibility that people in their twenties often feel during this period.[13] The sociologist Michael Rosenfeld claims that young people use this life stage to build up their personal and professional networks, setting up support systems and friendship groups that will nourish them even if they put off marriage.[14]

The compression of social life was not only imposed from above; young adults also constrained and protected themselves on their own volition, albeit in different ways, with varying levels of intensity, conservatism, and concern. This variation generated significant stress and conflict. Young adults who had always been relatively carefree in their social lives quickly became circumspect and judgmental. Some found themselves critically assessing which of their friends were "COVID safe" and which were reckless, making decisions about who to hang out with, confide in, or cut off based on whether they wore a mask, went to parties, or kept distant. Some became angry and disappointed by friends who violated health guidelines, or at those who followed the rules too closely, or at those who just didn't seem to be paying attention. Others discovered that they were now outcasts, sanctioned and estranged from friends who deemed them irresponsible or untrustworthy where COVID was concerned.

Anxieties about contracting and transmitting the coronavirus led the young adults we interviewed to engage in a process I call "social pruning," whereby they cut ties with some friends and strengthened bonds with others, reconfiguring their networks to protect themselves and their families.

The young adults we interviewed reported that when the shutdowns began the main site of their social activities quickly moved online. They grew even more tethered to their phones and social media platforms, more caught up in the cyclone of digital drama—He said what? Is she at a party? Am I the only one staying home?—that, inevitably, got under their skin. Some young people moved to states where the economy and social life remained more open, places like Florida and Texas. Those who stayed in New York City felt the door slam on their physical existence, their worlds reduced to small, suffocating apartments. Instead of basing friendships on the things they did together, they bonded by sharing sacrifices. The fun part of being young and in the city was gone. In the summer, when the lockdown eased, young adults found themselves scrutinizing each other's activities and searching for a comfort zone. A Snapchat story of a backyard barbecue, an Instagram post of a trip to Mexico (or even just over the bridge to Manhattan), or an invitation to participate in any of the above—these were suddenly shocking proof of *something*, although it was hard to pin down exactly what. Everyone's behavior was loaded with new significance: wearing masks, attending parties, taking risky jobs, or eating indoors became emblems of politics and personal values. Everyone became a judge.

Jamie, a twenty-five-year-old actor, thought of these divisions in concrete terms. "I definitely have categories of friends now that I didn't have before," he explained. "Most of my close friends are [behaving] how I am behaving, trying to be a 'good person' I guess. . . . I have a category of friends that are behaving mostly good but some of them do some things that I don't agree with . . . and I'm not the type of person who will forget that. And then I have a category of friends that I might never hang out with again because they behaved so poorly in my view. With a lot of those people, I was drifting apart from them anyway."

Some felt that they had new appreciation for the relationships they already had, like with their family or partners. Others shared that they now choose their friends more carefully, and let go of some connections that no longer feel genuine or necessary. More, still, had trouble understanding the new chasms that separated them from friends, partners, or family members. Some explained the sudden disconnect as a mismatch of values, such as whether to put one's community or personal life first. Jamie described it as a "willful ignorance" that shone a light on people's personal values "in more ways than just COVID." Others simply chalked it up to selfishness or stupidity. Whatever it was, these differences felt real enough to divide and define relationships. A few people reported that their oldest and closest friendships were the ones that changed most drastically, or even fell apart.

When the pandemic hit, Cindy's social life did a U-turn. She was twenty-four, going to school in Manhattan, playing on a sports team, attending study groups in the library, and meeting up with friends whenever she had a spare moment. "I was very much living for New York City. Interacting with strangers, being on the subway, [enjoying] random stuff like people holding the door for each other," she explained. Everything changed in February, when she flew back from Italy on a packed plane after receiving, on that same day, a notification that the coronavirus had been detected outside of China. She got sick soon after she returned. Really sick. Cindy spent the first two weeks of the new semester in bed with a fever and a cough so bad it scared her. "You know when you're sick when you're like, six or something and you think you're gonna die?" she asked. "It was that kind of sick." Looking back, she's positive that she had COVID-19. But at the time there were no tests available, and no one knew how to diagnose the disease. At urgent care, the doctor told Cindy she needed sleep and Tylenol. But she was so winded that she couldn't get down the stairs to let her dog outside. She had groceries left outside her apartment, and hired someone to come walk her dog. By the time Cindy recovered, she only had a few days in class before her school announced that they would be going remote for the next few weeks. They never went back. By mid-March Cindy had moved out of her apartment in the city and into her childhood bedroom upstate. She missed the energy of her daily life, the company of classmates and friends. "It was a no-end-in-sight kind of feeling," she recalled. "I felt like my life was wasting away. I was like, I want to see my friends, I want to do things, I want to work!"

At first, she felt lucky that two of her oldest friends lived just down the street, having moved back into their parents' homes as well. They would go for walks every day, letting their dogs play in the grass by the middle school they'd all attended. It felt safe since they were only at home with their families. But as spring turned to summer and her friends started feeling more lenient about socializing, Cindy's feeling of security dissipated. She started skipping their daily walks and turning down invitations to meet for dinner. She felt a pit in her stomach when she saw their social media. "One girl posted a video from this party with her boyfriend and her huge family. They were all dancing and barbecuing and stuff. It was the beginning of May and it was still so scary. It was like, we're going into the grocery store in staggered lines and you want to go to a party like this?"

Eventually, Cindy confronted them. "There was definitely a minor rift in our friendship when I told them I didn't want to see them anymore because they were being reckless," she reported. One of her friends didn't speak to her for a month. Cindy felt like she was doing the right thing, but it was hard to know that it meant growing apart from her good friends. She expressed a feeling that was common among the young adults we interviewed, a fear that avoiding people and social gatherings made them uncool or just different from others their age. "I was the weenie that wouldn't hang out and risk my dad's life by going to a pool party or something," she said. "It definitely made me feel like a weirdo. Like a super-cautious, why-are-you-being-so-dramatic kind of weirdo." But what felt even worse to Cindy was the growing suspicion that her friends might not be who she thought they were. "I definitely got the 'ick,'" she explained. "They were being irresponsible and I was like, we've been friends for twenty years, why are you acting like this? How could you be so irresponsible?" Inevitably, Cindy and her two friends severed ties.

With social pruning, we learned, some bonds grew stronger. Successful relationships provided protections that were otherwise hard to come by: comfort, understanding, support. Young adults consistently told us that the pandemic made them want fewer but closer friends and companions, connections with people who will stand by them and stick around. Fortunately for Cindy, another old friend, Sarah, had also moved back home for the pandemic, and the two of them had the same ideas about how to stay safe. When Cindy stopped seeing her two neighbors, she and Sarah got even closer, bonding during their masked, and slightly distanced, nightly walks. "Sarah's been my best friend since I was like, five, so if she had differed from me on this thing, I might think differently about her," Cindy confessed. Instead, they became more intimate than ever. "We were the weirdos that refused to go do anything."

A few months later, when the other two girls called them to apologize for their arrogance, admitting that they had both tested positive for COVID and passed it on to their families (none of whom had serious symptoms), Cindy and Sarah responded sympathetically. Privately, though, they felt a little vindicated. "I wasn't going to say 'I told you so,'" Cindy said, "but in the end they knew I was right."

When we spoke to Cindy, in February of 2021, she wasn't sure if she would rebuild the friendships she had lost in the pandemic, if her network would ever be as complete. Many young adults we interviewed reported feeling a deep sense of social loss from the pandemic, and a related anxiety that their friends, their community, may not come back. "Some people I was really close with and now I don't know what it's gonna look like going forward," Jamie, the twenty-five-year-old actor, wondered. "Like, will they come to my wedding? I don't know. It's stuff like that that makes me sad for sure." Craig, the twenty-three-year-old "theater dude," used to thrive on the collective, creative energy in his school arts scene. He and his friends would gravitate to university lounges or hit the park nearby to brainstorm ideas for plays or TV pilots. But now, he says, it's all moved online to Twitter, "which sucks and I hate it!" Craig misses the excitement of being with them, of never knowing who would show up, what they would come up with, what could happen in a space full of people with ideas and energy and life. "I don't feel like I've lost all my friends, but any semblance of community that I had, I don't really feel that anymore," he said. "That's sad, you know?"

Cindy had similar feelings. She told us that the only reason she met her best friend in college is that every day, the first thing she would do in class was ask Cindy if she could borrow a pen. It quickly became a running joke between them. But one day, Cindy got to class and found a new box of pens waiting on her desk. The two burst out laughing, and they've been close ever since. It's the surprising and small interactions like this that Cindy misses, and she's worried that they'll be hard to revive when the pandemic ends.

. . .

Yasmina, a twenty-one-year-old at a Jesuit college, told us that she's done with fleeting friendships, and is focusing on the people in her life whose ambitions, interests, and goals align with hers. "I kind of see who's in my life permanently, and I see who is in my life temporarily. . . . I find it a lot harder to maintain more of those surface-level connections with people." Leticia, also a twenty-one-year-old at the Jesuit college, said, "I'm more picky with who I relate to. I started to hang out only with specific people that were my really close friends. I try to avoid socializing with people that are not going to form long-lasting relationships with me." Both Yasmina and Leticia are spending more time with their romantic partners. Yasmina believes that going through the pandemic together made her relationship stronger. It was their hardest year ever, she said, but they survived. For Leticia, her close bond with her boyfriend, whom she had been casually seeing before the pandemic, is in part a result of the months where they were unable to do anything other than text and video call. "I liked the fact that we were just talking for like three months," she said. When they finally were able to go on actual dates ("mostly getting takeout and sitting in his car!"), she was comforted knowing they had cultivated trust and friendship first. "We were just there for each other," Leticia said. "That's all I needed."

In many cases, young people's need for intimacy in the pandemic intensified and accelerated their relationships. Some couples made big leaps at the outset of the crisis, deciding to quarantine together even though they had never cohabitated. Others jumped into a serious relationship during the peak pandemic months. Although online dating remained popular during the lockdown, surveys showed that levels of casual sex and hooking up declined.[15] Instead, young adults said they wound up reconnecting with people they had casually dated but not given much thought to before the lockdowns, and some rekindled romances that they thought had flamed out. A random Facebook message or Instagram DM from a mutual friend or a former hookup which they might otherwise have ignored was suddenly an opportunity for excitement, and possibly more. Cindy's now-boyfriend "slid into" her Instagram DMs after waiting five years for his shot. He had tried, unsuccessfully, to ask her out during their freshman year of college when they lived in the same dorm. She never thought twice about him. "As far as the pandemic goes, he got lucky with this one because I don't know if otherwise I would have been like, yeah sure I'll drive two hours to see you in my old college town and eat takeout in your living room by ourselves."

Dating during the pandemic required new decisions and compromises: young adults awkwardly discussed the date of their last negative test, the last person they had "hung out" with, whether they had socialized in indoor settings, wore a mask. Before the pandemic, most of them had lived in a dating world where casual encounters are widely accepted and culturally emphasized, where you never really know if someone you're dating is dating someone else, too. Now everything requires full disclosure and careful negotiation. Or at least that's what people want from a potential companion; what they have actually done, one never knows.

Radical uncertainty, the impossibility of knowing or understanding foundational issues about how to stay safe or sustain relationships or predict what school or work or your hometown would look like in the future, addled the minds of the young adults we interviewed. Few felt settled before the pandemic, but they could predict which career paths were open and reachable, what kind of financial support or debt they would carry, the horizon for their next phase of development if not beyond. They struggled with acute shocks: the sudden surge in COVID deaths, the quarantines and lockdowns, the recession, the moves back into childhood homes. But they also felt an underlying dread of long-lasting crises in personal, political, and economic life. All that was solid really had melted into air. Stress, anxiety, depression suffused their environment. As several studies have established, mental health problems during the pandemic were higher among young adults than any other group.[16] Our interviews help uncover what those problems felt like, and how young people managed them as they struggled to get by.

Craig, the twenty-three-year-old who now dreams of busking his way across the country, was a few weeks away from graduation when his college went remote. He packed his things and flew home to his family's house in Southern California without knowing whether or when he would return. At first, his childhood home seemed like an oasis. The virus was scarce in California. The weather was good. There was so much more space. But he wasn't prepared to walk into a household haunted by childhood grudges, lingering resentments, and emotional trip wires. "The whole thing turned into this pressure cooker," Craig told us. His stepbrother had always struggled with mental health issues. The confinement and anxiety sent him into a tailspin. "[It] erupted into this nightmare," Craig told us. His stepbrother began threatening violence, toward himself and toward other people in the family. Craig felt like he needed to protect himself. He found another place to live, stayed mostly indoors, did everything he could to avoid other people, and more to avoid his own inner fears. "I sort of emotionally just shut down, and I have been ever since."

Escaping himself proved more difficult than Craig anticipated. For three months straight, he found himself wondering: "Is this the end of everything? Are we ever going to have a future? Is anyone going to accomplish anything they ever wanted to accomplish? Is all of that over? I don't know what's going to happen, and I'm numb to everything at this point," he acknowledged. Desperate for relief, Craig made it back to New York during the summer, beckoned by a steep drop in the rental market and an invitation from a college friend. It felt good to be there, but he fretted over conflicts that were popping up across the U.S. at the time, from the police attacks on Black Lives Matter activists to the armed protests over mask mandates. "Jesus Christ, it will shake your faith in people," Craig said. "Seeing the anti-mask thing going around, it's so disturbing." Now, he said, "I value stability less than I ever did. It's something that I no longer really expect or necessarily want, feeling stable and like I know what's going to happen."

Gabriella, on the other hand, was tired of the instability. When the pandemic hit, she was twenty-four and six months pregnant, taking six classes at a large public college in Brooklyn and working thirty hours a week at a pharmacy. Before COVID, Gabriella knew what her life was supposed to look like. She and her husband had settled into a Brooklyn apartment; she was about to finish her degree in early childhood education, and she felt prepared for motherhood. "When everything shut down and became chaotic, it was traumatizing and scary. I didn't know what to feel or what was the right thing to do." The pharmacy told her she was an essential worker but couldn't get her a face mask. Her husband, a police officer, was even more exposed. Every day, Gabriella left her house feeling scared of what the virus could do to her or to her unborn daughter. When she was eight months pregnant, Gabriella's boss allowed her to stay home and rest. Instead, she drove upstate to help care for her parents and her grandmother, all of whom had tested positive for COVID. Gabriella and her ten-year-old sister, who had no symptoms, quarantined in a small rental apartment with little to no cell reception or internet. Within days, both of them had caught the virus, too.

Luckily, no one in the family got dangerously sick, but that didn't stop Gabriella from developing anxiety. "I felt like my body was shutting down on me. I had to just sit down and take a breath." Her baby's arrival was magical. Naturally, it also ushered in a new wave of stress and fear. Back home, in Brooklyn, she had an infant and the weight of the world on her shoulders. She had planned on sleeplessness, changing diapers, and feeding, but not on quarantines, physical distancing, and sanitizing, or on feeling scared of all the places where she had become a regular, including the pharmacy and the grocery store. Worse, Gabriella told us, she grew afraid of her own stress and anxiety, because she knew it was bad for the baby, and bad for herself. She couldn't wait for her daughter to be able to play with other kids someday. There's a great playground nearby, a park, good schools. She hoped they would become safe again, that soon the children in her neighborhood wouldn't have to wear a mask.

Priya, who wore a mask everywhere, had always felt the burden of responsibility. She lives with her parents, both taxi drivers, her brother, and her cousins on the border of Long Island and Queens. There is a gendered division of domestic labor in her

family, and, as in most American families before and during the
pandemic, the women take on the lion's share of the burden.[17]
Everyone in the apartment works long hours, and Priya, a few
weeks from graduation at the public university in March 2020,
told us that she had been doing most of the family's cooking and
cleaning since she was eleven. "I had to take on a lot of responsibilities that were unfair for my age, but I had no other choice."
She took pride in her work ethic and her accomplishments. She
was an editor at the campus paper, an intern, a success in every
way. "I had my life together," Priya said. "Then this happened."

Although her parents kept driving their taxis, Priya couldn't
help feeling that preserving their health was her responsibility. It
was as if their roles changed, and suddenly she was the parent.
"It was just so anxiety-inducing. I felt like I was the person that if
somebody got sick, it was my fault," she told us. "One wrong mistake on my part and my parents could get sick and never recover."
She was constantly imploring them to wear their masks, wash their
hands longer, get tested when they could. "I had to walk behind
them like they were toddlers sometimes." At school, her workload
somehow intensified. At one point, she was doing a big research
paper on the juvenile justice system and she suddenly felt like the
ceiling would collapse. "I sat down at the dining room table to
write my paper, and I just started crying. I was like, this is just so
much. I'm the youngest person in the house, I shouldn't be the
one having to take care of everybody." But there was no escape.

Priya worried that this feeling might never go away, that
the mental toll it's taken will damage her permanently. "I've
already started to block out some of the memories. There were
way too many times when I was just so hopeless, points of like,
true despair, where I was like, this is never going to end and I
don't know what's going to happen. Will anything get better ever
again?" Priya couldn't help but feel a sense of unfairness. She had
done so much to prepare for her future, diligently cultivating a
life path. Now it was blocked, as was her understanding of who
she was and what would happen next. "I'm very much a planner,"
she told us. "It makes me anxious not to be able to see into the
future. It terrifies me, knowing that I may leave college and not
know what to do."

Previous crises, including wars, economic depressions, and epidemics, have had a powerful impact on the development of those who survived them, particularly young adults and adolescents.[18] It is too early to predict how the COVID-19 pandemic will shape today's young adults. We do not yet know how long the disease will circulate and mutate, how many more people will get critically ill or die, whether and how different industries, cities, nations, and societies will bounce back. But there is no question that young adults who lived through it endured exceptionally high levels of stress and anxiety, and that their experiences will have a lasting impact on their development.

We already have good research on the factors that made some young adults suffer more acutely during the pandemic, and hints at what made others more resilient. One particularly informative study, conducted by psychologists in Europe, draws on research from a twenty-year cohort study of young people who participated in several waves of assessments, one every few years, from 2004 through the first year of the COVID crisis.[19] "The largest risk factor for emotional distress during COVID-19 was previous emotional distress," the authors found. Social stressors that young adults experienced before the pandemic, such as being bullied or feeling excluded, made people more susceptible to trauma from the new disruptions. So, too, did economic distress that some—but not all—young people endured. "Economic downturn changes young adults' future outlook," they write, "including their visions and hopes for their professional and economic futures." Migrants, who were more likely to be separated from family during the pandemic, faced higher risks of emotional distress; women did also, likely because of more exposure to stressors during childhood. For American observers, the main limitation of this study is that the subjects were far less likely to experience severe COVID or the death of a family member than people in the U.S., for the simple reason that the U.S., by comparative standards, had so much trouble controlling the disease.

In crucial ways, the pandemic stalled young adults on their paths toward adulthood. It disrupted, delayed, and in some cases terminated their formal educations. It lowered their likelihood of getting married and having children. It stalled their careers. It's remarkable, how frequently the young adults we interviewed insisted that the pandemic had forced them to grow up quickly—a cost whose significance is hard to measure, but whose impact is surely profound. "When this started, I was young and rambunctious," Cindy recounted. "I was running around New York City and doing all the things I wanted. Now I wake up and I eat my granola, I read my book, and I'm like, all right, what's on the news today? I feel like an old person, just wasting away in my house." Keisha's experience was similar. "A lot of time has passed," she remarked. "Before this whole thing started, I was just carefree. I feel like I'm getting older—mentally older, more mature." Keisha also felt that the plague year had taken a toll on her body. "I'm twenty-four, but my back is eighty years old!" Natalie, who spent much of the pandemic taking care of a sibling with a severe chronic illness, sounded a similar note. "I've always been mature," she told us. "But now I'm even more so. I always joke that I'm twenty-two going on forty." Justine, who's still in college, said, "That's it. You're not a teenager no more! You're not a kid no more—that's all my parents tell me. This is the real world. Now I really have to start growing up."

The emotional impact of this fast, forced transition to adulthood varied across the college-educated young people we interviewed. Some fixated on the things they lost: the carefree party culture, the casual and low-stakes relationships, the faith in institutions, the belief, now shattered, that their parents could support them, that political leaders could protect them, that other members of their society would look out for each other when their lives were on the line. "I have no faith in anything anymore, and that's sort of a nightmare," Craig said. "I've been feeling nihilistic. I don't know what to believe in." Many mourned the loss of freedom and independence. Moving back in with their parents or being separated from the social world felt like a step back from the self-reliance and self-knowledge they had been cultivating since they moved out. In ordinary times, college-educated young adults in America spend their twenties and some of their thirties in an "age of self-focus," a period of "in-between-ness" where they make decisions without parents or teachers as ringleaders, and without the accountability of having a child or a spouse.[20] The pandemic made them accountable to everyone, and forced them to take on responsibilities beyond their years.

We heard several variations on this idea that the pandemic has been a lesson in the nature of life's fundamental uncertainty, of how little is guaranteed. Several of the young adults we interviewed reported enduring an "identity crisis" during the initial plague year, in which they took stock of their pre-COVID ambitions and realized that they would likely be incompatible with the post-COVID world. The pandemic—along with climate change, threats to democracy, and attacks on long-taken-for-granted civil rights—made young adults worry that their future possibilities are dwindling, that their lives will be more turbulent than they had expected. Some expressed an unshakable fear that, when the pandemic is finally over, they will never get where they want to be.

Nearly every college-educated young adult we interviewed reported experiencing heartbreakingly painful and difficult problems during the pandemic: The deaths of friends and family members. Jobs terminated. Sacred rituals and pivotal events canceled. Relationships severed. Stress, anxiety, depression, and worse. But it was striking to hear so many young adults report feeling "lucky" or "fortunate." Before Craig narrated his path from optimism to nihilism, security to anxiety about the physical health of his family and his own mental health, we asked how he was doing. "I'm actually having a pretty good pandemic," was his immediate response.

In his study of the children of the Great Depression, Glen Elder Jr. found that Americans who grew up in the 1930s made similar comparative judgments to describe their experiences, reporting that, " 'Conditions were not as bad for us as they were for other families,' or 'They were worse,' or 'We were all in the same boat.' "[21] It's possible that sentiments like these stem from self-protective impulses that the sociologist Stanley Cohen called "states of denial," in his account of how individuals and societies deal with profound suffering.[22] But perhaps they come from something more humane and hopeful: an appreciation for one's own life and resilience during a historic period of death and devastation, a sense that, no matter how difficult today is, tomorrow they can find a better path.

CHAPTER 16

American Anomie

In May 2020, Hamlet Cruz-Gomez became a father. The timing wasn't perfect. Ideally, he would have spent the weeks before
his daughter's birth with his wife, Angelica, enjoying some quiet
moments of nesting, seeing close friends and family, and preparing
their home for the baby's arrival. But Cruz-Gomez, aged twenty-
five, was a radiological technician at Montefiore Hospital, in the
Bronx, which made him an essential worker. As the virus surged
through New York City, Cruz-Gomez dutifully commuted to the
hospital, and spent his days surrounded by death and disease. To
protect Angelica and the baby, he self-isolated, returning home
just in time to join them for the delivery. Despite the pandemic,
it was a joyous and hopeful time.[1]

On the afternoon of June 30, Cruz-Gomez drove his Honda
CR-V to Queens to do some grocery shopping for the family. The
timing could not have been worse. Around noon, Ramon Pena,
a thirty-seven-year-old from the Bronx, stole a box truck in the
Jamaica neighborhood, where its driver was making deliveries.
According to investigators, Pena began driving the truck at break-
neck speed, traveling up to fifty miles per hour on the busy city
streets. "A delivery truck matching the stolen vehicle's description was later seen striking in excess of 20 parked and moving
cars—some of them occupied and causing injuries—along Hum-

boldt and Metropolitan avenues in both Queens and Brooklyn," the District Attorney's Office reported. The truck ran through a series of red lights and shifted into the wrong side of the street, tearing through the city until it T-boned Cruz-Gomez's Honda as he pulled out of the Metro Mall parking lot, crashing into the driver's side of the vehicle. Pena jumped out of the truck and ran to a nearby subway station, where police apprehended him. Cruz-Gomez was transported to the Elmhurst General Hospital, where he went into cardiac arrest and died.[2]

Two days later, the Queens District Attorney's Office charged Pena with murder in the second degree, manslaughter in the second degree, assault in the first degree, felony assault in the second degree, grand larceny in the third degree, leaving the scene without reporting a death, and various traffic violations. If convicted of all charges, he faced twenty-five years to life in prison. "This kind of senseless mayhem is unacceptable and will not be tolerated in Queens County," said Melinda Katz, the DA.[3] Local officials promised to crack down.

Senseless mayhem was rising throughout New York City and across the United States during the late spring and summer of 2020—on roads and highways, parks and public plazas, even in the privacy of family homes. The social upheaval from the first wave of COVID—the generalized anxiety, the extended lockdowns, the school closures, the prohibition on gatherings, the contentious disputes over mask mandates, the incendiary feuds between two political blocs in a nation where the reds and the blues had come to see each other as mortal enemies—had sparked a surge of destructive behavior. It didn't happen immediately. Overall, crime in the U.S. went down between March and July 2020, but then things changed dramatically. The CDC reported a "record increase" in homicides during 2020. In the protests for Black Lives Matter, vandals shattered the glass storefronts of upscale commercial establishments throughout the country, creating a landscape of disorder and decay. Domestic violence spiked to alarming levels, as did alcohol and drug use, as well as lethal overdoses.[4] Gun sales soared.[5] Carjackings and hate crimes increased sharply.[6] Businesses selling essential medical supplies engaged in price gouging.[7] Cybercrime skyrocketed.[8] In America, reckless driving, resulting in a rash of fatal accidents like the one that killed Hamlet Cruz-Gomez, and, in more typical cases, the deaths of unlucky pedestrians, was particularly widespread.[9]

In the media, journalists often attributed this spike in destructive behavior to stress, alienation, anomie, and isolation, all of which unmoored Americans and left them in a disordered, dysregulated social world. "We're social beings, and our isolation is changing us," wrote Olga Khazan in *The Atlantic.* "The pandemic loosened ties between people: Kids stopped going to school; their parents stopped going to work; parishioners stopped going to church; people stopped gathering, in general. . . . In the past two years, we have stopped being social, and in many cases we have stopped being moral, too."[10] The problem with this argument is that nearly every nation experienced changes in social life that were similar to what happened in the U.S. during 2020. In most of Europe and Asia, the lockdowns and distancing mandates were far more severe than they were in America; stress and anxiety were high as well. Yet no European or Asian society saw rates of destructive behavior rise at anywhere near the American level. In fact, the reverse happened: most of them witnessed a remarkable decline in violent crime.

Consider, for instance, the most extreme expression of antisocial violence: homicide. In typical years, homicides rates are far higher in the U.S. than in Australia, Europe, and Asian nations—not because Americans commit more crimes (they don't), but because guns are so readily available.[11] That matters for understanding trends from year to year, because it takes a lot of additional murders to change the overall rate in the U.S., whereas in other places relatively small increases can make a big difference. This makes it all the more significant that, in the United States, the homicide rate spiked by 30 percent between 2019 and 2020, the highest single-year increase in more than a century.[12] By contrast, England and Wales experienced a 12 percent drop in homicides during the first pandemic year.[13] Australia's homicide rate fell by 3 percent, Taiwan's by 15 percent, and Hong Kong's by 9 percent.[14] In Canada, homicides went up by roughly 7 percent (partly attributable to twenty-two deaths in one mass-shooting incident).[15] In South Korea, the homicide rate stayed constant.[16]

It's tempting to say that America's extraordinary surge in homicides during 2020 is simply due to the prevalence of guns and the rise in gun sales. Guns, no doubt, are a big part of the story, but access to firearms can't explain why another form of violence, reckless driving, rose so much higher in the U.S. than in comparable nations. Despite a substantial drop in traffic deaths during the first months of the pandemic, America's rate of traffic fatalities rose by more than 7 percent in 2020, fueled by a wave of terrible crashes as the economy opened and drivers returned to the roads.[17] Nothing like this happened in Europe. In Great Britain, for instance, the Department of Transport reported a 17 percent drop in road deaths between 2019 and 2020, identical to the decline across nations in the European Union.[18] In South Korea, traffic accidents resulting in death or serious injury fell more than 10 percent, the most significant reduction since the government began keeping statistics.[19] Hong Kong's traffic fatalities fell 10 percent, too.[20] Canada experienced a more modest, 1 percent decrease in vehicular fatalities, but it did experience a 12 percent drop in serious injuries.[21] Australia, too, reported a small decline.[22]

When it comes to violent and antisocial behavior during the first year of the pandemic, America is truly exceptional. The question is why.

The answers involve both deep-seated and contingent factors. According to one school of thought, the nation's culture was formed through and durably shaped by violence. This is the core claim of the American Studies scholar Richard Slotkin, whose trilogy on myths of the frontier in the United States argues that anxieties about Indigenous people, whom colonial settlers sought to dominate and exterminate, became moral justifications for all kinds of brutality that have shaped American norms and institutions.[23] The social psychologist Richard Nisbett makes a similar argument about the legacy of slavery, particularly in the South and West of the U.S. Slavery, Nisbett explains, required white people to engage in—and legitimate—violent suppression of other human beings. The result, he claims, was the rise of a regional culture in which "violence is a natural and integral part."[24] Naturally, proponents of this view would suggest, the tendency toward brutality expressed itself in 2020, when the nation came under duress.

To the "culture of violence" argument, another, more prominent line of thinking insists the social disintegration that America experienced in 2020 is rooted in the nation's individualistic—if not hyper-individualistic—cultural values. Social distance and extreme individuation in the pandemic undercut solidarity, and, as the Wharton economist Marshall Meyer argues in an article about fatal car crashes on "Hobbesian highways," turned everyday life on America's roads into a war of "all against all."[25] There is, in fact, ample evidence that American culture is unusually individualistic. "In American culture, the ultimate source of action, meaning, and responsibility is the individual rather than the group," writes the U.C. Berkeley sociologist Claude Fischer. "Cross-national polling suggests that Americans are likelier than other Westerners to understand the world in terms of independent, self-reliant individuals" who are responsible for their own fate. For evidence, he points to the World Values Survey, which asks people "how much freedom of choice and control you feel you have over the way your life turns out." Americans, Fischer reports, "were far likelier, at 44 percent, to rate their freedom and control at 9 or 10 on the scale than were residents of any of 10 other large, industrial, Western democracies."[26] Materially, and even morally, Americans see themselves as on their own.

But not entirely. American individualism, as observers from Alexis de Tocqueville to Robert Bellah have pointed out, has always lived in tension with another powerful strain of national culture, voluntarism.[27] Americans are more likely than Europeans to join civic organizations and belong to religious congregations. They're more likely to get married and have children. They identify with and express strong commitments to their own social group.[28]

These "paradoxes of American individualism" (to use Fischer's term) make it difficult to predict how the U.S. will respond to any given stress or crisis. But even if America's orientation toward individualism were more straightforward, linking an underlying cultural tendency—be it violence or self-reliance—to specific pandemic conduct wouldn't be fully satisfying. Culture can predispose people to certain kinds of action, but the real challenge is to show why particular behaviors emerge at some times and places yet not others. In the case of the U.S., for instance, America's underlying proclivities for violence don't explain why homicides dropped so precipitously in the decades leading up to the pandemic. Nor does America's love of individualism account for the nation's occasional outpourings of collectivism and solidarity. Understanding the surge in violent, antisocial behavior during the pandemic requires identifying more proximate forces that shaped Americans' feelings and beliefs when the crisis started, the conditions that helped turn the outbreak of COVID into a massive upheaval, resulting in anomie.

Even without the pandemic, the United States was destined to experience a tumultuous 2020. That November, the country would hold one of the most important elections in the nation's history, and also one of the most contentious. Polarization was tearing at the social fabric. Democrats, increasingly, claimed that Republicans were undermining democratic norms and destroying democratic institutions, gaming the political system to promote their own party's power regardless of the civic price. Republicans, increasingly, believed that Democrats were against freedom, capitalism, and America itself. In a survey conducted by the Pew Research Center during September 2019, 75 percent of Democrats said they considered Republicans to be "closed minded," while roughly 70 percent of Republicans said they considered Democrats to be "unpatriotic" and "closed minded."[29] When, that December, the House of Representatives voted to impeach President Trump, the mutual disdain intensified. The Senate began its first impeachment trial in January 2020, and Republicans, who held the majority, quickly acquitted him. That left American voters to choose whether Trump would remain in office, when they went to polls in November. In the long campaign year that followed, people on both sides of the partisan divide came to believe that the republic itself was at risk.

The right, led by Trump's strongman approach to political power,[30] asserted its right to defend the country by any means necessary. Violence, in Trump's worldview, was legitimate if the occasion called for it, even if there was not a direct physical threat. From 2015, when Trump began his campaign for the 2016 election, through the pandemic, journalists documented scores of occasions when the president himself encouraged hate groups and the use of political violence to achieve his objectives.

At first Trump's calls for brutality were mainly directed at activists who disrupted his rallies. In 2015, Trump's security guards removed a Black man who yelled "Black lives matter" during his speech. "Maybe he should have been roughed up, because it was absolutely disgusting what he was doing," Trump declared. At an event in Iowa in 2016, Trump told the crowd about rumors that protesters might throw tomatoes at the stage. "If you see somebody getting ready to throw a tomato, knock the crap out of them, would you? Seriously. Just knock the hell out of them," he said. "I promise you, I will pay for the legal fees. I promise. There won't be so much of them because the courts agree with us." In Las Vegas, he called attention to a protester, saying, "I'd like to punch him in the face," before reminiscing about the time when violence was accepted. "We're not allowed to punch back anymore. I love the old days. You know what they used to do to guys like that when they were in a place like this? They'd be carried out on a stretcher, folks."[31] One month before the election, he was caught on camera bragging about committing sexual assault. "Grab 'em by the pussy," he advised the television personality Billy Bush in a discussion about how to treat attractive women. "You can do anything."[32]

These threats and incitements did more than pump up the crowd at Trump's rallies; they also gave rise to a significant increase in violent behavior. Epidemiologists discovered that cities where Trump held rallies experienced, on average, 2.3 additional assaults on the day of the event than on an ordinary day. The study, published in the journal *Epidemiology*, involved analyzing crime trends during campaign rallies organized by both Trump's and Hillary Clinton's campaigns. Clinton's rallies, the authors found, had no discernible effect on local crime rates. Trump's, however, consistently resulted in bloodshed.[33]

Once Trump took office, his advocacy of hate groups and

provocations of violence expanded into new domains. He repeatedly referred to mainstream journalists as peddlers of "fake news"
and accused them of being "enemies of the people." He called
for police to be more violent with suspects, gushing about the
times "when you see these towns and when you see these thugs
being thrown into the back of a paddy wagon, you just see them
thrown in, rough, I said, please don't be too nice. Like when you
guys put somebody in the car and you're protecting their head,
you know, the way you put their hand over, like, don't hit their
head and they've just killed somebody. Don't hit their head. I
said, you can take the hand away, okay?" Trump called for more
cruel treatment of undocumented immigrants, and instituted a
policy of forcibly separating children from their parents, a blatant
violation of human rights. After one of the participants in a white
supremacist rally in Charlottesville, Virginia, drove his car into a
crowd of protestors, killing Heather Heyer, a thirty-two-year-old
local woman, and injuring several others, Trump refused to cat-
egorically condemn the rally, and instead insisted that there were
"good people" marching, too.[34]

America has a long tradition of sustaining small militias, and
their right to bear arms is protected by the Constitution. But
Trump offered more praise and admiration for militant extremist groups than any president in modern U.S. history, despite the
fact that several federal agencies, including the FBI, the Department of Homeland Security, the Department of Justice, and the
Government Accountability Office, warned that white supremacist extremism and far-right groups posed—as a joint intelligence bulletin from the Federal Bureau of Investigation and the
Department of Homeland Security put it—a "persistent threat
of lethal violence."[35] The number of active hate groups soared to
record levels during the Trump presidency, the Southern Poverty
Law Center reports, peaking at more than one thousand in 2018
and remaining near "historic highs" through 2020.[36]

Although several major news media outlets condemned these
practices, conservative outlets, including the Fox News network
and a bevy of radio stations, podcasts, and websites, embraced
Trump's strongman approach. Moral outrage about the loss of

American greatness. Resentment of the "soft" political leaders whose policies weakened us, with footage of violent acts committed during progressive protests playing in the background. The promise to seize power and reassert control. Pundits and politicians mimicked Trump in substance and style, with frequent displays of masculinity and bravado. On social media, the pages of right-wing groups filled with chatter from people pledging to fight back against everyone who threatened them, whether migrants or minorities, environmentalists, democratic socialists, or just plain liberals. The left responded, albeit in far smaller numbers, with antifa organizing to combat white nationalists, fascists, and authoritarians when they marched on American streets.

At a moment when avoiding crisis required social cohesion and collective action, Americans got radicalized. Consider Daniel Presti's experience on Staten Island. The government asked him to sacrifice his small business in the name of public health, but instead of public funds and assistance, he got a cold shoulder and threats of punishment if he violated the rules. Presti felt abandoned by the state and society, an outcast, if not a stranger in his own land. It seemed like other people mattered, but not him or his family. He thought the social compact had been violated, and the more time he spent watching right-wing cable news channels and engaging with social media groups dedicated to whipping up outrage, the more certain he was about the need to fight back. It helped that so many other people living around him shared his worldview, and that activists as well as national political leaders—including the president—endorsed protests against governors, and in some cases, outright violence.

The pandemic created a new field of battle, and new sources of conflict as well. Predictably, Trump directed the first wave of blame and anger at China, with rhetoric that stirred up anti-Asian sentiment and, as human rights groups warned, helped spark a wave of racist violence. Next, the White House cast doubt on the scientific assessments of federal medical and public health leaders, questioning their claims about the danger of the new coronavirus and suggesting unproven, alternative pharmaceutical cures for the disease. During the first year of the pandemic, the Trump administration and its political allies came to advocate and model a distinctive approach: instead of coordinated collective action, Americans would largely be free to do as they pleased.

President Trump's April 3 initial statement about the CDC's mask guidelines was the most significant event in the evolution of this laissez-faire policy. By announcing the CDC's recommendation that Americans wear masks in public, and immediately saying, "I'm choosing not to do it," the president was encouraging each individual to decide what they would or would not do.[37] The principle applied to nearly everything in the pandemic: Whether to distance. What medications to use. Testing. Tracing. Ultimately, and perhaps most consequentially, whether to take a vaccine.

In states run by Democratic governors who imposed more stringent public health regulations, conservatives organized fierce campaigns against lockdowns and mask mandates. Right-wing groups rallied at statehouses and city halls across the country. Some protesters openly carried firearms, and occasionally things turned violent. In mid-April, the Michigan Freedom Fund, a conservative group partly funded by Secretary of Education Betsy DeVos, organized the first major anti-lockdown rally in America. They returned on April 30, when the state assembly voted to extend Michigan's state of emergency. "Dozens of men with assault rifles filled the rotunda and approached the barred doors of the legislature," *The New Yorker* reported. "Facing a police line, they bellowed, 'Let us in!'"[38]

Political leaders in other democratic societies took a different approach. In Australia, conservative prime minister Scott Morrison insisted that "there are no blue teams or red teams . . . there are no more unions or bosses. There are just Australians now, that's all that matters."[39] When Morrison implemented new social and economic restrictions in early April 2020, he spoke before Parliament and appealed to the nation's commitment to public health, the common good, and the shared fight against a common threat, not to each individual's right to do as they please.

> We are not a coerced society. We act through our agreement and our willful support of the national interest,

through our many institutions, including this Parliament and the many others around this country. And we will not surrender this. . . . Our sovereignty is demonstrated by the quality of life we afford Australians, with world class health, education, disability, aged care, and a social safety net that guarantees the essentials that Australians rely on. We will not surrender this. And above all, our sovereignty is sustained by what we believe as Australians, what we value, and hold most dear, our principles, our way of doing things. We will never surrender this. So make no mistake, today is not about ideologies. We checked those at the door. Today is about defending and protecting Australia's national sovereignty. It will be a fight. It will be a fight we will win. But it won't be a fight without cost, or without loss. Defending our sovereignty has always come at a great cost, regardless of what form that threat takes, and today will be no different. So today, we will agree to pay that price, through the important measures we will legislate today. But today, as a government, I want to commit to all Australians, as prime minister, that once we have overcome these threats, and we will, we will rebuild, and we will restore, whatever the battle ahead takes from us.[40]

Most Western leaders used similar rhetoric to promote social cohesion, mutual responsibility, and shared purpose during the first year of the pandemic. In a speech in late March, Canadian prime minister Justin Trudeau justified social restrictions as a way of protecting vulnerable citizens and essential workers: "If you choose to get together with people or go to crowded places, you're not just putting yourself at risk. You're putting others at risk, too. Your elderly relative who's in a senior home. Your friend with a preexisting condition. Our nurses and doctors on the frontlines. Our workers stocking shelves at a grocery store. They need you to make the right choices. They need you to do your part."[41] Even Boris Johnson, who initially advocated a more individualistic approach to the pandemic, adopted the language of common cause in battle after a surge of cases in the U.K.: "In this fight we can be in no doubt that each and every one of us is directly enlisted. Each and every one of us is now obliged to join together to halt the spread of this disease, to protect our NHS [National Health Service], and to save many, many thousands of lives. And I know that as they have in the past so many times, the people of this country will rise to that challenge. And we will come through it stronger than ever. We will beat the coronavirus and we will beat it together. And therefore, I urge you at this moment of national emergency to stay at home, protect our NHS, and save lives."[42]

Political leaders in democratic societies cannot dictate how people behave in a crisis, of course, and it would be as unfair to attribute all of America's social violence to the strongman president as it would be to attribute the cooperation in Australia and Canada to their prime ministers' pleas for unity and understanding. But officials, as stacks of social science research show, play an influential part in shaping opinion and directing action during moments of uncertainty. They have an outsized role in defining the situation for the media and citizens. They have unmatched power in setting the agenda for policymakers and framing public debate.[43] Substantively, Trump's COVID rhetoric undermined whatever chance Americans had to find grounds for solidarity. In a plausible, counterfactual reality, a strongman like Trump might have attempted to unify the country with language about a common enemy and a great fight, using the military metaphors that worked so well for conservatives like Morrison and Johnson. Instead, he delegated responsibility to each state and citizen. The government would make essential investments in bailing out the economy and subsidizing vaccine production, both on an unprecedented scale. But for decisions about how to manage the virus, Americans were on their own.

Now the combination of elements that ate away at America's weakened social bonds becomes more visible. An underlying culture of individualism and self-reliance, along with a predisposition toward violence, fed into a political climate marked by distrust and division. The president, who wielded unusual power and influence in the state of pandemic emergency, urged citizens to distrust scientific experts and gave tacit permission to ignore public health guidelines that they disliked.[44] His supporters, in the media and in other political offices, endorsed this view. What's more, they tolerated—and in some cases even advocated—violent opposition to mask mandates, business closures, public lockdowns, and other regulations said to be "tyrannical" violations of individual rights. In this context, hostility flourishes. People lose confidence in the idea of civil society. They survive by looking out for themselves.

The stories of people like Nuala O'Doherty and mutual aid groups like the COVID Care Neighbor Network serve as stark reminders that American society did not dissolve during 2020. In small towns, suburbs, and urban neighborhoods across the country, community organizations stepped up to support people in need. But Americans proved more adept at bonding with those who shared their worldviews, political affiliations, and identities than at bridging divisions with those who were different. As the nation barreled toward the presidential election, what Americans held in common was disdain for the other side.

A shared emotional state—marked by fear, hatred, resentment, indignation, and rage—stoked the flames of American fury, accelerating the trend toward anomic violence.[45] The president, with his menacing displays of outrage and threats to exact revenge on his adversaries, reset the nation's emotional register during the years leading into the pandemic. The media, attuned to the popular appeal of angry voices decrying purportedly evil acts, amplified the hostile tone. Whereas, in other historical moments, Americans tended to avoid politics and contentious confrontations, in 2020, they were looking for reasons to act out.[46] Americans decorated their cars and trucks with the words of warfare. On roadways, bumper stickers with a rattlesnake and the message "Don't Tread on Me" proliferated, as did those with "Come and Take It" printed below a cannon or an AR-15. "Not My President" was a common message on the vehicles of the president's critics, as were "TRE45ON" and "Resist." It's no accident that they drove with more reckless aggression, too.

In universities, conservative and moderately liberal students complained that "cancel culture" had created a climate of fear on campus, shutting down possibilities for open expression, let alone productive debate. One politically progressive young adult we interviewed told us how his "woke" peers had intimidated and silenced him, even as he participated in BLM marches. "I've seen people sharing Christopher Dorner memes, idolizing him. He was that ex-cop in L.A. who went on a killing spree and shot LAPD officers and their families as a way to clear his name. A lot of people I know kind of see him as a hero. But it's weird because, in a way, I am cop-spawn. My grandpa was a Border Patrol agent, and whatever security I have in this world is built on that. I guess I'm a piece of shit, too, then. And it's very strange to think that I'm a legitimate target to those people because my grandpa was a cop, you know?"

The de-pacification of everyday life extended to nearly every place where people from different sides of the social divide intermingled. In shopping centers, conservatives openly mocked mask wearers for their passive obedience, while liberals shouted down those with bare faces for recklessly endangering everyone nearby. Occasionally, these disputes resulted in violence, sometimes in homicidal attacks. In school districts, financially secure parents who could work remotely and support their children with online education dismissed the concerns of working-class families who needed classrooms to reopen so they could make ends meet. On airlines, "unruly passengers" became a scourge for flight attendants and fellow travelers. Fights over mask mandates were the most common source of trouble, because an outspoken subset of fliers insisted on removing their face covering after takeoff. But other problems, including passengers who flew despite having COVID and transmitted the virus to those in their vicinity, turned air travel into a stressful and antisocial experience. The closer Americans came to those who were not part of their own communities, the more they wanted to stay apart.

Epilogue

In the story that Americans often tell themselves, the United States is a great democratic society. Since World War II, when the U.S. played a decisive role in defeating the Nazis and fascists, Americans have also taken to calling their nation the "leader of the free world."[1]

The truth has always been more complicated. For centuries, the U.S. afforded the franchise to only a select group of citizens. Women did not win the right to vote until 1920, when Congress ratified the Nineteenth Amendment. Before the Voting Rights Act of 1965, Blacks who tried to vote were often subjected to poll taxes, literacy tests, bureaucratic obstacles, and violent suppression. Even after that victory, Black voters have faced undue barriers at polling places, including disproportionately long wait times and unfounded charges of voter fraud.[2]

The American record on leading the free world is equally checkered. The U.S. fought against authoritarianism in some places, such as Germany and the Soviet Union, but tolerated and even supported it in others, including Spain, Argentina, and Paraguay. In several Latin American nations, from Guatemala to Chile, the U.S. helped armed rebels and military insurgents overthrow democratically elected government leaders.[3] Dictatorships were acceptable, as long as rulers catered to American interests. Freedom, like democracy, was a conditional good.

As an alarming number of Americans saw it, both freedom and democracy were at risk in the closing months of 2020. That November, U.S. voters would elect their next president, either Donald Trump or Joe Biden, and decide whether Republicans or Democrats would control Congress. For party leaders, the stakes were unprecedented. "Democracy is on the ballot," Biden cautioned. During a town hall event in Pennsylvania, the Democratic nominee told the audience that Trump's failure to handle the pandemic had deprived Americans of basic liberties: "You lost your freedom because he didn't act. The freedom to go to that ballgame, the freedom for your kid to go to school, the freedom to see your mom or dad in the hospital. The freedom just to walk around your neighborhood, because of failure to act responsibly."[4]

Trump issued similar warnings. "The Democrats want to take away your guns, they want to take away your health care, they want to take away your vote, they want to take away your freedom. They want to take away everything," he said—first before his impeachment trial, and with variations on the theme at campaign events throughout 2020. "We can never let this happen."[5]

Voting—the physical act of registering, getting a ballot, marking it up, submitting it, and ensuring that it is counted accurately—has always been a contested process in American elections. The pandemic introduced new problems and intensified others. What kinds of accommodations should states make for citizens who wanted to exercise their franchise but were worried about catching the coronavirus in public settings? How much should governments promote and invest in alternatives to the conventional system of voting in a designated polling place, such as drop boxes or mail-in ballots? What did state and local officials need to do to make sure the ballots they received and the counting systems they employed were safe and secure?

For state and local election managers, infectious disease control was by no means the only challenge. Throughout 2020, President Trump used the power of his office to raise questions about the legitimacy of the electoral process—just as he had done during and after the 2018 midterms. In July 2020, when states were building out plans for expanded early voting and drop box programs, he suggested that the nation postpone the election and allow him to remain in office for an extended term. "With Universal Mail-In Voting (not Absentee Voting, which is good), 2020 will be the most INACCURATE & FRAUDULENT Election in history," Trump tweeted. "It will be a great embarrassment to the USA. Delay the Election until people can properly, securely and safely vote???" No president in American history had called for suspending an election, and Trump's idea got little support, not even from Republicans who otherwise followed his lead.

Although Trump stopped pushing to delay the election, he doubled down on claims that Democrats would do everything possible to manufacture votes in contested swing states and steal the election, hacking software, tampering with electronic counting systems, encouraging supporters to cast multiple ballots, urging noncitizens to vote. The opposition party, he insisted, was exploiting the pandemic to seize control of the country against the public's wishes. In August, when polls showed him trailing Biden by a wide margin, he declared that "the only way we're going to lose this election is if the election is rigged."[6]

Democrats had their own concerns about a rigged election. Like the president, they worried about mail-in voting, but while Trump warned that the U.S. Postal Service (USPS) would allow a host of illegal ballots to change the outcome, Democrats worried that it would do the opposite, delaying delivery so that ballots could not be tallied in time. The primary source of this concern was Louis DeJoy, a Republican "mega-donor" whom Trump appointed postmaster general despite his complete lack of experience with the USPS or any other public agency. In late summer 2020, DeJoy, intent on cutting the cost of operations, implemented sweeping changes that resulted in significant service delays. The timing of these interventions—in the middle of a pandemic, and just weeks before an election in which millions of Americans would vote by mail—invited suspicion. "Is Trump's New Post Office Chief Trying to Rig the Election?" a *Guardian* headline asked.[7]

In August, DeJoy announced he would suspend some of the new operating procedures, but his political adversaries were dubious. Later that month, the House of Representatives held a public hearing on "Protecting the Timely Delivery of Mail, Medicine, and Mail-In Ballots," at which Democrats grilled the postmaster general about his apparent political motivations and introduced a $25 billion bill to restore postal service to the delivery standards it maintained before his tenure.[8] In September, a federal judge in Washington blocked DeJoy from making additional modifications. "It is easy to conclude that the recent Postal Services' changes is an intentional effort on the part of the current Administration to disrupt and challenge the legitimacy of upcoming local, state, and federal elections," wrote U.S. district judge Stanley Bastian. The policies, he added, seemed geared toward "voter disenfranchisement."[9]

Roughly 155 million Americans, two thirds of all eligible citizens, voted on November 3, 2020, the highest turnout in the twenty-first century.[10] Disenfranchisement did not seem to be a major problem, but denialism did. Elections are ritual occasions, and one of the sacred moments in American presidential contests happens when the outcome becomes certain and the losing candidate calls the winner to concede. For decades, this has been the first step in a process that is also a hallmark of American democracy and a long-standing source of national pride: the peaceful transition of power. In 2020, however, Trump made no such call. Instead, his advisers contacted Fox News executives and influential journalists, demanding that they retract their projections. Jared Kushner called Rupert Murdoch, but he could not persuade him to help. At 2:30 a.m. on November 4, Trump declared the election results in Arizona a "fraud," called for officials to stop counting ballots, and said the Supreme Court should decide the winner.[11]

At 11:24 a.m. on November 7, CNN became the first major news network to project that Biden would be the winner.[12] Others, including the right-wing network Fox News, quickly followed. Biden had won close races in pivotal states such as Arizona, Georgia, Michigan, Nevada, Pennsylvania, and Wisconsin. He took the popular vote by nearly seven million, and won 306 Electoral College votes compared to Trump's 232. It was, by any measure, a decisive victory. But the president refused to accept the result. Within hours, Trump took to social media and declared himself the victor. "I WON THIS ELECTION, BY A LOT!" he tweeted, along with a statement that the race was "far from over."[13] "They stole it from me," he told the head of the Republican National Committee. "I'm just not going to leave."[14] In the following weeks, Trump and his allies filed sixty-two lawsuits in state and federal courts, all part of a sweeping effort to overturn the election results in the states that he lost. By early January 2021, all but one inconsequential case had failed. The president was unmoved by the decisions. "This Fake Election can no longer stand," he tweeted in December, when the only procedure remaining was for Congress to formally count the Electoral College results, on January 6, 2021. "Get moving Republicans."[15]

In the closing days of 2020, Republicans across America did exactly that.

On December 30, 2020, more than 3,800 Americans died of COVID, making it the most lethal day of the first pandemic year. That same day, China reported zero COVID deaths, and its reported seven-day average for COVID deaths was zero as well.[16] In fact, since March 2020, China, with more than 1.4 billion people, had consistently reported between zero and one COVID deaths per week at the national level. Despite being the site of the first coronavirus outbreak, China claimed that its total COVID mortality in 2020 was under five thousand. Researchers from outside the country doubted the accuracy of these numbers, but their limited access to reliable Chinese health statistics make it difficult to know what really happened. Analyses of excess deaths during 2020 and 2021 published in *The Lancet* and in *Nature*, for instance, yielded excess death numbers for China that varied by 400,000.[17]

For Chinese health officials, the number to keep in focus during the closing months of 2020 was zero, for its ambitious, and exacting, Zero COVID policy. "The current strategic goal is to maintain no or minimal indigenous transmission of SARS-CoV-2 until the population is protected through immunisation with safe and effective COVID-19 vaccines, at which time the risk of

COVID-19 from any source should be at a minimum," wrote a team of scholars led by the Chinese Center for Disease Control and Prevention in July 2020. "China's containment effort has strikingly curtailed morbidity and mortality from COVID-19 and stopped community transmission."[18] Their challenge was to continue blocking transmission in future outbreaks, no matter how contagious the variant. Critics worried about the human costs of these measures. How long could Chinese people remain locked down in their homes and shut out of social and cultural activities? The nation was by no means democratic, but there was a limit to what Chinese citizens would accept.

In November 2022, Chinese activists initiated a remarkable series of protests over the government's ill-fated efforts to maintain Zero COVID for good. For nearly three years, residents of China had endured long bouts of home confinement, with mandatory COVID tests for everyone who wanted to enter a public space. Now a vocal social movement refused. In cities across the country—Urumqi, Shanghai, Chengdu, Wuhan, and Beijing, where the cost of dissent could be frighteningly high—people marched for hours in the cold, chanting "We want freedom!" and demanding change.[19] On December 7, the Chinese government backed down in surprisingly abrupt fashion, opening schools that had suspended in-person classes, ending obligatory testing, and allowing travelers to return without lengthy quarantines. The public reaction was euphoric but short-lived. Lacking protection from messenger RNA (mRNA) vaccines or previous exposures to COVID, the Chinese population was primed for infection and vulnerable to severe disease. Within weeks, case levels were soaring, emergency care centers were beyond capacity, and dead bodies—visible from satellite images but not in official statistics—were piling up around medical facilities and funeral homes. In mid-January 2023, Beijing reported that China had experienced sixty thousand COVID deaths in the five weeks since it rolled back the Zero COVID restrictions; outside observers estimated that the actual toll was several times higher, in the hundreds of thousands, if not more.[20] A top Chinese health official suggested that more than one billion people had been infected since the state rolled back its restrictions, and in mid-February 2023, four separate academic research groups estimated that between one million and 1.5 million people had died of COVID since the pandemic began.[21]

China's case numbers remained high through the Lunar New Year celebrations, when Chinese people embraced the opportunity to travel around the country and visit relatives again. By the time the surge subsided, it was hard to avoid the conclusion that China's public health, in 2023, looked far more like America's in 2020 than officials would admit. China's leader, Xi Jinping, had found a way to contain and control the disease temporarily, albeit at the expense of Chinese liberty and collective life. But his fantasy of evading the crisis proved unrealistic. The strongman could not protect the nation, no matter what story he told.

In Australia, policy measures during the last months of 2020 sparked controversy, too. Thanks to strong public health interventions, including strict limitations on travel and social gatherings, 2020 had been the least deadly year in recent history. The Australian Institute of Health and Welfare reported roughly eight thousand fewer deaths in 2020 than in 2019, and both men and women experienced their highest-ever life expectancy—the very opposite of trends in the U.S.[22]

Preserving life in a global pandemic, however, was not enough to satisfy everyone. Lockdowns, a growing number of Australians complained, induce a heavy social and economic toll, and some states were using them too much. In Victoria, they were so limiting, and so long-lasting—the government had imposed an initial lockdown from March 30 to May 11, and a second lockdown from July 7 to October 26—that some who initially supported the measures questioned whether the cure was more damaging than the disease. By fall, hundreds of people began defying the rules on gathering in public, taking to the streets and calling for a sweeping reopening. Their message was amplified by groups promoting anti-vaccine messages and COVID conspiracy theories. Police responded by invading the home of one prominent movement activist and arresting others who promoted demonstrations online.[23] Advocates for civil liberties had long considered Australia "one of Earth's freest societies"; now they were questioning its commitment to basic human rights.[24]

In England, critics of public health restrictions had also questioned the government's commitment to civil liberties during 2020. Compared to Australians, British people had extraordinary freedom to interact and circulate. So, too, did the coronavirus, which is one reason why, that December, the Delta variant of COVID arrived in the United Kingdom from India, where it was first identified earlier that month. Delta was more than twice as contagious as previous variants, and more likely to result in hospitalization.[25] England, in part because of its resistance to limiting economic activity and social gatherings, had been one of the most dangerous places to be during the first year of the pandemic. Its 85,000 excess deaths ranked third-highest among all nations, behind the U.S. and Italy; its per capita excess mortality ranked ninth.[26] People were already angry and exhausted from the year of sacrifice, suffering, and political instability. With the Christmas and New Year's holidays coming, millions had planned travel to visit with friends and family. Now everything was in jeopardy again.

In a press conference on December 19, Prime Minister Boris Johnson announced that cases of Delta were surging in parts of London, the South East and East of England, and he introduced new restrictions in each of these "tier 4" hot spots. "Residents in those areas must stay at home, apart from limited exemptions set out in law. Non-essential retail, indoor gyms and leisure facilities, and personal care services must close. . . . People should not enter or leave tier 4 areas, and tier 4 residents must not stay overnight away from home."[27]

Johnson was well aware that these measures would be unpopular. "I know how much emotion people invest in this time of year, and how important it is for grandparents to see their grandchildren, and for families to be together," he said. "We are sacrificing our chance to see loved ones this Christmas, so we have a better chance of protecting their lives so we can see them at future Christmases."[28] If Johnson was hopeful that England would soon "beat back" and "defeat" the virus, it was because on December 8, the country became the first place in the Western world to begin using a clinically approved COVID vaccine.[29] Within ten days, more than 350,000 people had already received their first dose, and the government planned a mass vaccination campaign for the months ahead. "There is now hope—real hope—that we will soon be rid of this virus," Johnson proclaimed. "We will reclaim our lives."

In America, there was also real hope about being rid of the virus. The U.S. had not done much right during the first year of the pandemic, but developing safe and powerful new vaccines to protect against COVID within one year of its emergence was a landmark achievement, one of the greatest in the history of medical science. Like most great successes, the vaccine had many parents, including the scientists who spent decades experimenting with mRNA technology, pharmaceutical corporations that supported their research, and the U.S. federal government, which invested $14 billion in Operation Warp Speed, a public-private partnership (with, it became clear, a name that would not inspire confidence in those who were anxious about the risks of new pharmaceutical interventions) designed to accelerate the production of COVID vaccines and treatments.

At times, Trump took credit for the remarkably fast rollout of COVID vaccines in America. "You saw that very few people thought that this was possible," he said. "People that aren't necessarily big fans of Donald Trump are saying, 'Whether you like him or not, this is one of the greatest miracles in the history of modern-day medicine' or any other medicine—any other age of medicine."[30] According to a report by the House Select Subcommittee on the Coronavirus Crisis, members of the Trump administration pressured the Food and Drug Administration to issue an emergency use authorization for distribution of the COVID vaccine before the presidential election in November, ostensibly in hope of getting a political bump.[31] When they failed, and Trump lost the election, the president's enthusiasm for the vaccine diminished.

On December 14, Sandra Lindsay, a nurse at New York's Long Island Jewish Medical Center, became the first American to receive the vaccine outside of a medical trial. CNN televised the vaccination live, and Governor Andrew Cuomo streamed it at his news conference. More than five hours later, at 2:24 p.m., Trump tweeted, "First Vaccine Administered. Congratulations USA! Congratulations WORLD!" Most of the president's tweets that day, however, were dedicated to overturning the election. At 1:57 p.m.: "Why did the Swing States stop counting in the middle of the night? @MariaBartiromo Because they waited to find out how many ballots they had to produce in order to steal the Rigged Election. They were so far behind that they needed time, & a fake water main break, to recover!" At 2:38 p.m.: "Swing States that have found massive VOTER FRAUD, which is all of them, CAN-NOT LEGALLY CERTIFY these votes as complete."[32] Trump also used Twitter to announce that Jeff Rosen, a deputy attorney general who, the president hoped, would support his efforts to remain in office, would replace Bill Barr as attorney general, because earlier that day Barr announced his plan to resign.

The night before the vaccine rollout, the Trump administration did make one significant announcement about its participation, and its message foreshadowed the ideological message that conservatives would maintain for the remainder of the pandemic. Originally, the White House had announced that officials from all three branches of government would receive their first doses of the vaccine around December 14. But at the last minute, the president insisted on a change. "People working in the White House should receive the vaccine somewhat later in the program, unless specifically necessary," he tweeted. "I have asked that this adjustment be made. I am not scheduled to take the vaccine, but look forward to doing so at the appropriate time. Thank you!"[33]

Trump, who survived a severe case of COVID in October 2020, may have had good personal reasons to delay getting inoculated; he likely had antibodies from the recent infection, and was at relatively low risk of disease two months later. His decision, however, affected all White House staff, regardless of their previous exposure to the virus, and it was widely interpreted as an expression of uncertainty about the new vaccine. After all, the president and his senior health advisers had spent the better part of the year vilifying "deep state" scientists and questioning their judgment about how to cure or prevent transmission of COVID.[34] Moreover, the White House, despite its financial support for Operation Warp Speed, had refused Pfizer's urgent request for the government to purchase 100 million doses of its vaccine in October, and now the federal government did not have enough doses to supply the entire population at risk right away. Was there a reason they were preventing White House staff from getting shots in the first stage of the mass vaccination campaign, and not ordering enough doses for everyone who needed them? Surely, prominent conservative pundits declared, it was because the Trump administration did not believe it was safe.

For much of 2020, right-wing activists had been preparing the groundwork for a fight against vaccine mandates in America. Some promoted disinformation, insisting, for instance, that the vaccines were killing or sterilizing recipients, that they caused people to shed COVID and transmit it to unvaccinated people, or that they contained microchips that the government would use to track everyone foolish enough to get inoculated. The latter theory circulated so widely that roughly one in five Americans believed it is "definitely true" or "probably true" that "the U.S. government is using the COVID-19 vaccine to microchip the population."[35] Others claimed that, for ideological reasons, health officials were pushing unproven vaccines and withholding support for "miracle drugs" such as ivermectin that—as Dr. Pierre Kory told the Senate's Homeland Security Committee—were proven to prevent transmission and severe illness "in nearly all" who take it.[36] Another faction objected to a state-sponsored vaccine campaign on libertarian grounds, arguing that all individuals had the right to choose whether to get inoculated. "Where is 'my body, my choice' when it comes to this?" asked Dr. Jane Orient, executive director of an organization that opposes vaccine mandates, and an advocate for treating COVID with hydroxychloroquine.[37] Powerful Republicans in Congress embraced these positions. Trump, always eager to appear on national television, refused to get inoculated on camera. Among conservatives, skepticism about the vaccine grew.

There are legitimate reasons to be concerned about the risks of a vaccine made with new technology. In America, where the

government, universities, and the medical industry have a history
of experimenting on vulnerable populations and racial minorities, the skepticism is especially well founded. But much of the
opposition to the COVID vaccine was rooted in bad faith. On
social media, vaccine disinformation circulated widely, and misinformation became a regular feature of right-wing cable news.
Some of the disinformation came from Russian bots and troll
farms, which, along with Russia's foreign broadcast network, RT,
had a well-documented record of promoting anti-vaccine sentiment to destabilize democratic societies.[38] But Americans produced a staggering amount of it—not only in groups dedicated to
political conversations, either. Rumors about the hidden agendas
of government officials and the corrupt profiteering of global
pharmaceutical companies penetrated social media groups dedicated to popular culture, parenting, diet, and sports. Some went
viral, and none more so than Dr. Judy Mikovits's short video
Plandemic, which warns that "at least 50 million Americans would
die, probably from the first dose," if the government mandated
vaccination.[39] Just as, in the middle of 2020, ideological divisions
shaped Americans' beliefs about which medications for COVID
were more or less effective, at the end of 2020, party affiliation
was already determining whether people would get a shot. The
result was an unusual, if not distinctively American, phenomenon: in a nation where lifesaving vaccines would soon be widely
available, nearly half the population was prepared to turn them
down.[40]

Historically, epidemics and pandemics have sparked major transformations in states and societies. Sometimes, they lead to dramatic improvements in public health, scientific progress, and
public goods; sometimes, though, they induce little more than
pain, suffering, and loss. In the fifteenth century, a number of
Mediterranean governments developed legislation banning commerce with traders from areas with clusters of plague. In Italian
states, the medical historian Mark Harrison writes, leaders broke
from the traditional view that infectious disease was a "blight of
God," and developed new state agencies "to administer quaran-

tine and lazarettos, in the belief that plague was a contagious disease that could be prevented by thwarting its transmission."[41]

In the seventeenth century, European cities reeling from
deadly outbreaks of infectious diseases such as plague, cholera,
and smallpox appointed public authorities to devise quarantine
and isolation measures; in the early eighteenth century, several
new American port cities followed suit, in hope of preventing
international transmissions. During 1793, a yellow fever epidemic in Philadelphia killed roughly one in ten residents of what
was then America's largest metropolis, and caused nearly half of
the population to flee. The crisis convinced the founding fathers,
including George Washington, Thomas Jefferson, and Alexander
Hamilton, that more outbreaks could cripple the young nation
and end the democratic experiment before it had time to develop.
In response, President John Adams introduced plans to impose
strict quarantines during future epidemics and Congress passed
the Act for the Relief of Sick and Disabled Seamen, which eventually developed into what is now the national Public Health Service.[42] Across the fledgling nation, a public health infrastructure
began to take shape.

The nineteenth century, the Yale public health scholar
Charles-Edward Winslow argued, marked the world's "great
sanitary awakening."[43] By then, medical researchers had established the links between crowding, pollution, exposure to waste,
and disease. "Illness came to be seen as an indicator of poor social
and environmental conditions," reports the Institute of Medicine, the health arm of the National Academy of Sciences, and
this new perspective inspired a shift in public policy. "Protecting health became a social responsibility. Disease control continued to focus on epidemics, but the manner of controlling turned
from quarantine and isolation of the individual to cleaning up
and improving the common environment. And disease control
shifted from reacting to intermittent outbreaks to continuing
measures for prevention." Cities began decontaminating drinking water, removing dead animals from the streets, and collecting garbage more aggressively. "With sanitation, public health
became a societal goal and protecting health became a public
activity."[44] It also became a cause for new forms of diplomacy.

The first International Sanitary Conference, held in Paris during 1851, established a framework for cooperation around infectious disease containment, even among competing states.[45]

Not all pandemics come with silver linings. The Great Influenza outbreak of 1918–19 was, as the historian Alfred Crosby put it, "the greatest failure of medical science in the twentieth century or, if absolute numbers of the dead are the measure, of all time."[46] The flu killed some 50 million people, 675,000 of whom lived in the U.S., and infected roughly one fifth of the human population. But the disaster took place in the shadow of the First World War, and, as Crosby writes, it "has never inspired awe, not in 1918 and not since, not among the citizens of any land and not among citizens of the United States."[47] What changed after the pandemic? Governments around the world built up their public health agencies and invested in research on influenza. In 1919, leaders of Red Cross societies in the U.S., Britain, France, Italy, and Japan convened in Cannes, where a group that included Nobel laureates and scientific luminaries created an international health organization to help monitor and manage medical crises that became the precursor to the WHO.[48] "But all of this is minor compared to what has been done since to fight threats such as polio, heart disease, and cancer, and the effort was uncoordinated and underfinanced and feeble." Far from transforming states and societies, Crosby concludes, "it did not spur great changes in the structures and procedures of governments, armies, corporations, or universities. It had little influence on the course of political or military struggles."[49] Instead of looking inward to see how they could do better, most Americans "let the pandemic slip their minds."[50]

Since the middle of the twentieth century, new threats, including both nuclear weapons and novel infectious diseases such as Ebola, HIV/AIDS, and SARS, have shaped the political imagination, inspiring the advent of what the anthropologists Stephen Collier and Andrew Lakoff call "vital systems security."[51] Under this regime, cities, nations, and nongovernmental agencies invest in programs that anticipate novel emergencies and model possible responses. Disease surveillance is crucial to this project, as is international data sharing and cooperation, through agencies such as the WHO. It involves enhancing "preparedness," with stockpiles of medication and personal protective equipment, and strategic risk communication. Information technology, pharmaceutical innovation, critical infrastructure, and logistics play essential roles. As the concept suggests, this new security regime prioritizes "vital systems," and requires governments to maintain them in the face of catastrophic threats. Human health is predicated on "resiliency," which has become a core objective of public policy, but so, too, is another sacred value: the flow of global commodities and the preservation of economic life.

The coronavirus pandemic of 2020 induced some notable breakthroughs. Improved technologies for remote work and school allowed people to remain productive without leaving their homes. National governments in affluent societies injected unprecedented amounts of money into the economy, shoring up businesses and staving off poverty with extraordinary success. "Warp speed" government investments in medical science accelerated the pace of pharmaceutical development, allowing mRNA vaccines, which had been used experimentally but never approved for the public, to hurtle past regulatory hurdles and into people's arms.

None of these changes, however, was an unalloyed good. The rise of remote work and online education was a boon for the technology sector and delivery businesses, but it proved devastating for downtowns and city centers, and its impacts on human health and happiness are decidedly mixed. Going remote was especially difficult for working mothers, who wound up doing the majority of their family's additional domestic labor, supervising their children in internet classrooms, and doing their ordinary jobs—often all at once. "Other countries have safety nets," the sociologist Jessica Calarco argued, "America has women." For millions, remote work meant absorbing an overwhelming load of intense, often intimate labor, and women left their paying jobs in droves.[52]

Public spending to bail out corporations and workers also had uneven effects. Some countries, including the U.S., made filing for and receiving benefits far easier for large companies than for small businesses and families, resulting in widespread feelings of injustice and, for people like Daniel Presti, a sense that the system was rigged. The vaccine rollout was even more manifestly unequal. Wealthy nations in the Global North had the resources and institutions required to secure the scarce new medical commodity—and commodity is what the vaccine was. Developing nations in the Global South did not. The virus was poised to continue spreading, mutating, and evolving until every society was inoculated. But the world's most powerful governments did little to make that happen. By the end of 2020, the virus was on the move, too.

By 2023, the pandemic was responsible for roughly 7 million reported deaths, and 20 million excess deaths, worldwide.[53] The U.S. registered more than one million COVID deaths and more than 1.7 million excess deaths. "When compared to other countries and adjusted for population size," the Kaiser Family Foundation found, in its study of "premature mortality" during the crisis, "the U.S. had the highest excess mortality rate among similarly large and wealthy countries for the period 2020–2021. . . . In addition the U.S. also saw a higher rate of death among younger people, and thus a larger increase in premature deaths per capita than peer countries."[54]

In America, however, the recurrent surges of death and disease from the coronavirus did little to move public sentiment about how to build a better country. In the first stage of the pandemic, the goal of saving lives above all other considerations justified sweeping emergency measures, such as lockdowns and border closures and prohibitions on gatherings of all kinds. The initial global response, as Didier Fassin argues, established a new moral economy, with "values and affects, obligations, and norms" based on the imperative to protect the vulnerable, at virtually any cost. But by the end of 2020, a rising number of Americans believed that—or, more accurately, acted as if—they had sacrificed enough. People seemed unmoved by reports of catastrophic mortality that, in other times, would surely have caused outrage and anxiety. Instead of calling for new public health measures, Americans grew numb to the carnage, content to accept their neighbors' suffering and loss. Their sense of mutual responsibility diminished as steadily as their life expectancy dropped. It was less a Hobbesian war of "all against all" than a cold war of collective attrition, marked by subversion, propaganda, hostility, and threats in American communities, and expressed each day in the coroner's office, one solitary death at a time.

"2020," the historian Adam Tooze writes, was "a comprehensive crisis of the neoliberal era . . . the end of an arc whose origin is to be found in the 1970s," when free markets and hyper-individualism became the organizing principles for a new world order.[55] It was also, researchers at the University of Cambridge's Centre for the Future of Democracy conclude, a crisis for populists and populism. "Individual populist leaders exhibit declining approval ratings, electoral support for populist parties is falling, and most tellingly of all, public approval for core populist ideas—such as belief in 'will of the people' or that society is divided between ordinary people and a 'corrupt elite'—has fallen dramatically."[56] It's true that neoliberalism and populism failed, catastrophically, during the first year of the great coronavirus pandemic. Leaders who stood for either, or, as in the U.S. and England, both of these forms of political organization, promoted policies that increased the human toll of COVID. Trump lost the 2020 election in America, due largely to concerns about his leadership in the pandemic. Two years later, Boris Johnson was forced to resign because of the parties he threw while England was under lockdown, and Jair Bolsonaro was defeated at the polls. But neoliberalism itself looks likely to survive the calamity, and populist authoritarianism appears more resilient than the scholars at Cambridge suggest.

Social solidarity, however, took a critical blow during the pandemic. The political and ideological divisions that separated Americans before the crisis did not doom the country to a fractious or embattled experience. In the first months of the crisis, as social scientists from Stanford University found, affective polarization— "the extent to which partisans feel more negatively towards the opposing party than toward their own"—did not increase. As the economist Matthew Gentzkow reports, "affective polarization in fact fell significantly with the onset of the pandemic," leading the research team to issue the "cautiously optimistic conclusion that the coronavirus may have brought partisans together in the face of a common threat."[57] At the local level, too, Americans banded together to help each other get through their darkest moments. Mutual aid networks sprouted up across the country, in states red and blue, as did food pantries, community refrigerators, and little free libraries. For those who committed themselves to these collective, grassroots projects, cautious optimism about social cohesion seemed warranted, too.

By late summer, though, hardly anyone in the U.S. maintained hope that the nation would come together. As the pandemic evolved and intensified, Americans with different political allegiances fought over nearly every basic issue, from face masks to medications, school closures to open sidewalks, mutual obligations to individual rights. Not every divided nation experienced this level of conflict. In a survey conducted in September 2020, for instance, a majority of respondents in Denmark, Sweden, South Korea, and Australia—all countries with contentious politics and fiercely contested elections—said that their nation "is now more united than before the coronavirus outbreak." In the next tier of countries, which included France, Germany, Japan, and the U.K., between 39 and 47 percent of respondents felt the same way. The United States was the one clear outlier in the study, in a class by itself. A mere 18 percent of Americans said the nation "is now more united than it was before the coronavirus outbreak"[58]—and for a good reason: its social bonds were broken.

Recall that the U.S. has long ranked among the world's most individualistic societies. It's a nation where people believe that they, not the state or society, are responsible for their own wellbeing, where control is an unqualified virtue, and personal freedom is paramount.[59] Americans are also joiners, eager to participate in voluntary organizations and loyal to their chosen groups. But they can be harsh and judgmental of those who make other choices or identify with different people. In the years leading up to the pandemic, they had come to perceive those affiliated with the opposing political party as "immoral" and as "enemies." By the end of 2020, these sentiments had become pervasive.[60] Pundits and professors warned that the nation might be heading toward civil war.

No democratic society can survive without a healthy supply of social solidarity. When they lose it, the wealthy run away with the nation's riches and leave the poor homeless and destitute, health disparities widen across the social classes, racial segregation accelerates and distrust rises, the social order snaps. During plagues and pandemics, solidarity becomes all the more essential.[61] Commitment to the common good, and not only to our own individual interest, is what keeps us from hoarding medicine, toughing out a cold in the workplace, or sending a sick child to school. It's what compels us to let a ship of stranded people dock in our safe harbors, to knock on our older neighbor's door.

Crises, we know, can be switching points for states and societies. No matter how poorly suited the nation's political leaders were for the challenge, or how polarized its people had grown, there was at least a chance that the pandemic would help the U.S. rediscover its better, more collective self. That did not happen.

For now, at least, the U.S. appears ready to treat the plague of 2020 just as it did the Great Influenza, as a nonevent, a "forgotten pandemic" whose impact is perplexingly diminutive given the scale of death and disruption it caused.[62] "By the end of 2021," writes Atul Gawande, "Americans were dying three years sooner, on average, than they were before COVID-19, with life expectancy falling from 79 years to 76 years."[63] By 2023, more Americans had died of COVID after 2020 than they had during the first year of the outbreak, and as many as 94 percent of the U.S. population had contracted the disease.[64] "216,617 children lost a co-residing caregiver to COVID-19; 77,283 lost a parent and more than 17,000 children lost the only caregiver with whom they lived" reports a study led by the policy scholar Dan Treglia. In New York City, nearly 9,000 children experienced a parent dying of COVID.[65] For them, as for so many other Americans, moving on from the pandemic was no easy task.

On May 11, 2023, the U.S. allowed its COVID-19 public health emergency declaration to lapse, signaling the official end of the pandemic crisis. In the media, a handful of medical leaders and policy experts called for the nation to begin preparing for the next catastrophe, but few political leaders were rallying to revive the nation's public health. As the country geared up for the 2024 elections, the will not to know about COVID-19 or the social conditions that made it so devastating had taken over American political culture. "The Mask Mandates Did Nothing," a *New York Times* headline in February 2023 declared, despite the fact that scientific research showed no such thing. Ron DeSantis, a favorite to challenge Trump for the Republican presidential nomination, was one of many political leaders who characterized the entire public health response to COVID—from masks to lockdowns and vaccination campaigns—as dangerously misguided. "Power-hungry elites tried to use the coronavirus to impose an oppressive biomedical security state on America, but Florida stood as an impenetrable roadblock to such designs," he boasted.[66] Democrats, wary of being associated with coronavirus restrictions, tried to avoid the topic. Denial was everywhere. So, too, was the threat of another crisis, including one that concerned a growing number of epidemiologists: an even deadlier pandemic, this one from a mutant strain of H5N1, otherwise known as avian flu.

Although the calendar has turned, the story of 2020 is far from over, and its potential to move us in new directions is not yet tapped dry. The pandemic, writes Arundhati Roy, "is a portal, a gateway from one world into the next."[67] Today, there is little question that the next world is coming. The "American Century" is over. Democratic societies throughout the world are teetering. Authoritarians are amassing power. The fight for racial justice and social equity is intensifying. The planet is melting, the ground giving way beneath our feet.

The greatest challenge of this moment is to find a new vision for the world that's emerging, a better way to inhabit the places we've inherited or built. 2020 has helped us see things more clearly, but ultimately our fate depends on whether we can imagine something better and create a path that leads there. Our time is precious.

APPENDIX

A NOTE ON THE RESEARCH

Public issues are always experienced in deeply personal terms; neither society nor individuals can be understood in isolation. We live in an age of technocratic knowledge, and today, with oceans of big data available for analysis, the "super crunchers" and "quants" urge us to be skeptical of stories about small-scale human experiences and events. Statistics, it is true, can be extraordinarily powerful. For some kinds of knowledge, they're indispensable, and here I use them to establish a variety of facts about what happened, where, why, and to whom, in 2020. That said, sometimes statistics can be dangerously misleading, particularly when they are used as political weapons to define reality in contentious situations, or when the phenomenon they're trying to measure is difficult to count and observe. The most sophisticated techniques for data analysis we have are useless, and even misleading, if the numbers they contain are based on half-truths or lies.

Coronavirus cases and fatalities are not easy to verify and record in official statistics, which means most governments have likely undercounted its prevalence. For the first several months of 2020, few nations had enough tests to confirm that a person had been infected. Later, even in places where assays were readily available, countless people who caught the virus were asymptomatic and didn't think to get tested, while others with symptoms opted to avoid a formal exam and let the illness run its course. COVID deaths were more likely to get counted. But in many places, there was a significant gap between official COVID deaths, for which there was a specific diagnosis and mortality attribution, and the "excess deaths," a measure of the disparity between the typical mortality level in a given time frame and the actual number who died during that same period in a time of heightened risk. During 2020 and 2021, as an influential study in *The Lancet* showed, governments around the world reported 5.94 million COVID deaths, but the excess death level was 18.2 million, more than three times higher than the official toll.[1]

COVID statistics from 2020 are even more unreliable in places where governments actively manipulated COVID data to downplay the number of cases, improve their public image, or advance their own agendas. China was slow to report the initial outbreak of the novel coronavirus, and outside observers insist that it dramatically underreported COVID mortality throughout the pandemic.[2] Researchers from the Institute for Health Metrics and Evaluation at the University of Washington singled out Brazil, India, Mexico, and the United States for "likely wide variances between officially reported covid deaths and actual fatalities." Ron DeSantis, the Republican governor of Florida, and Andrew Cuomo, the Democratic governor of New York, were accused of "cooking the books" on COVID deaths in their states to make it look like they managed the crisis more successfully than they did.[3] The Trump administration rerouted hospital data on COVID patients from the CDC to the White House, so that it could assert control over vital information and justify whichever policy prescriptions it preferred.[4]

The controversies over basic biopolitical data from 2020 make it all the more important to heed the late sociologist C. Wright Mills's call for research that examines individual struggles in fine detail as well as larger societal trends. "No social study that does not come back to the problems of biography, of history and of their intersections within a society has completed its intellectual journey," Mills insisted.[5] For that reason, this book looks just as closely at the lived experiences of individuals trying to get by and protect the people around them as at the large-scale trends that we can chart on a graph. There are numbers and there are narratives, and by alternating between them we get a depth of knowledge about the world that would otherwise be impossible to reach.

From the moment I heard about the new coronavirus that was circulating across the planet, I knew that social forces beyond the purview of medical science would determine its impact and course. The question was how to study them. Within a few months of its emergence, COVID-19 had become a global phenomenon. There was no way to construct a standard survey that could capture all the problems that surfaced as the viral emergency evolved, and no way to track its social life in every place it touched.

I decided to approach it on two tracks. First, I designed a series of sociological research projects that would assess relatively large-scale questions about important variations in the pandemic experience. These included a series of comparative analyses: How did two sets of nation-states—China and Taiwan (the Republic of China), and the liberal Anglo-Saxon countries Australia, the United States, and the United Kingdom—respond to the initial outbreak of COVID-19, and why were their public health strategies so different? How did trust—of government, scientists, and other citizens—affect the capacity of states and societies to protect themselves? Why, in some places, did face masks become loaded objects that triggered cultural, political, and physical conflict, while in others they were used widely, with little controversy or debate? What made social distancing so difficult? Why did violence and antisocial behavior spike in the U.S. but decline in most other societies? What made some poor urban neighborhoods so much more vulnerable to COVID fatalities than others that are demographically similar? How did some nations manage to build trust in government, science, and fellow citizens during 2020, while others went in the opposite direction? How, exactly, did race matter in the pandemic? How were young adults and people living alone affected by the sudden changes in their social conditions? What could members of communities do to help each other survive?

To answer these questions, I assembled a research team (consisting of sociology students and a postdoctoral fellow trained in communications) and conducted a set of formal studies, some quantitative, some qualitative, with strategic samples that would allow us to understand a range of experiences for people involved in different situations. Most of these studies involved doing in-depth interviews, and the restrictions of the pandemic required that the majority of these be done remotely, via phone or Zoom. Collectively, we conducted more than 230 interviews, and we assigned pseudonyms to the participants, as is conventional in social science research at this scale.

The second track of my investigation was quite different. When the pandemic began, I was working on a profile of a landscape architect for *The New Yorker*, and learning to appreciate Mills's insight about the value of history and biography in sociological research. I decided that I would place the life stories of a select number of people at the heart of *2020*, with an "intensity sample" of someone from each borough of New York City. There were several reasons for focusing on the place where I have lived and worked for the past twenty years, in addition to the fact that I was there when everything started. For much of 2020, New York City was the epicenter of the pandemic, with more confirmed COVID-19 cases and deaths than any other metropolis. It is also, and not unrelatedly, among the most global of cities, with more than three million immigrants (out of a total population of 8.5 million) and a constant circulation of people and goods from throughout the world. But if New York City contains the universe, it also shuffles or, alternatively, segregates everyone within it, creating what the urban sociologist Robert Park once described as "a mosaic of little social worlds which touch but do not interpenetrate."[6] From this mosaic, I would search for people and places whose experiences spoke to larger sociological trends.

There is, of course, no single person whose narrative perfectly characterizes their neighborhood, no one place that typifies the borough or city at large. The people I decided to profile are obviously not a representative sample of anything, and their accounts of what happened during 2020 should not be read as such. Instead, they are included in this book because they experienced, with an intensity that allows for unusual insight, something powerful and important that shaped the social life of the pandemic. Each of the people profiled here was willing to participate in the project, speaking with me at length, all on multiple occasions and some repeatedly over the course of a year. I emailed or read every subject the quotes I would use from our interviews as well as the surrounding text, and allowed them to change the wording or clarify their meaning. (I did the same with Benjamin Bier, whose story opens the book.) With their permission, I use their real names in my reporting.

The act of selecting individuals to profile was driven by my own analysis of which issues and conditions in each borough would be best illuminated through the lens of history and biography, and by the fortune of finding people who wanted to share. In Manhattan, my initial objective was to identify someone who had grappled with the challenge of school closures, since there are 1.1 million children in New York City public schools, and teaching them at home meant upending the social order. As an elementary school principal in Chinatown, May Lee had to manage far more than the transition to remote education. She also had to protect her community from a surge in anti-Asian violence and discrimination, and defend herself against another potentially lethal disease.

In the Bronx, where the city's Black, Latino, and low-income populations are concentrated, my goal was to find someone on the front lines of the battle against COVID, someone so caught up in the pandemic vortex that their story would bring the social drama to life. Sophia Zayas, a Bronx native who was serving as the borough's regional representative for the governor during 2020, may as well have come from a casting agency. Through her family, her neighborhood, her job, and, ultimately, her body, she inhabited the pandemic fully, and in a way that reveals how much the Bronx endured.

Staten Island is, by far, the whitest and most politically conservative borough in New York City, a place where people are often skeptical about state regulations and wary of excessive government intervention, where few are shy about speaking their mind. Although the borough is famous for its large population of police and firefighters, it also has a healthy share of small business owners and local entrepreneurs, and most of them struggled to get by when the city shut down. I wanted to find someone who lived and worked at the crux of all of this, and when I read a newspaper story about Daniel Presti and the fight to keep Mac's Public House open despite the local lockdowns, I knew I had found my ideal subject. Presti's story seemed particularly important, because his experience—feeling mistreated, abandoned, stigmatized, and then punished by the government—was so common during the pandemic, in right-leaning parts of New York as in Republican districts throughout the U.S. His transformation from a relatively apolitical local businessman to a radicalized right-wing activist was part of a social change that needs to be understood in more personal and human terms than our conventional political rhetoric allows. Presti is the only person in this book who stopped responding to my messages during the research process, but he remained a public personality, speaking out at conservative rallies and using social media to warn about the dangers of public health mandates and other restrictions. I promised that I would tell his story faithfully, so that readers could appreciate his perspective and also learn about his legal vindication.

In Queens, I searched for someone who lived in the cluster of crowded immigrant neighborhoods that experienced a dire surge of cases and fatalities during the initial outbreak, and also for someone who went to great lengths to help their neighbors survive. In the early stages of my research on how people in this part of Queens were responding to the virus, I started following mutual aid networks on social media and reaching out to leaders of community organizations. The name that kept coming up was Nuala O'Doherty, a retired prosecutor and candidate for local office who had just started the COVID Care Neighbor Network from her home in Jackson Heights. O'Doherty was as busy as anyone in New York City, but she squeezed me into her schedule for long conversations and helped me get to know the area firsthand.

In Brooklyn, I looked for someone whose fate was explicitly shaped by the borough's race and class dynamics. I came across Enuma Menkiti, a Black woman who worked in a local charter school and was married to a Black man who worked as a corrections officer at Rikers Island, through an interview that she did with the Brooklyn Public Library. When I contacted her for an introductory conversation, she told me about her children being kicked out of their progressive home day care because the leaders viewed her husband, an essential worker, as a disease vector, and also about how people in her social network helped her find high-quality health care when she contracted COVID. Her experiences were at once uniquely personal and indicative of universal trends.

Once I had found someone from each borough, I reviewed the themes their stories would likely address and considered which significant topics their biographical profiles would not cover. Two stood out as essential: the experience of losing a family member to COVID and struggling to mourn them due to restrictions on social gatherings, and the experience of breaking out of pandemic lockdowns to participate in Black Lives Matter protests. Sandra Bloodworth, director of the Metropolitan Transportation Authority's Arts & Design department, showed me the image of Thankachan Mathai from the MTA's memorial, Travels Far, which she helped organize. Her colleagues introduced me to Mathai's son, Mathews, who generously offered an account of his family's devastating year. Sandra and Mathews never met or spoke to each other, but together they told a necessary story about work, death, grief, and memory. I can't imagine not including them in this book. I feel the same way about Brandon English, whose story I found through Olutoyin Demuren, a research assistant on this project who did interviews with people who participated in Black Lives Matter protests. English, like so many people in New York City, witnessed unnerving levels of death and violence during 2020. But his story is here because he dedicated himself to something vital, the project of achieving justice, and repairing the world.

ACKNOWLEDGMENTS

I got a lot of help on this one—most notably, from the people who shared their time and their stories. Thank you to May Lee, Sophia Zayas, Daniel Presti, Nuala O'Doherty, Enuma Menkiti, Brandon English, Mathews Thankachan, Sandra Bloodworth, and Benjamin Bier, each of whom figures prominently here, and to the hundreds of people who participated anonymously in the sociological research projects that ground this book.

Isabelle Caraluzzi was about to graduate from NYU and begin a dream job in Italy when the pandemic started. The coronavirus didn't care about anyone's plans, though, and it forced her to pivot. She took a chance on this project, moved back to New York, and quickly became an ace assistant, collaborator, and friend. I could not have done this book without her. I'm particularly appreciative of the interviews that Isabelle conducted for the chapter "Growing Up." She is now a doctoral student at NYU Sociology, and I can't wait to see what she does next.

I feel similarly about a number of other students and early career scholars who collaborated on *2020*. Melina Sherman joined the team as a postdoctoral fellow and did excellent research on the digital life of the pandemic. Jennifer Leigh, a doctoral student in sociology, conducted interviews and helped analyze data about the experiences of people living alone. Selections from work I did with both Melina and Jennifer appear here. Parts of the chapter "Trust" were previously published in Eric Klinenberg and Melina Sherman, "Face Mask Face-Offs: Culture and Conflict in the COVID-19 Pandemic," *Public Culture* 33, no. 3 (2021): 441–66. Parts of the chapter "Home Alone" were previously published in

Eric Klinenberg and Jenny Leigh, "On Our Own," *Social Problems* (2023). I thank the publishers, Duke University Press and Oxford University Press, for permission to reuse this material here.

NYU Sociology doctoral students Michelle Cera, Olutoyin Demuren, Jocelyn Pak Drummond, and Sejin Um also made important contributions. Michelle and Sejin conducted interviews for a study about the meanings of masks. Olu interviewed people who got involved in Black Lives Matter protests. Jocelyn crunched the numbers so we could see how New York City neighborhoods fared during the initial surge. I got a further boost from NYU undergraduates. Julia Kempton deserves special recognition for the depth and intelligence of her research memos on a range of topics, from nursing homes and prisons to international public health policies. Jasmine Kwak, Sophia Santaniello, Manning Snyder, and Jacob Mulliken (a student at Brown) did standout work as well.

None of this would have been possible without the generous support of two funders. The Robert Wood Johnson Foundation not only provided the major grant I needed to build a team and launch this project in spring 2020, but also offered substantive feedback along the way. Thanks to Lori Melichar and Sharon Roerty for leading this effort. I was fortunate to receive the Knight Foundation's Public Spaces Fellowship just before the pandemic started. Although we were unable to do the work we originally planned, Lily Weinberg and her colleagues were open to my change in direction. I'm grateful.

For more than twenty years now, I've received steady support from New York University. The Institute for Public Knowledge and the Department of Sociology are special places, and colleagues from both have shaped everything I do. Lindsey Edwards, Ingrid Gould Ellen, Jacob Faber, Jeff Manza, Harvey Molotch, Dana Polan, Eyal Press, Rowan Ricardo Phillips, and Matthew Wolfe offered incisive feedback on various parts of *2020*. Beyond NYU, Eric Bates, David Grazian, Ariel Kaminer, David Kirkpatrick, Andrew Lakoff, Patrick LeGales, Dylan McCormick, Patrick Sharkey, Stephanie Staal, and Rona Talcott lent their editorial eyes to these pages, too.

Andrew Miller, my true editor, made this book infinitely better. He asked tough but essential questions and offered fresh perspectives on debates I'd settled prematurely. Andrew was a wise, spirited companion through a crisis that proved longer and more challenging than either of us anticipated. My thanks to Andrew, Tiara Sharma, Reagan Arthur, Fred Chase, Nicole Pedersen, and the entire crew at Alfred A. Knopf for bringing this book to life. I'm also appreciative of Nicole Pasulka, my exacting fact-checker. Nicole did everything possible to verify the claims made here; any remaining mistakes are mine.

I made no mistakes when I decided to work with Elyse Cheney and her team at the Cheney Agency, including Beniamino Ambrosi, Grace Johnson, and Isabel Mendia. From the outset, Elyse insisted that this book would be worth the effort, even if it meant thinking incessantly about a pandemic that so many others tried to ignore or forget. As always, she was right.

To the extent that my mind did wander off the subject of 2020 during these past few years, I have my family to thank. Kate, Lila, Cyrus: None of you ever anticipated how much time we would spend together as the world around us trembled and cracked. It's impossible to overstate how much I've depended on your love and laughter through all of this. The singing. The soccer. The long walks with Coco. The cooking. The eating. The excursions. The games. Thank you for being everything to me. This book is dedicated to you.

NOTES

PROLOGUE BREATHE

1. On the relationship between inequality and exposure to the coronavirus and COVID, see Steven Thrasher, *The Viral Underclass* (New York: Celadon, 2022).
2. Lauren Smiley, "27 Days in Tokyo Bay: What Happened on the *Diamond Princess*," *Wired*, April 30, 2020.
3. See Chris Baraniuk, "What the *Diamond Princess* Taught the World About COVID-19," *BMJ* 369 (2020), https://doi.org/10.1136/bmj.m1632.
4. Hitoshi Oshitani, "What Japan Got Right About COVID-19," *New York Times*, January 24, 2022.
5. Kenji Mizumoto et al., "Transmission Potential of the Novel Coronavirus (COVID-19) Onboard the *Diamond Princess* Cruise Ship, 2020," *Infectious Disease Modelling* 5 (2020): 264–70.
6. Thomas Fuller et al., "21 Coronavirus Cases on Cruise Ship Near California," *New York Times*, March 6, 2020.
7. Catherine Kim, "The Trump Administration Doesn't Yet Have a Plan to Handle *Grand Princess* Coronavirus Cases, Officials Say," *Vox*, March 8, 2020.
8. Donald Trump (@realDonaldTrump), "We have a perfectly coordinated and fine tuned plan at the White House for our attack on CoronaVirus," Twitter, March 8, 2020. 8:45 a.m.
9. Kim, "The Trump Administration Doesn't Yet Have a Plan to Handle *Grand Princess* Coronavirus Cases, Officials Say."
10. Mario Koran, "From Paradise to Coronavirus: The *Grand Princess* and the Cruise from Hell," *The Guardian*, March 14, 2020.
11. Abigail Weinberg, "Total Isolation. No Testing. Communication Breakdown. Inside the Coronavirus Cruise Ship Evacuation," *Mother Jones*, March 13, 2020.
12. Mark Berman and Faiz Siddiqui, "*Grand Princess* Passengers Were Quarantined on Bases. How Many Actually Have Coronavirus Will Remain a Mystery," *Washington Post*, March 23, 2020.

13. Ibid.
14. Émile Durkheim, *Suicide* (New York: Free Press, 1951). See especially Chapter 5, "Anomic Suicide."

CHAPTER ONE "IT WAS A BATTLE" (MAY LEE)

1. Sarah Kramer, "Three Generations Under One Roof," *New York Times*, September 23, 2011.
2. Yanzhong Huang, "The SARS Epidemic and Its Aftermath in China: A Political Perspective," in *Learning from SARS: Preparing for the Next Disease Outbreak: Workshop Summary* (Washington, DC: National Academies Press, 2004).
3. David L. Roberts, Jeremy S. Rossman, and Ivan Jarić, "Dating First Cases of COVID-19," *PLOS Pathogens* 17, no. 6 (2021).
4. Wenjun Wang et al., "Using WeChat, a Chinese Social Media App, for Early Detection of the COVID-19 Outbreak in December 2019: Retrospective Study," *JMIR mHealth and uHealth* 8, no. 10 (2020).
5. Kimmy Yam, "Anti-Asian Hate Crimes Increased by Nearly 150% in 2020, Mostly in N.Y. and L.A., New Report Says," NBC News, March 9, 2021.
6. Ayal Feinberg, "Hate Crimes Against Asian Americans Have Been Declining for Years. Will the Coronavirus Change That?," *Washington Post*, April 13, 2020.
7. Ann Dornfeld, "All Seattle Public Schools Closed for at Least Two Weeks Starting Thursday Due to Coronavirus Outbreak," KUOW Public Radio, March 11, 2020.
8. Greg B. Smith, "How NYC Schools Officials Played Down the COVID-19 Threat," *The City*, May 11, 2020.
9. Eliza Shapiro, "New York City Public Schools to Close to Slow Spread of Coronavirus," *New York Times*, March 15, 2020.
10. *New York City's Digital Divide: 500,000 NYC Households Have No Internet Access When It Is More Important Than Ever Before*, New York: Citizens' Committee for Children of New York, 2021.
11. Ibid.
12. Mark Lieberman, "Schools Should Prepare for Coronavirus Outbreaks, CDC Officials Warn," *Education Week*, February 25, 2020.
13. Valerie Strauss, "Senators Press Betsy DeVos on Education Department's Coronavirus Response," *Washington Post*, March 10, 2020.
14. Smith, "How NYC Schools Officials Played Down the COVID-19 Threat."
15. Ibid.
16. Annalise Knudson, "Schools Closed: Here's Where NYC Students Can Get Free Meals," *SI Live*, March 22, 2020.
17. "De Blasio Sounds Confident Note on Opening Schools, as Majority Plan In-Person Learning," NBC News New York, August 10, 2020.
18. United States Centers for Disease Control and Prevention, *Delay or Avoid-*

ance of Medical Care Because of COVID-19–Related Concerns—United States, June 2020; Mark É. Czeisler et al., Morbidity and Mortality Weekly Report 69: 1250–57, Washington, DC: CDC, September 2020.

19. Eliza Shapiro, Dana Rubinstein, and Emma G. Fitzsimmons, "New York City Delays Start of School to Ready for In-Person Classes," New York Times, September 1, 2020.

CHAPTER TWO   INITIAL RESPONSE

1. Zaheer Alam, "The First Fifty Days of COVID-19," Elsevier Public Health Emergency Collection (2020): 1–7; Jeanna Bryner, "1st Known Case of Coronavirus Traced Back to November in China," Live Science, March 14, 2020.

2. Carl Zimmer, Benjamin Mueller, and Chris Buckley, "First Known Covid Case Was Vendor at Wuhan Market, Scientist Says," New York Times, November 18, 2021.

3. Michael Worobey, "Dissecting the Early COVID-19 Cases in Wuhan," Science 6572, no. 374 (2021): 1202–4.

4. Ibid.; Chaolin Huang et al., "Clinical Features of Patients Infected with 2019 Novel Coronavirus in Wuhan, China," The Lancet 395, no. 10223 (February 2020): 497–506.

5. Guobin Yang, The Wuhan Lockdown (New York: Columbia University Press, 2020), p. 10.

6. Disease Outbreak News: COVID-19 China, Geneva: World Health Organization, January 2020.

7. Jon Cohen, "Chinese Researchers Reveal Draft Genome of Virus Implicated in Wuhan Pneumonia Outbreak," Science Insider, January 11, 2020.

8. WHO Statement on Novel Coronavirus in Thailand, Geneva: World Health Organization, January 2020.

9. Susie Neilson and Aylin Woodward, "A Comprehensive Timeline of the Coronavirus Pandemic at 1 Year, from China's First Case to the Present," Business Insider, December 2020. For Taiwan, see Shao-Chung Cheng et al., "First Case of Coronavirus Disease 2019 (COVID-19) Pneumonia in Taiwan," Journal of the Formosan Medical Association 3, no. 119 (2020): 747–51.

10. Greg Hunt, First Confirmed Case of Novel Coronavirus in Australia, Government of Australia, Minister for Health and Aged Care, January 2020, https://www.health.gov.au/ministers/the-hon-greg-hunt-mp/media/first-confirmed-case-of-novel-coronavirus-in-australia; Ryan Rocca, "Canada's 1st Confirmed COVID Case Was Reported in Toronto 2 Years Ago Today," Global News Canada, January 2022, https://globalnews.ca/news/8536383/canadas-1st-covid-case-confirmed-2-years-ago/; David Reid, "UK Confirms Its First Coronavirus Cases," NBC News, January 2020, https://www.cnbc.com/2020/01/31/uk-confirms-two-cases-of-coronavirus.html.

11. See Howard Markel et al., "Nonpharmaceutical Interventions Implemented by US Cities During the 1918–1919 Influenza Pandemic," JAMA 298/6

(2007): 644–54. One of the most important studies of the Great Influenza pandemic of 1918–19, this paper shows how the timing and duration of public health interventions across U.S. cities shaped mortality. The paper's core finding, which has significant implications for COVID-19 response, is that there is "a strong association between early, sustained, and layered application of non-pharmaceutical interventions and mitigating the consequences of the 1918–1919 influenza pandemic in the United States."

12. Didier Fassin, "The Moral Economy of Life in the Pandemic," in Didier Fassin and Marion Fourcade, eds., *Pandemic Exposures: Economy and Society in the Time of Coronavirus* (Chicago: Hau, 2022), pp. 155–75.

13. Sheila Jasanoff et al., *Comparative Covid Response: Crisis, Knowledge, Politics (An Interim Report)* (Cambridge: Harvard School of Government, 2020).

14. World Health Organization (@WHO), "FACT: #COVID19 is NOT airborne. The #coronavirus is mainly transmitted through droplets generated when an infected person coughs, sneezes or speaks," Twitter, March 28, 2020, 2:44 p.m. As of May 2023, the WHO's tweet had attracted 38,600 retweets and 43,200 likes.

15. Gaston Bachelard, *The New Scientific Spirit* (Boston: Beacon Press, 1934; 1984).

16. See Gil Eyal, *The Crisis of Expertise* (Cambridge, UK: Polity Press, 2019).

17. John Horgan, "Will COVID-19 Make Us Less Democratic and More Like China?," *Scientific American*, April 2020.

18. Danielle Allen, *Democracy in the Time of Coronavirus* (Chicago: University of Chicago Press, 2022).

19. Global Health Security Index, "About," GHS Index, https://www.ghs index.org/about/. The medical anthropologist Andrew Lakoff argues that the GHSI was not really designed to measure the preparedness of wealthy, developed nations. Instead, it was set up as part of the WHO's International Health Regulations project of improving "core capacities" of global health security in poor countries, so that donor nations had a tool of evaluation to assess improvement. See Andrew Lakoff, "Preparedness Indicators: Measuring the Condition of Global Health Security," *Sociologica* 15, no. 3 (2021): 25–43.

20. Andrew Lakoff, "Preparing for the Next Emergency," *Public Culture* 19, no. 2 (2007): 247–71.

21. There is a logic for selecting these nations. During the pandemic, policy analysts often argued that countries in East Asia were to contain the virus because they relied on authoritarian political control and widespread cultural dispositions that discouraged dissent. The differences between the "Two Chinas" show that there is more to it than that. Similarly, the vast sociological literature on welfare states and political culture generally groups together the Anglo nations, including Australia, the U.K., and the U.S., in a narrow set of countries where liberalism reigns, social protections are modest, and government regulation is limited. All three were led

by conservative national governments when the pandemic started, and seem poised to respond in similar fashion. But the surprising variation among them points to crucial and consequential differences in the politics of public health.

22. Yang, *The Wuhan Lockdown*, p. 3.
23. Ibid., p. 4.
24. Andrew Green, "Li Wenliang," *The Lancet* 10225, no. 395 (2020): 682.
25. Edward Wong, Julian E. Barnes, and Zolan Kanno-Youngs, "Local Officials in China Hid Coronavirus Dangers from Beijing, U.S. Agencies Find," *New York Times*, August 19, 2020 (updated September 17, 2020).
26. Katherine Mason, "Reflecting on SARS, 17 Years and Two Flu-Like Epidemics Later," *Somatosphere* (blog), March 16, 2020.
27. Richard McGregor, "China's Deep State: The Communist Party and the Coronavirus," *Lowy Institute*, July 2020.
28. Selam Gebrekidan et al., "Ski, Party, Seed a Pandemic: The Travel Rules That Let COVID-19 Take Flight," *New York Times*, September 30, 2020.
29. Frank Snowden, *Epidemics and Society: From the Black Death to the Present* (New Haven: Yale University Press, 2019), pp. 455–56. See also Frank Snowden, "Emerging and Reemerging Diseases: A Historical Perspective," *Immunological Review* 225, no. 1 (2008): 9–26.
30. Paul Farmer, "Social Inequalities and Emerging Infectious Diseases," *Emerging Infectious Diseases* 2, no. 4 (1996): 259–69.
31. Robert Webster, "Wet Markets—A Continuing Source of Severe Acute Respiratory Syndrome and Influenza?," *The Lancet* 363, no. 9404 (2004): 234–36.
32. Yang, *The Wuhan Lockdown*, p. 15.
33. Ibid., pp. 14–16.
34. Marisa Taylor, "Exclusive: U.S. Slashed CDC Staff Inside China Prior to Coronavirus Outbreak," Reuters, March 25, 2020.
35. Lawrence Wright, "The Plague Year," *The New Yorker*, January 4/11, 2021.
36. World Health Organization (@WHO), "Preliminary Investigations Conducted by the Chinese Authorities Have Found No Clear Evidence of Human-to-Human Transmission of the Novel #Coronavirus (2019-nCoV) Identified in #Wuhan, #China," Twitter, January 14, 2020, 6:18 a.m.
37. Yanan Wang and Ken Moritsugu, "Human-to-Human Transmission Confirmed in China Coronavirus," *AP News*, January 20, 2020.
38. "Five Million People Left Wuhan Before the Lockdown: Where Did They Go?," China Global Television Network, January 27, 2020.
39. Shengjie Lai et al., "Effect of Non-Pharmaceutical Interventions to Contain COVID-19 in China," *Nature* 585 (2020): 410–13.
40. Javier Hernández, "China Spins Coronavirus Crisis, Hailing Itself as a Global Leader," *New York Times*, February 28, 2020.
41. *CECC Held a Press Conference and Announced Its Latest Understanding on Developments of the Epidemic, While Urging Citizens to Refrain from Sharing*

Unsubstantiated Information and Hearsay, Government of Taiwan, Ministry of Health and Welfare, December 2019.

42. C. Jason Wang et al., "Response to COVID in Taiwan," *JAMA* 323, no. 14 (2020): 1341–42.

43. Ying-Hen Hsieh et al., "SARS Outbreak, Taiwan, 2003," *Emerging Infectious Diseases* 10, no. 2 (2004): 201–6.

44. *SARS Experience*, Government of Taiwan, Ministry of Health and Welfare, May 2020.

45. *Formalized the Definition of Coronavirus Cases and Reporting & Handling Procedures*, Government of Taiwan, Ministry of Health and Welfare, January 2020.

46. Chih-Wei Hsieh et al., "A Whole-of-Nation Approach to COVID-19: Taiwan's National Epidemic Prevention Team," *International Journal of Political Science* 42, no. 3 (2021): 300–315.

47. Wang et al., "Response to COVID in Taiwan."

48. Cheryl Lin et al., "Policy Decisions and Use of Information Technology to Fight COVID-19, Taiwan," *Emerging Infectious Diseases*, 26, no. 7 (2020): 1506–12.

49. "Taiwanese Man to Be Fined for Not Reporting Viral Symptoms," *Focus Taiwan CNA English News*, January 25, 2020.

50. Lin et al., "Policy Decisions and Use of Information Technology to Fight COVID-19, Taiwan."

51. Rory Daniels, "Taiwan's Unlikely Path to Public Trust Provides Lessons for the US," Brookings Institution, September 15, 2020.

52. Lauren Gardner, "Update January 31: Modeling the Spreading Risk of 2019-nCoV," Johns Hopkins Center for Systems Science and Engineering, January 31, 2020.

53. Lin et al., "Policy Decisions and Use of Information Technology to Fight COVID-19, Taiwan."

54. Tsung-Mei Cheng, "How Has Taiwan Navigated the Pandemic?," *Economics Observatory*, December 2021; Chih-Wei Hsieh et al., "A Whole-of-Nation Approach to COVID-19," 300–315.

55. Hsiang-Yu Yuan et al., "Assessment of the Fatality Rate and Transmissibility Taking Account of Undetected Cases During an Unprecedented COVID-19 Surge in Taiwan," *BMC Infectious Diseases* 22, no. 1 (2022): 1–11.

56. Note that Taiwan is not an OECD nation, but the analysts compared it to OECD countries. See Cheng, "How Has Taiwan Navigated the Pandemic?"

57. Data are from the Johns Hopkins Coronavirus Resource Center, accessed on February 17, 2023, https://coronavirus.jhu.edu/data/mortality.

58. Katharine Murphy, "Dear Michael McCormack: The Only 'Raving Lunatics' Are Those Not Worrying About Climate Change," *The Guardian*, November 11, 2019.

59. Waleed Aly, "Carefree Larrikin Is a Myth. Australians Are Obedient to Authority," *Sydney Morning Herald*, December 17, 2020.

60. Guardian Staff and Australian Associated Press, "Coronavirus: Foreign Arrivals from Mainland China Will Not Be Allowed into Australia, Scott Morrison Says," *The Guardian*, February 1, 2020.

61. Colin Dwyer, "Australia, New Zealand Closing Borders to Foreigners in Bid to Contain Coronavirus," NPR, March 2020.

62. Grace Tobin, "Coronavirus Fires Up Production at Australia's Only Medical Mask Factory," ABC News Australia, March 26, 2020.

63. Melbourne Law School, "VIDEO: COVID-19—What Is Australia's National Cabinet?," University of Melbourne, April 2020.

64. *Australian Health Protection Principal Committee (AHPPC) Advice to National Cabinet on 24 March 2020*, Canberra: Department of Health, March 24, 2020.

65. Colin Packham and Byron Kaye, "Australia Faces New Restrictions as Coronavirus Cases Jump," Reuters, March 23, 2020.

66. Reuters Staff, "Australia Strengthens Self Isolation Rules for Returning Citizens as Coronavirus Spreads," Reuters, March 26, 2020.

67. Damien Cave, "A Lucky Country Says Goodbye to the World's Longest Boom," *New York Times*, March 27, 2020.

68. Colin Packham and Jonathan Barrett, "Growth in Australia Coronavirus Cases Slows, but Experts Urge Caution," Reuters, March 30, 2020.

69. Damian Cave, "The Secret Powers of an Australian Prime Minister, Now Revealed," *New York Times*, August 16, 2022.

70. Abbie Bray, "Good Morning Britain Flooded with Almost 300 Ofcom Complaints After Piers Morgan 'Mocks Chinese People,'" *Metro UK*, January 22, 2020.

71. Sam Phan, "The Coronavirus Panic Is Turning the UK into a Hostile Environment for East Asians," *The Guardian*, January 27, 2020.

72. "Coronavirus Will Be Here for Some Months, Says Health Secretary," BBC, February 3, 2020.

73. *Prime Minister's Statement on Coronavirus (COVID-19): 9 March 2020*, London: Office of the Prime Minister, March 2020.

74. "Explainer: 'Nudge Unit,'" Institute for Government, March 2020.

75. Benjamin Mueller, "As Europe Shuts Down, Britain Takes a Different, and Contentious, Approach," *New York Times*, March 13, 2020.

76. UK Behavioural Scientists, "Open Letter to the UK Government Regarding COVID-19," March 2020.

77. Mark Landler and Stephen Castle, "Behind the Virus Report That Jarred the U.S. and the U.K. to Action," *New York Times*, March 23, 2020.

78. Ed Yong, "The U.K.'s Coronavirus 'Herd Immunity' Debacle," *The Atlantic*, March 2020.

79. Mark Landler and Stephen Castle, "Britain Placed Under a Virtual Lockdown by Boris Johnson," *New York Times*, March 23, 2020; "Coronavirus: Strict New Curbs on Life in UK Announced by PM," BBC, March 24, 2020.

80. Angela Dewan and Sarah Dean, "Coronavirus Strikes UK Prime Minister Boris Johnson, His Health Secretary and His Chief Medical Adviser," CNN, March 27, 2020.
81. "Coronavirus: Boris Johnson Moved to Intensive Care as Symptoms Worsen," BBC, April 7, 2020.
82. Nick Paton Walsh and Mick Krever, "The UK's 'Coronavirus Dashboard' May be Under-Reporting Deaths Significantly," CNN, April 7, 2020.
83. "UK Has Second-Highest Coronavirus Death Toll in Europe, New Figures Show," CNBC, April 29, 2020.
84. See the BBC's coverage of the House of Commons report: Nick Triggle, "Covid: UK's Early Response Worst Public Health Failure Ever, MPs Say," BBC, October 12, 2021; and UK House of Commons, Health and Social Care, and Science and Technology Committees, *Coronavirus: Lessons Learned to Date*, Report no. 6, London: September 2021.
85. Nicholas Fandos and Michael D. Shear, "Trump Impeached for Abuse of Power and Obstruction of Congress," *New York Times*, December 18, 2019.
86. Ibid.
87. Matthew Belvedere, "Trump Says He Trusts China's Xi on Coronavirus and the US Has It 'Totally Under Control,'" CNBC, January 22, 2020.
88. Bob Woodward, *Rage* (New York: Simon & Schuster, 2020), p. 17.
89. Philip Bump, "What Trump Did About Coronavirus in February," *Washington Post*, April 20, 2020.
90. Ibid., p. 22.
91. Isaac Stanley-Becker and Laura Sun, "Senior CDC Official Who Met Trump's Wrath for Raising Concerns About Coronavirus to Resign," *Washington Post*, May 7, 2021.
92. Philip Bump, "What Trump Did About Coronavirus in February," *Washington Post*, April 20, 2020.
93. Bruno Latour, *Down to Earth: Politics in the New Climate Regime* (Medford, MA: Polity Press), p. 3.
94. Ibid., p. 7.
95. Jon Cohen, "The United States Badly Bungled Coronavirus Testing—But Things May Soon Improve," *Science*, February 28, 2020.
96. Andrew Jacobs, Matt Richtel, and Mike Baker, "'At War with No Ammo': Doctors Say Shortage of Protective Gear Is Dire," *New York Times*, March 19, 2020.
97. Ibid.
98. Kerry Breen, "NYC Hospital Responds to Photos of Nurses Wearing Trash Bags as Gowns," *Today*, March 27, 2020.
99. Jeanne Whalen et al., "Scramble for Medical Equipment Descends into Chaos as U.S. States and Hospitals Compete for Rare Supplies," *Washington Post*, March 24, 2020.
100. Neil Irwin, "Coronavirus Shows the Problem with Trump's Stock Market Boasting," *New York Times*, February 26, 2020.

101. Pippa Stevens, Maggie Fitzgerald, and Fred Imbert, "Stock Market Live Thursday: Dow Tanks 2,300 in Worst Day Since Black Monday, S&P 500 Bear Market," CNBC, March 12, 2020.

102. "Trump Declares National Emergency over Coronavirus," BBC, March 13, 2020.

103. Dan Mangan, "Trump Issues 'Coronavirus Guidelines' for Next 15 Days to Slow Pandemic," CNBC, March 16, 2020.

104. Caitlin McCabe, Anna Hirtenstein, and Chong Koh Ping, "Dow Plummets Nearly 3,000 Points as Virus Fears Spread," *Wall Street Journal*, March 16, 2020.

105. Catie Edmondson, "5 Key Things in the $2 Trillion Coronavirus Stimulus Package," *New York Times*, March 25, 2020.

106. Sarah Mervosh, Denise Lu, and Vanessa Swales, "See Which States and Cities Have Told Residents to Stay at Home," *New York Times*, April 20, 2020.

107. Maggie Haberman and David Sanger, "Trump Says Coronavirus Cure Cannot 'Be Worse Than the Problem Itself,'" *New York Times*, March 23, 2020.

108. Chris Cillizza, "The Florida Governor Just Got Called Out over His Handling of Coronavirus," CNN, March 23, 2020.

109. Griff Witte, "South Dakota's Governor Resisted Ordering People to Stay Home. Now It Has One of the Nation's Largest Coronavirus Hot Spots," *Washington Post*, April 13, 2020.

110. Will Feuer, "US Coronavirus Cases Top 200,000 as Virus Spreads and Testing Ramps Up," CNBC, April 1, 2020.

111. Kevin Liptak et al., "Trump Says He Wants the Country 'Opened Up and Just Raring to Go by Easter,' Despite Health Experts' Warnings," CNN, March 24, 2020.

112. Aaron Rupar, "Trump's Dangerous 'LIBERATE' Tweets Represent the Views of a Small Minority," *Vox*, April 17, 2020.

113. Mike Pence, "There Isn't a Coronavirus 'Second Wave,'" *Wall Street Journal*, June 16, 2020.

CHAPTER THREE "TWENTY-FOUR HOURS A DAY" (SOPHIA ZAYAS)

1. *At Novel Coronavirus Briefing, Governor Cuomo Announces State Is Partnering with Hospitals to Expand Novel Coronavirus Testing Capacity in New York*, video, audio, photos, and rush transcript, New York State Office of the Governor, March 2, 2020.

2. Ross Barkan, "A Brief History of the Cuomo–de Blasio Feud," *The Nation*, April 17, 2020.

3. Ezra Klein, "Coronavirus Will Also Cause a Loneliness Epidemic," *Vox*, March 12, 2020.

4. Catherine K. Ettman et al., "Prevalence of Depression Symptoms in US Adults Before and During the COVID-19 Pandemic," *JAMA Network Open* 3, no. 9 (2020).

5. Alison Abbott, "COVID's Mental-Health Toll: How Scientists Are Tracking a Surge in Depression," *Nature*, February 3, 2021.

6. Luis Ferré-Sadurní and Joseph Goldstein, "1st Vaccination in U.S. Is Given in New York, Hard Hit in Outbreak's First Days," *New York Times*, December 14, 2020.

7. *Governor Cuomo and Mayor de Blasio Announce Mass Vaccination Site at Yankee Stadium to Open Friday*, New York State Office of the Governor, February 3, 2021.

8. Troy Closson, "Vaccination Rate Lags in N.Y.C. as Disparities Persist," *New York Times*, May 6, 2021; Mihir Zaveri, "New ZIP Code Data Reflects Disparities in N.Y.C.'s Vaccination Effort, Officials Say," *New York Times*, February 16, 2021. By May 2021, less than 30 percent of the Bronx population had been fully vaccinated: Rocco Vertuccio, "Bronx Vaccination Rates Still Lowest in the City," *New York 1 News*, May 13, 2021.

CHAPTER FOUR   TRUST

1. Gil Eyal, *The Crisis of Expertise* (Cambridge, UK: Polity Press, 2019), p. 43.

2. Paul Karp and Ben Doherty, "Coronavirus: Mass Events and Foreign Travel Should Be Cancelled, Says Australian Government," *The Guardian*, March 13, 2020.

3. Luke Henriques-Gomes, "Australians' Trust in Governments Surges to 'Extraordinary' High Amid Covid," *The Guardian*, December 16, 2020.

4. "Scott Morrison Defends Decision to Attend Rugby League Game During Coronavirus Outbreak—Video," *The Guardian*, March 13, 2020.

5. Caroline Overington, "Scott Morrison Enjoying a Beer at the Footy While Victorians Grapple with COVID Lockdown Is Not a Good Look," *Australian*, July 12, 2020; Max Laughton, " 'I'm Still Going to the Footy': ScoMo's Weird Take After Announcing Crowd Ban Plan," Fox Sports, March 13, 2020.

6. David Speers, "Scott Morrison's 'F-Word' Misread the Public Mood on the Coronavirus Pandemic," ABC News, March 14, 2020.

7. Ibid.

8. Dawn Kopecki, "CDC Recommends Canceling Events with 50 or More People for the Next Eight Weeks Throughout US," CNBC, March 16, 2020.

9. "March 2020: Dr. Anthony Fauci Talks with Dr. Jon LaPook About COVID-19," *60 Minutes*, YouTube video, 1:27, March 8, 2020, https://www.youtube.com/watch?app=desktop&v=PRa6t_e7dgI&ab_channel=60Minutes.

10. Karl Weick and Kathleen Sutcliffe, *Managing the Unexpected: Resilient Performance in an Age of Uncertainty* (Hoboken, NJ: John Wiley & Sons, 2011). Also see Chris Ansell and Arjen Boin, "Taming Deep Uncertainty: The Potential of Pragmatist Principles for Understanding and Improving Stra-

tegic Crisis Management," *Administration & Society* 51, no. 7 (2017): 1079–1112.

11. P. Sol Hart, Sedona Chinn, and Stuart Soroka, "Politicization and Polarization in COVID-19 News Coverage," *Science Communication* 42, no. 5 (2020): 679–97; Julie Jiang et al., "Political Polarization Drives Online Conversations About COVID-19 in the United States," *Human Behavior and Emerging Technologies* 2, no. 3 (2020): 200–211.

12. Tamara Qiblawi and Caroll Alvardo, "Ukrainian Males Aged 18–60 Are Banned from Leaving the Country, Zelensky Says in New Declaration," CNN, February 25, 2022.

13. Led By Donkeys (@ByDonkeys), " 'Follow the rules,' " Twitter, May 25, 2022, 11:54 a.m.

14. Daisy Fancourt, Andrew Steptoe, and Liam Wright, "The Cummings Effect: Politics, Trust, and Behaviours During the COVID-19 Pandemic," *The Lancet* 396, no. 10249 (2020): 464–65.

15. Ibid.

16. Adrian O'Dowd, "COVID-19: Johnson Is on Back Foot over Next Steps to Control Pandemic," *BMJ* 369 (2020): m2152.

17. Jen Gaskell, et al., "Public Trust and COVID-19," *Trustgov*, July 29, 2020.

18. "Partygate: A Timeline of the Lockdown Gatherings," BBC News, May 19, 2022; Mark Landler, Stephen Castle, and Megan Specia, "Johnson Says He's Humbled by 'Partygate' Report but Will Go On," *New York Times*, May 25, 2022.

19. William Booth and Karla Adam, "U.K. 'Partygate' Investigation Ends with 126 Fines, No Further Citations for Boris Johnson," *Washington Post*, May 19, 2022.

20. Martin Farrer, " 'Failure of Leadership': What the Papers Say About Johnson and the Sue Gray Partygate Report," *The Guardian*, May 25, 2022.

21. "Romania: Ministers Flout Protective Measures," *Euro Topics*, June 2, 2020.

22. German Lopez, "Why New York Has 14 Times as Many Coronavirus Deaths as California," *Vox*, April 13, 2020.

23. Ibid.

24. *CDPH Guidance for the Prevention of COVID-19 Transmission for Gatherings*, California Department of Public Health, Health and Human Services Agency, September 2020.

25. *Guidance for Private Gatherings*, California Department of Public Health, Health and Human Services Agency, October 2020.

26. Miriam Pawel, "Opinion: Gavin Newsom, What Were You Thinking?," *New York Times*, November 25, 2020.

27. Tejal Rao, "Why Was Newsom's French Laundry Moment Such a Big Deal? Our California Restaurant Critic Explains," *New York Times*, September 14, 2021; Taryn Luna, "Photos Raise Doubts About Newsom's Claim That Dinner with Lobbyist Was Outdoors Amid COVID-19 Surge," *Los Angeles Times*, November 18, 2020.

28. "California Gov. Newsom Announces New COVID-19 Restrictions," ABC News San Diego, November 16, 2020.

29. Pawel, "Opinion: Gavin Newsom, What Were You Thinking?"

30. "Tucker Carlson: Gavin Newsom's French Laundry Birthday Dinner Goes Beyond Mere Hypocrisy," Fox News, November 18, 2020.

31. Meghan Roos, "What the French Laundry Has to Do with Gavin Newsom's Recall Election," *Newsweek*, September 9, 2021.

32. Carla Marinucci, "French Laundry Snafu Reignites Longshot Newsom Recall Drive," *Politico*, November 25, 2020; Mark DiCamillo, "Voters Now Much More Critical of Governor Newsom's Performance," University of California Berkeley, Institute of Governmental Studies, Release #2021-01.

33. Jill Cowan, "How Much Was Spent on the Recall? One Estimate: Nearly Half a Billion Dollars," *New York Times*, September 15, 2021.

34. Dali L. Yang, "Wuhan Officials Tried to Cover Up COVID-19—and Sent It Careening Outward," *Washington Post*, March 10, 2020.

35. Uri Friedman, "The Coronavirus-Denial Movement Now Has a Leader," *The Atlantic*, March 27, 2020.

36. Natalie Colarossi, "8 Times World Leaders Downplayed the Coronavirus and Put Their Countries at Greater Risk for Infection," *Business Insider*, April 11, 2020; "Governor Cuomo Admits to Withholding Nursing Home Deaths," BBC News, February 16, 2021.

37. Sarah Evanega et al., *Coronavirus Misinformation: Quantifying Sources and Themes in the COVID-19 "Infodemic,"* New York: Cornell University, The Cornell Alliance for Science, 2020; *Novel Coronavirus(2019-nCoV) Situation Report #13*, Geneva: World Health Organization, February 2020, p. 2.

38. See Bob Woodward, *Rage* (New York: Simon & Schuster, 2020), p. 17.

39. Donald Trump (@realDonaldTrump), "we now have the lowest Fatality (Mortality) Rate in the World," Twitter, July 6, 2020, 4:17 p.m.

40. Christian Paz, "All the President's Lies About the Coronavirus," *The Atlantic*, November 2, 2020.

41. Evanega et al., *Coronavirus Misinformation: Quantifying Sources and Themes in the COVID-19 "Infodemic."*

42. Lauren Egan, "Trump Calls Coronavirus Democrats' New Hoax," NBC News, February 28, 2020.

43. Sheera Frenkel, "The Most Influential Spreader of Coronavirus Misinformation Online," *New York Times*, July 24, 2021.

44. Barbara Feder Ostrov, "Cue the Debunking: Two Bakersfield Doctors Go Viral with Dubious COVID Test Conclusions," *Cal Matters*, April 27, 2020.

45. Quint Forgey, "'Fauci's a Disaster': Trump Attacks Health Officials in Fiery Campaign Call," *Politico*, October 19, 2020.

46. Kate Bennett and Evan Perez, "Nation's Top Coronavirus Expert Dr. Anthony Fauci Forced to Beef Up Security as Death Threats Increase," CNN, April 2, 2020.

47. Aaron Blake, "Republicans' Disregard for Doctors on the Coronavirus," *Washington Post*, December 7, 2021.

48. Kevin Vallier, "Why Are Americans So Distrustful of Each Other?," *Wall Street Journal*, December 17, 2020.

49. Cailey Griffin and Amy Mackinnon, "Report: Corruption in U.S. at Worst Levels in Almost a Decade," *Foreign Policy*, January 28, 2021.

50. Kevin Vallier, *Trust in a Polarized Age* (New York: Oxford University Press, 2021).

51. Vallier, "Why Are Americans So Distrustful of Each Other?"

52. "Partisan Antipathy: More Intense, More Personal," Pew Research Center, October 10, 2019.

53. Wendy Wang, "The Partisan Marriage Gap Is Bigger Than Ever," *The Hill*, October 27, 2020.

54. Cass Sunstein, *#Republic: Divided Democracy in the Age of Social Media* (Princeton: Princeton University Press, 2016).

55. Levi Boxell, Matthew Gentzkow, and Jesse M. Shapiro, "Is the Internet Causing Political Polarization? Evidence from Demographics," National Bureau of Economic Research, Working Paper no. 23258 (2017).

56. Beth Simone Noveck et al., "The Power of Virtual Communities," GovLab at NYU Tandon School of Engineering, February 2021.

57. Sarah Perez, "Coronavirus-Related Facebook Support Groups Reach 4.5M in US as Misinformation and Conspiracies Spread," *TechCrunch*, April 21, 2020.

58. Saiful Islam et al., "COVID-19–Related Infodemic and Its Impact on Public Health: A Global Social Media Analysis," *The American Journal of Tropical Medicine and Hygiene* 103, no. 4 (2021): 1621.

59. Rebecca Storen and Nikki Corrigan, *COVID-19: A Chronology of State and Territory Government Announcements (Up Until 30 June 2020)*. Parliament of Australia, Department of Parliamentary Services, Research Paper Series, 2020–21, Canberra, October 2020.

60. Michael McGowan, "Where 'Freedom' Meets the Far Right: The Hate Messages Infiltrating Australian Anti-Lockdown Protests," *The Guardian*, March 25, 2021.

61. Damien Cave, "How Australia Saved Thousands of Lives While Covid Killed a Million Americans," *New York Times*, May 15, 2022.

62. Ibid.

63. Ibid.

CHAPTER FIVE "NOTHING LEFT TO LOSE" (DANIEL PRESTI)

1. Bill de Blasio (@BilldeBlasio), "Since I'm encouraging New Yorkers to go on with your lives + get out on the town despite Coronavirus, I thought I would offer some suggestions. Here's the first: thru Thurs 3/5 go see "The Traitor"

@FilmLinc. If "The Wire" was a true story + set in Italy, it would be this film," Twitter, March 2, 2020, 8:16 p.m.

2. New York Times Editorial Board, "New York City to Close Schools, Restaurants and Bars," *New York Times*, March 15, 2020.

3. Dana Rubinstein and Scott Piccoli, "N.Y.C. Enters Phase 4, but Restaurants and Bars Are Left Behind," *New York Times*, July 20, 2020.

4. Tanay Warerkar, "A Timeline of COVID-19's Impact on NYC's Restaurant Industry," *Eater*, December 30, 2020.

5. John Del Signore, "State Cracks Down on Staten Island Tavern Declaring Itself an 'Autonomous Zone' Free from COVID Restrictions," *Gothamist*, November 29, 2020.

6. George Joseph, "'Autonomous Zone' Bar Owner Allegedly Drove into Sheriff's Deputy While Evading Arrest. DA Doesn't Seek Bail," *Gothamist*, December 8, 2020.

7. Ganesh Setty and Leah Asmelash, "A Staten Island Bar Manager Hit a Deputy with His Car While Trying to Escape Arrest, NYC Sheriff's Office Says," CNN, December 7, 2020.

8. Kevin Sheehan, Tina Moore, and Aaron Feis, "Lawyer Says Sheriff Allegedly Rammed by NYC Bar Owner's SUV Is Lying About Broken Legs," *New York Post*, December 7, 2020.

9. Daniel Presti (@DannyPresti), "It's just about time to nut up or shut up here in NYC. We're going to find out who really wants to fight for their freedom and what you're willing to sacrifice. This is where we make our stand. I'm all in," Twitter, August 21, 2021, 8:41 a.m.; Daniel Presti (@DannyPresti), "School is about to start here in NY soon. If your child is healthy and you are complying with sending them in with masks, you are part of the problem. Don't tell me there are no options. We all have a choice . . . Fight back," Twitter, August 30, 2021, 1:44 p.m.

10. Frank Donnelly, "In Latest Battle with City, Grant City Bar's Manager and His Lawyer File Suit, Alleging Defamation and False Imprisonment," *SILive*, July 9, 2021.

11. Kimiko de Freytas-Tamura, "A Hospital Finds an Unlikely Group Opposing Vaccination: Its Workers," *New York Times*, August 22, 2021.

12. Daniel Presti (@DannyPresti), "I am neither left nor right. Start seeing the problems we have in life are manufactured from government, and its both sides. How many more judges have to rule against us? How many more rigged elections do we have to witness? It's all decided ahead of time. Until we all say No.," Twitter, September 16, 2021, 4:55 p.m.

13. Donnelly, "In Latest Battle with City, Grant City Bar's Manager and His Lawyer File Suit, Alleging Defamation and False Imprisonment."

14. Daniel Presti (@DannyPresti), "NYC is on the verge of collapse," Twitter, October 20, 2021, 11:44 a.m.

15. Leeroy Johnson (@LeeroyPress), "At the protest against mandates held by the #FDNY at Gracie Mansion In NYC, the home of Mayor Bill De Blasio.

Danny Presti from Mac's public house in Staten Island. Protesters brought bags of Garbage to Gracie Mansion and left it at the Doorstep of Mayor De blasio #NYC #NY," Twitter, October 28, 2021, 1:57 p.m.

16. Luis Ferré-Sadurní and Jonah E. Bromwich, "Andrew Cuomo Is Charged in Sexual Misconduct Complaint," *New York Times*, October 28, 2021.

17. Daniel Presti (@DannyPresti). "Too many people still think we worry about dying from covid," Twitter, October 4, 2021, 9:01 a.m.

CHAPTER SIX THE MEANING OF MASKS

1. Paula Trubisky, Stella Ting-Toomey, and Sung-Ling Lin, "The Influence of Individualism-Collectivism and Self-Monitoring on Conflict Styles," *International Journal of Intercultural Relations* 15, no. 1 (1991): 65–84, https://doi.org/10.1016/0147-1767(91)90074-Q.

2. In a paper about culture and mask use during the COVID-19 pandemic, a group of American and Chinese scholars led by the MIT social psychologist Jackson Lu explains that "people in collectivistic cultures are more likely to agree with statements like 'I usually sacrifice my self-interest for the benefit of my group' and 'My happiness depends very much on the happiness of those around me,' whereas people in individualistic cultures are more likely to agree with statements like 'I often do my own thing' and 'What happens to me is my own doing.'" Jackson Lu, Peter Jin, and Alexander S. English, "Collectivism Predicts Mask Use During COVID-19," *Proceedings of the National Academy of Sciences* 118, no. 23 (2021): e2021793118.

3. Jordan Sand, "We Share What We Exhale: A Short Cultural History of Mask-Wearing," *Times Literary Supplement*, May 1, 2020.

4. Christos Lynteris, "Plague Masks: The Visual Emergence of Anti-Epidemic Personal Protection Equipment," *Medical Anthropology* 37, no. 6 (2018): 442–57.

5. K. F. Cheng and P. C. Leung, "What Happened in China During the 1918 Influenza Pandemic?," *International Journal of Infectious Diseases* 11, no. 4 (2007): 360–64.

6. Christine Hauser, "The Mask Slackers of 1918," *New York Times*, August 3, 2020.

7. Brian Dolan, "Unmasking History: Who Was Behind the Anti-Mask League Protests During the 1918 Influenza Epidemic in San Francisco?," *Perspectives in Medical Humanities* (2020).

8. Yella Hewings-Martin, "How Do SARS and MERS Compare with COVID-19?," *Medical News Today*, April 10, 2020.

9. Ellen Nakashima, "SARS Signals Missed in Hong Kong," *Washington Post*, May 20, 2003.

10. *How SARS Changed the World in Less Than Six Months*, World Health Organization, News Bulletin 81/8, 2003.

11. Ibid.

12. Ibid.
13. Gil Eyal, "Futures Present: The Pandemic and the Crisis of Expertise," New School India China Institute, January 27, 2021.
14. Ebony Bowden and Bruce Golding, "Trump Administration Weighs Legal Action over Alleged Chinese Hoarding of PPE," *New York Post*, April 5, 2020; Yanqiu Rachel Zhou, "The Global Effort to Tackle the Coronavirus Face Mask Shortage," *US News*, March 18, 2020.
15. "Japan to Give Two Masks Each to 50 Million Households to Fight Virus," *Japan Times*, April 2, 2020.
16. E. Tammy Kim, "How South Korea Solved Its Face Mask Shortage," *New York Times*, April 1, 2020.
17. Jacqueline Howard, "WHO Stands by Recommendation to Not Wear Masks If You Are Not Sick or Not Caring for Someone Who Is Sick," CNN, March 31, 2020.
18. *Disease Outbreak News, Pneumonia of Unknown Cause—China*, World Health Organization, January 5, 2020.
19. *Disease Outbreak News, COVID-19—China*, World Health Organization, January 12, 2020.
20. *Newsroom Questions and Answers, Emergencies: International Health Regulations and Emergency Committees*, World Health Organization, December 19, 2019.
21. *Statement on the First Meeting of the International Health Regulations (2005) Emergency Committee Regarding the Outbreak of Novel Coronavirus (2019-nCoV)*, World Health Organization, January 23, 2020.
22. Michael Collins, "The WHO and China: Dereliction of Duty," Council on Foreign Relations, February 27, 2020.
23. *Statement on the Second Meeting of the International Health Regulations (2005) Emergency Committee Regarding the Outbreak of Novel Coronavirus (2019-nCoV)*, World Health Organization, January 30, 2020.
24. Deborah Netburn, "A Timeline of the CDC's Advice on Face Masks," *Los Angeles Times*, July 27, 2021.
25. Jon Cohen, "Not Wearing Masks to Protect Against Coronavirus Is a 'Big Mistake,' Top Chinese Scientist Says," *Science*, March 27, 2020.
26. Robert Tait, "Czechs Get to Work Making Masks After Government Decree," *The Guardian*, March 30, 2020.
27. Antonia Noori Farzan, "A Border City Is Handing Out $1,000 Fines for Those Who Don't Cover Their Faces," *Washington Post*, April 3, 2020.
28. Jacqueline Howard, "WHO Stands by Recommendation to Not Wear Masks If You Are Not Sick or Not Caring for Someone Who Is Sick," CNN, March 31, 2020.
29. Abby Goodnough and Knvul Sheikh, "C.D.C. Weighs Advising Everyone to Wear a Mask," *New York Times*, March 31, 2020.
30. Neeltje van Doremalen et al., "Aerosol and Surface Stability of SARS-CoV-2 as Compared with SARS-CoV-1," *New England Journal of Medicine* 382 (2020): 1564–67.

31. Colin Dwyer and Allison Aubrey, "CDC Now Recommends Americans Consider Wearing Cloth Face Coverings in Public," NPR, April 3, 2020.

32. "Donald Trump Coronavirus Briefing Transcript April 3: New CDC Face Mask Recommendations," *Rev*, April 3, 2020.

33. Dominique Petruzzi, "To What Extent Are Face Masks Effective for Preventing the Spread of Coronavirus?," *Statista*, February 2, 2022.

34. Dan Diamond, "Pence Flouts Hospital Policy, Goes Maskless in Mayo Clinic Visit," *Politico*, April 28, 2020.

35. Jun Lang, W. W. Erickson, and Z. Jing-Schmidt, "#MaskOn! #Mask Off! Digital Polarization of Mask-Wearing in the United States During COVID-19," *PLOS ONE* 16, no. 4 (2021): e0250817.

36. Claudia Deane, Kim Parker, and John Gramlich, "A Year of U.S. Public Opinion on the Coronavirus Pandemic," Pew Research Center, March 5, 2021.

37. Vicky McKeever, "Most Brits Just Won't Wear Face Masks—Here's Why," CNBC, July 15, 2020.

38. Chris Anderson and Sara Hobolt, "No Partisan Divide in Willingness to Wear Masks in the UK," London School of Economics, November 18, 2020.

39. Candice Jaimungal, "Mask Mandates Remain Popular Among Most Americans," YouGov, July 30, 2020.

40. Émile Durkheim and Marcel Mauss, *Primitive Classification* (Chicago: University of Chicago Press, 1963), pp. 17–18.

41. Renyi Zhang et al., "Identifying Airborne Transmission as the Dominant Route for the Spread of COVID-19," *PNAS* 117, no. 26 (May 2020): 14857–63.

42. Apoorva Mandavilli, "W.H.O. Finally Endorses Masks to Prevent Coronavirus Transmission," *New York Times*, June 5, 2020.

43. "Tucker Carlson: The Cult of Mask-Wearing Grows, with No Evidence They Work," Fox News, October 13, 2020.

44. "Howard Plays Viral Videos of People Refusing to Wear a Face Mask," *The Howard Stern Show*, YouTube video, 3:17, June 16, 2020, https://www.youtube.com/watch?v=7dFz4sJ5RPs.

45. "Home Depot Face Mask Dispute Turns Violent," *NowThisNews*, YouTube video, 3:35, July 9, 2020, https://www.youtube.com/watch?v=u0F8_hIitpU.

46. "Video Shows Customer's Racist Mask Rant After Refusing to Cover Her Face in California Starbucks," NBC News, YouTube video, 1:22, October 20, 2020, https://www.youtube.com/watch?v=nZOh5bjYi0U.

47. "Lyft Passenger Goes on Racist Rant . . . After Being Asked to Wear a Mask," TMZ, June 19, 2020.

48. "Customer Is Kicked Out of Costco for Refusing to Wear a Mask," *The Daily Mail*, Facebook, May 21, 2020. https://www.facebook.com/watch/?v=688506455271433.

49. "Personal Measures Taken to Avoid COVID-19," YouGov, March 17, 2020.

50. Michael McGowan, "How Victoria's Covid Lockdown Protests Are Galvanising Australia's Right," *The Guardian*, September 18, 2020; Nicole Bogart, "Anti-Mask Rallies Held Across Canada Despite Increased Support for Mandatory Masks," CTV News, July 20, 2020; "Coronavirus: Thousands Protest in Germany Against Restrictions," BBC News, August 1, 2020.

51. Peter Wade, "Trump Campaign Staff: 'You Get Made Fun of If You Wear a Mask,'" *Rolling Stone*, July 10, 2020; Daniel Victor, Lew Serviss, and Azi Paybarah, "In His Own Words, Trump on the Coronavirus and Masks," *New York Times*, October 2, 2020.

CHAPTER SEVEN   "SOMETHING'S MISSING IN MY SOUL"
(ENUMA MENKITI)

1. Michael Winerip and Michael Schwirtz, "Rikers: Where Mental Illness Meets Brutality in Jail," *New York Times*, July 14, 2014.

CHAPTER EIGHT   THE PROBLEM OF DISTANCING

1. Gagandeep Kaur, "Banished for Menstruating: The Indian Women Isolated While They Bleed," *The Guardian*, December 22, 2015.

2. Eugenia Tognotti, "Lessons from the History of Quarantine, from Plague to Influenza A," *Emerging Infectious Diseases* 19, no. 2 (2013): 254–59.

3. Tara John and Ben Wederman, "Italy Prohibits Travel and Cancels All Public Events in Its Northern Region to Contain Coronavirus," CNN, March 8, 2020.

4. Aude Mazoue, "In Pictures: A Look Back, One Year After France Went into Lockdown," France 24, March 17, 2021.

5. Robert Glass et al., "Targeted Social Distancing Design for Pandemic Influenza," *Emerging Infectious Diseases* 12, no. 11 (2006): 1671–81.

6. Howard Markel, Harvey B. Lipman, and Alexander Navarro, "Nonpharmaceutical Interventions Implemented by US Cities During the 1918–1919 Influenza Pandemic," *JAMA* 298, no. 6 (2007): 644–54.

7. *Transcript for CDC Media Telebriefing: Update on 2019 Novel Coronavirus (2019-nCoV)*, Atlanta: U.S. Department of Health and Human Services, Centers for Disease Control and Prevention, 2020.

8. Ibid.

9. Noah Higgins-Dunn and Will Feuer, "Cuomo Orders Most New Yorkers to Stay Inside—'We're All Under Quarantine Now,'" CNBC, March 20, 2020.

10. "Coronavirus Updates from March 28, 2020," CBS News, March 28, 2020; Bill Mahoney and Josh Gerstein, "Rhode Island Ends Specific Restrictions on New Yorkers—By Making Them National," *Politico*, March 29, 2020.

11. Wei Lyu and George L. Wehby, "Shelter-in-Place Orders Reduced COVID-19 Mortality and Reduced the Rate of Growth in Hospitaliza-

tions," *Health Affairs* 39, no. 9 (2020); Charles Courtemanche et al., "Strong Social Distancing Measures in the United States Reduced the COVID-19 Growth Rate," *Health Affairs* 39, no. 7 (2020); Oguzhan Alagoz et al., "Effect of Timing of and Adherence to Social Distancing Measures on COVID-19 Burden in the United States: A Simulation Modeling Approach," *Annals of Internal Medicine* 174, no. 1 (2021): 50–57.

12. André Aleman and Iris Sommer, "The Silent Danger of Social Distancing," *Psychological Medicine* (July 6, 2020): 1–2; Katie Lewis, "Psychotherapy COVID-19: Preliminary Data on the Impact of Social Distancing on Loneliness and Mental Health," *Journal of Psychiatric Practice* 26, no. 5 (2020): 400–404; Esther Crawley et al., "Wider Collateral Damage to Children in the UK Because of the Social Distancing Measures Designed to Reduce the Impact of COVID-19 in Adults," *BMJ Paediatrics Open* 4, no. 1 (2020); Per Engzell, Arun Frey, and Mark Verhagen, "Learning Loss Due to School Closures During the COVID-19 Pandemic," *Proceedings of the National Academy of Sciences* 118, no. 17 (2021).

13. Pamela E. Klassen, "Why Religious Freedom Stokes Coronavirus Protests in the U.S., but Not Canada," *The Conversation*, May 2020.

14. As of April 2022, two men had pled guilty to charges in the case and two men had been acquitted. Neil MacFarquhar, "Member of Extremist Group Pleads Guilty in Michigan Governor Kidnapping Plot," *New York Times*, January 27, 2021; Mitch Smith, "Two Men Acquitted of Plotting to Kidnap Michigan Governor in High-Profile Trial," *New York Times*, April 8, 2022.

15. Farhad Manjoo, "I Traced My COVID-19 Bubble and It's Enormous," *New York Times*, November 20, 2020.

16. Kevin Quealy, "The Richest Neighborhoods Emptied Out Most as Coronavirus Hit New York City," *New York Times*, May 15, 2020.

17. "Over 333,000 New Yorkers Have Left City Since COVID Pandemic Began in March," *CBS New York*, January 8, 2021.

18. The Department of Homeland Security text is here: U.S. Department of Homeland Security, Cybersecurity & Infrastructure Security Agency, *Memorandum on Identification of Essential Critical Infrastructure Workers During COVID-19 Response*, Washington, DC, March 2020. Also see Andrew Lakoff, "'The Supply Chain Must Continue': Becoming Essential in the Pandemic Emergency," *Items*, November 2020.

19. Ayman El-Mohandes et al., "COVID-19: A Barometer for Social Justice in New York City," *The American Journal of Public Health* 110, no. 111 (2020): 1656–58.

20. Y-H Chen et al., "Excess Mortality Associated with the COVID-19 Pandemic Among Californians 18–65 Years of Age, by Occupational Sector and Occupation: March Through November 2020," *PLOS ONE* 16, no. 6 (2021): e0252454.

21. On farmworker demographics, see U.S. Department of Agriculture, Economic Research Service, *Farm Labor*, Washington, DC, March 2022. On the

ethnicity of farm workers, see The National Center for Farmworker Health, *Agricultural Worker Demographics*, Texas, April 2018.

22. Eugene Scott, "Trump's Most Insulting—and Violent—Language Is Often Reserved for Immigrants," *Washington Post*, October 2, 2019.

23. *US: New Report Shines Spotlight on Abuses and Growth in Immigrant Detention Under Trump*, Human Rights Watch, New York, NY.

24. *United Farm Workers of America, Micaela Alvarado and Maria Trinidad Madrigal v. Foster Poultry Farms*, Superior Court of the State of California, County of Merced, December 18, 2020.

25. Josh Funk, "At Least 59,000 U.S. Meat Workers Caught COVID-19 in 2020, 269 Died," PBS News, October 27, 2021.

26. Chen et al., "Excess Mortality Associated with the COVID-19 Pandemic Among Californians 18–65 Years of Age, by Occupational Sector and Occupation: March Through November 2020."

27. Ibid.

28. Anna Wilde Mathews et al., "COVID-19 Stalked Nursing Homes Around the World," *Wall Street Journal*, December 31, 2020.

29. Edgardo Sepulveda, "A Comparison of COVID-19 Mortality Rates Among Long-Term Care Residents in 12 OECD Countries," *Journal of the American Medical Directors Association* 21, no. 11 (2020): 1572–74.

30. Mathews et al., "COVID-19 Stalked Nursing Homes Around the World."

31. Ibid.

32. A study by the International Long-Term Care Policy Network showed that nursing homes accounted for just 8 percent of South Korea's COVID deaths through July 9, 2020, a fraction of the proportion in every one of the twenty-seven other developed nations included in the analysis. Adelina Comas-Herrera et al., "Mortality Associated with COVID-19 Outbreaks in Care Homes: Early International Evidence," International Long-Term Care Policy Network, CPEC, London School of Economics, 2020.

33. Julie Ireton, "Canada's Nursing Homes Have Worst Record for COVID-19 Deaths Among Wealthy Nations: Report," CBC News, March 30, 2021; Canadian Institute for Health Information, "The Impact of COVID-19 on Long-Term Care in Canada: Focus on the First 6 Months," Ottawa, Ontario, 2020, p. 6. Note that the proportion of deaths in nursing homes may reflect an undercount of the total number of COVID deaths in Canada. By 2021, the excess death figures for Canada suggested that there were more community deaths than health officials had officially recorded. Nonetheless, no nation matched the disparity between nursing home and community deaths in Canada.

34. Nathan M. Stall et al., "For-Profit Nursing Homes and the Risk of COVID-19 Outbreaks and Resident Deaths in Ontario, Canada," medRxiv 2020.05.25.20112664.

35. Ibid.

36. Murray Brewster and Vassy Kapelos, "Military Alleges Horrific Conditions, Abuse in Pandemic-Hit Ontario Nursing Homes," CBC News Canada, May 26, 2020.
37. Dan Bilefsky, "31 Deaths: Toll at Quebec Nursing Home in Pandemic Reflects Global Phenomenon," *New York Times*, April 16, 2020.
38. Canadian Institute for Health Information, "The Impact of COVID-19 on Long-Term Care in Canada: Focus on the First 6 Months," p. 6.
39. Kelsey Johnson, " 'We Are Failing Our Grandparents' Canada's Trudeau Says as COVID-19 Hammers Nursing Homes," Reuters, April 2020.
40. Sepulveda, "A Comparison of COVID-19 Mortality Rates Among Long-Term Care Residents in 12 OECD Countries."
41. A study published in *JAMA Network Open* estimates that during 2020, 592,629 nursing home residents in the U.S. caught COVID, and 118,335 people died. In 2022, the White House acknowledged that mortality in American long-term-care facilities had topped 200,000. See K. Shen et al., "Estimates of COVID-19 Cases and Deaths Among Nursing Home Residents Not Reported in Federal Data," *JAMA Network Open* 4, no. 9 (2021): e2122885. See also "FACT SHEET: Protecting Seniors by Improving Safety and Quality of Care in the Nation's Nursing Homes," The White House, February 28, 2022.
42. Bryant Furlow, Carli Brosseau, and Isaac Arnsdorf, "Nursing Homes Fought Federal Emergency Plan Requirements for Years. Now, They're Coronavirus Hot Spots," *ProPublica*, May 29, 2020.
43. Yuan Zhang et al., "Working Conditions and Mental Health of Nursing Staff in Nursing Homes," *Issues in Mental Health Nursing* 37, no. 7 (2016): 485–92.
44. "Median Wages per Compensated Hour in U.S. Skilled Nursing Facilities as of 2018, by Occupation," *Statista*, March 7, 2022.
45. A group of UCLA and Yale economists who used geolocation data from mobile phones to track staff networks and labor patterns of American care workers during eleven weeks in 2020 found that during the pandemic, "nursing homes, on average, share connections with 7 other facilities" through their employees, and that about "49 percent of COVID cases among nursing home residents are attributable to staff movement between facilities." Keith Chen, Judith A. Chevalier, and Elisa F. Long, "Nursing Home Staff Networks and COVID-19," National Bureau of Economic Research, 2020.
46. Tanya Lewis, "Nursing Home Workers Had One of the Deadliest Jobs of 2020," *Scientific American*, February 18, 2021.
47. Gabriel Winant, "What's Actually Going On in Our Nursing Homes: An Interview with Shantonia Jackson," *Dissent Magazine*, Fall 2020.
48. Ibid.
49. Ibid.
50. Mathews et al., "COVID-19 Stalked Nursing Homes Around the World."

51. Vincent Mor et al., "Driven to Tiers: Socioeconomic and Racial Disparities in the Quality of Nursing Home Care," *The Milbank Quarterly* 82, no. 2 (2004): 227–56.

52. Derek Cantù, "Minority Residents in Illinois Nursing Homes Died of COVID-19 at Disproportionate Rates," NPR Illinois, May 3, 2021.

53. Rebecca J. Gorges and Tamara Konetzka, "Factors Associated with Racial Differences in Deaths Among Nursing Home Residents with COVID-19 Infection in the US," *JAMA Network Open* 4, no. 2 (2021): e2037431.

54. James S. House, Karl R. Landis, and Debra Umberson, "Social Relationships and Health," *Science* 241(1988): 540–45; Lisa Berkman and Thomas Glass, "Social Integration, Social Networks, Social Support, and Health," *Social Epidemiology* 1/6 (2000): 137–73; Ichiro Kawachi and Lisa Berkman, "Social Ties and Mental Health," *Journal of Urban Health* 78, no. 3 (2001): 458–67.

55. Christopher Cronin and William Evans, "Nursing Home Quality, COVID-19 Deaths, and Excess Mortality," *Journal of Health Economics* 82 (2022): 102592.

56. Michael Levere, Patricia Rowan, and Andrea Wysocki, "The Adverse Effects of the COVID-19 Pandemic on Nursing Home Resident Well-Being," *Journal of the American Medical Directors Association* 22, no. 5 (2021): 948–54.

57. Julie Ward et al., "COVID-19 Cases Among Employees of U.S. Federal and State Prisons," *American Journal of Preventive Medicine* 60, no. 6 (2021): 840–44.

58. Brendan Saloner, Julie Ward, and Kalind Parish, "COVID-19 Cases and Deaths in Federal and State Prisons," *JAMA* 324, no. 6 (2020): 602–3.

59. Neal Marcos Marquez et al., "Assessing the Mortality Impact of the COVID-19 Pandemic in Florida State Prisons," medRxiv: 2021.04.14 .21255512.

60. Maura Turcotte et al., "The Real Toll from Prison COVID Cases May Be Higher Than Reported," *New York Times*, July 7, 2021.

61. Ibid.

62. Paulina Villegas, "A Rikers Island Inmate with Coronavirus Was Granted Emergency Release. He Died That Afternoon," *Washington Post*, October 18, 2021.

63. Emily Widra and Dylan Hayre, "Failing Grades: States' Responses to COVID-19 in Jails & Prisons," Prison Policy Initiative, June 2020.

64. "California Profile," Prison Policy Initiative, 2022.

65. "Texas Profile," Prison Policy Initiative, 2022.

66. Widra and Hayre, "Failing Grades: States' Responses to COVID-19 in Jails & Prisons."

67. Didier Fassin, "The Moral Economy of Life in the Pandemic," in Didier Fassin and Marion Fourcade, eds., *Pandemic Exposures: Economy and Society in the Time of Coronavirus* (Chicago: Hau, 2022), p. 167.

CHAPTER NINE "THE BRIDGE" (NUALA O'DOHERTY)

1. Sara Krevoy, "MTA Shares Details of Queens Bus Network Redesign," *Queens Ledger,* December 30, 2019.
2. Ibid.
3. Jim Burke, "Op-Ed: MTA's Queens Bus Redesign Is Not Good for Jackson Heights," *StreetsBlog NYC,* January 7, 2020.
4. Michael Kimmelman, "Jackson Heights, Global Town Square," *New York Times,* August 27, 2020.
5. *Which Neighborhoods Have More Nearby Park Space Per Capita?,* New York City Independent Budget Office, July 15, 2020, accessed September 2, 2022.
6. *Overcrowding in New York City Community Districts,* New York: Institute for Children, Poverty & Homelessness, 2016.
7. Brigid Bergin, "Two COVID-19 Deaths at NYC Board of Elections, and More Than a Dozen Sickened," *Gothamist,* April 3, 2020.
8. Annie Correal and Andrew Jacobs, "'A Tragedy Is Unfolding': Inside New York's Virus Epicenter," *New York Times,* April 9, 2020.
9. Ibid.
10. Michael Rothfeld et al., "13 Deaths in a Day: An 'Apocalyptic' Coronavirus Surge at an N.Y.C. Hospital," *New York Times,* March 25, 2020.
11. Together We Can Community Resource Center Inc., COVID Care Neighbor Network, https://www.togetherwecanrc.org/covid-care-neighbor -network, accessed September 2, 2022.
12. Winnie Hu, "The Pandemic Gave New York City 'Open Streets.' Will They Survive?," *New York Times,* August 9, 2021.
13. Andrew Siff, "12-Year-Old Boy Pinned by Jeep in Front of Queens School: Police, Witnesses," NBC New York, March 28, 2019.
14. Gersh Kuntzman, "UPDATED: De Blasio Commits to 100 Miles of 'Open Streets,'" *StreetsBlog NYC,* April 27, 2020.
15. Gersh Kuntzman and Clarence Eckerson Jr., "WE FIRST! After Mayoral Announcement, Neighborhoods Demand Open Streets," *StreetsBlog NYC,* April 28, 2020.
16. Hu, "The Pandemic Gave New York City 'Open Streets.' Will They Survive?"
17. Ibid.
18. Gersh Kuntzman, "ANALYSIS: DOT Plan for 'Gold Standard' 34th Ave. Open Street Is a Step Forward, but Definitely Not a 'Linear Park,'" *StreetsBlog NYC,* October 19, 2021.

CHAPTER TEN NEIGHBORHOODS

1. "State of the City," New York University, Furman Center report, https://furmancenter.org/stateofthecity/view/state-of-new-yorkers-and -neighborhoods.

2. Michael Schwirtz and Lindsey Rogers Cook, "These N.Y.C. Neighborhoods Have the Highest Rates of Virus Deaths," *New York Times*, May 18, 2020.
3. Nancy Krieger et al., "Relationship of Political Ideology of US Federal and State Elected Officials and Key COVID Pandemic Outcomes Following Vaccine Rollout to Adults: April 2021–March 2022," *The Lancet Regional Health-Americas* 16 (2022): 100384. Krieger and her colleagues measure exposure to conservatism through three factors: the political ideology of congressional representatives, the level of support for COVID-19 relief bills, and the extent to which Republicans are represented in the area's political offices.
4. Valeria Mogilevich et al., "Corona Plaza Es Para Todos! Making a Dignified Public Space for Immigrants," Queens Museum, 2016.
5. Neighborhoods are often defined and measured differently by various agencies and researchers, and Corona is no exception. Here, the data I use for Corona are from the 11368 zip code, which is a common way to bound the area. Some researchers, including my colleagues at NYU's Furman Center, combine Corona with Elmhurst in a larger agglomeration. The data I cite on severe crowding in Corona refer to this combined pair.
6. "Neighborhood Profiles: Elmhurst-Corona," New York University, Furman Center report, https://furmancenter.org/neighborhoods/view/elmhurst -corona.
7. Previous studies have looked at different categories of occupations and industries to approximate a measure of either essential worker status or the ability to work from home. Jocelyn Drummond, a doctoral student in sociology at NYU who assisted me on the research in Queens, created a hybrid list of occupations that are both on the list of New York State essential businesses (from the state's Executive Order 202.6) and are less likely to be done at home. Using these data, we ranked all New York City zip codes to see which had the greatest share of essential workers who could not work at home, and Corona (zip code 11368) ranked first. See Jonathan Dingel and Brett Neiman, "How Many Jobs Can Be Done at Home?," National Bureau of Economic Research, Working Paper no. 26948 (2020).
8. Rivka Galchin, "A New Doctor Faces the Coronavirus in Queens," *The New Yorker*, April 20, 2020.
9. Michael Rothfeld et al., "13 Deaths in a Day: An 'Apocalyptic' Coronavirus Surge at an N.Y.C. Hospital," *New York Times*, March 25, 2020.
10. "Coronavirus, New York Hospitals," *New York Times*, May 14, 2020.
11. Bradley Jones, "The Changing Political Geography of COVID-19 Deaths over the Last Two Years," Pew Research Center, March 3, 2022.
12. Daniel Carrión et al., "Neighborhood-Level Disparities and Subway Utilization During the COVID-19 Pandemic in New York City," *Nature Communications* 12, no. 1 (2021): 1–10.
13. Serina Chang et al., "Mobility Network Models of COVID-19 Explain Inequities and Inform Reopening," *Nature* 589, no. 7840 (2021): 82–87.

14. Ibid.
15. Again, the data for Corona come from the 11368 zip code.
16. Here, as in Corona, I draw on one zip code, 11355, for data on Flushing. An adjacent zip code, 11354, is also often included in measures of the Flushing area, but for the sake of comparison I use only data from 11355 in this account. It's worth noting that the 11354 zip code had an extremely high COVID mortality rate during the first two months of the pandemic. One reason is that this area has an unusually large number of nursing homes, housing for the elderly, and very old residents; in fact, the proportion of residents aged eighty and above in zip code 11354 is nearly double the rate for the metropolitan area. This anomaly makes the 11355 zip code, where the population is relatively old but not nearly as old as in 11354, a better choice of comparison with Corona.
17. Census data show that Flushing has 2.9 residents per household, compared to 3.8 in Corona. https://censusreporter.org/profiles/86000US11355-11355/; https://censusreporter.org/profiles/86000US11368-11368/.
18. Vera Haller, "Downtown Flushing: Where Asian Cultures Thrive," *New York Times*, October 5, 2014.
19. Gil Eyal, *The Crisis of Expertise* (Cambridge, UK: Polity Press, 2019).
20. NYC Chinese Supermarket Closure March/April 2020, https://docs.google.com/spreadsheets/d/1zcMeOqeNeX0aeY807KESo2Ytq3sIaeCiKWfWOXRfbDQ/edit#gid=0.
21. Ann Choi and Josefa Velasquez, "Early Precautions Draw a Life-and-Death Divide Between Flushing and Corona," *The City*, May 3, 2020.
22. David Brand, "COVID-19 Has Killed More Than 200 People in 10 Queens Nursing Homes," *Queens Daily Eagle*, April 17, 2020.
23. Peter Kropotkin is credited with developing the term "mutual aid society" in a collection of essays, *Mutual Aid: A Factor of Evolution*, published in 1902. Kropotkin, a naturalist and anarchist philosopher, traces the roots of voluntary cooperation from animal species through a range of human societies, arguing that the tendency toward collectivism and mutual support is as much a driver of history as the tendency toward competition and conflict. "Sociability," he writes, "is as much a law of nature as mutual struggle. . . . [W]e maintain that under any circumstances sociability is the greatest advantage in the struggle for life. Those species which willingly or unwillingly abandon it are bound for decay." Peter Kropotkin, *Mutual Aid: A Factor of Evolution* (Montreal: Black Rose Books, 1902; 2021), Chapter 1. For a brief history of mutual aid groups and a how-to guide for those who want to build one, see Dean Spade, *Mutual Aid: Building Solidarity During This Crisis (and the Next)* (New York: Verso, 2020).
24. Quoctrung Bui and Emily Badger, "In These Neighborhoods, the Jobless Rate May Top 30 Percent," *New York Times*, August 5, 2020.
25. Kimiko de Freytas-Timura, "How Neighborhood Groups Are Stepping In Where the Government Didn't," *New York Times*, March 3, 2021.

CHAPTER ELEVEN "COVID WAS NOT
MY PRIMARY CONCERN" (BRANDON ENGLISH)

1. Ashley Southall, "Scrutiny of Social-Distance Policing as 35 of 40 Arrested Are Black," *New York Times*, May 7, 2020.
2. Ibid.
3. My account of what the police did to George Floyd relies on reporting by *The New York Times*, which reconstructed the event based on video evidence. See "How George Floyd Died, and What Happened Next," *New York Times*, May 19, 2020.
4. This quote, and the quotes from the report that follows, can be found on a website that archived the original www.insidempd.com statement: Minneapolis Police Department, *Investigative Update on Critical Incident*, John Elder, Report no. 20-140629, Minneapolis Police Department, 2020.
5. Ibid.
6. Elizabeth Alexander, "The Trayvon Generation," *The New Yorker*, June 15, 2020.
7. Ray Sanchez, Joe Sutton, and Artemis Moshtaghian, "4 Minneapolis Cops Fired After Video Shows One Kneeling on Neck of Black Man Who Later Died," CNN, May 26, 2020.
8. Ibid.
9. Ibid.; Derrick Bryson Taylor, "George Floyd Protests: A Timeline," *New York Times*, November 5, 2021.
10. "George Floyd: Timeline of Black Deaths and Protests," BBC, April 22, 2021.
11. Émile Durkheim, *The Elementary Forms of Religious Life*, translated by Karen E. Fields (New York: Free Press, 1912; 1995).
12. Tracey Porpora, "George Floyd Protests Continue Across U.S.; Another Planned for Sunday on Staten Island," *SILive*, May 31, 2020.
13. The Armed Conflict Location and Event Data project, in partnership with Princeton University's Bridging Divides Initiative, examined records of more than 10,600 demonstration events across the U.S. between May 24 and August 22, 2020. They report that, "Over 10,100 of these—or nearly 95%—involve peaceful protesters. Fewer than 570—or approximately 5%—involve demonstrators engaging in violence." *Demonstrations and Political Violence in America: New Data for Summer 2020*, Armed Conflict Location & Event Data Project, 2020.
14. Ali Watkins, Derek M. Norman, and Nate Schweber, "Shattered Glass in SoHo as Looters Ransack Lower Manhattan," *New York Times*, June 1, 2020.
15. *Demonstrations and Political Violence in America: New Data for Summer 2020*, Armed Conflict Location & Event Data Project.
16. Neil MacFarquhar, "Minneapolis Police Link 'Umbrella Man' to White Supremacy Group," *New York Times*, July 28, 2020.
17. Christine Ferretti, George Hunter, and Sarah Rahal, "Man Shot Dead,

Dozens Arrested as Protest in Detroit Turns Violent," *Detroit News*, May 29, 2020.

18. Michael Wilson, "Why Are So Many N.Y.P.D. Officers Refusing to Wear Masks at Protests?," *New York Times*, June 11, 2020.

19. Taylor, "George Floyd Protests: A Timeline."

20. "Bronx Neighborhood Profile," New York University, Furman Center.

21. Human Rights Watch, *"Kettling" Protesters in the Bronx: Systemic Police Brutality and Its Costs in the United States* (New York: Human Rights Watch, 2020); interview with Andom Ghebreghiorgis at 02:25 in Human Rights Watch, "US: New York Police Planned Assault on Bronx Protesters," September 30, 2020, video, 12:43. Much of the following section relies on reporting from Human Rights Watch.

22. Human Rights Watch, *"Kettling" Protesters in the Bronx.*

23. Human Rights Watch, "US: New York Police Planned Assault on Bronx Protesters."

24. Ibid.

25. Ibid.

26. Maria Cramer, "New York Will Pay Millions to Protesters Violently Corralled by Police," *New York Times*, March 1, 2023.

27. Thomas Sugrue (@TomSugrue), "As a historian of social movements in the U.S.," Twitter, June 6, 2020, 5:40 p.m.; Thomas Sugrue (@TomSugrue), "We have had some huge one-day demonstrations," Twitter, June 6, 2020, 5:45 p.m.; Thomas Sugrue (@TomSugrue), "But the two together—very unusual," Twitter, June 6, 2020, 5:46 p.m.

28. Larry Buchanan, Quoctrung Bui, and Jugal K. Patel, "Black Lives Matter May Be the Largest Movement in U.S. History," *New York Times*, July 3, 2020.

CHAPTER TWELVE   RACE

1. Boris Johnson (@BorisJohnson), "Over the last 24 hours I have developed mild symptoms and tested positive for coronavirus," Twitter, March 27, 2020, 7:15 a.m.

2. Kelley Benham French, "Coronavirus: We're in This Together," *USA Today*, April 9, 2020.

3. United Nations Department of Global Communications, *COVID-19 Photo Essay: We're All in This Together*, New York: Secretariat of the United Nations, 2020, https://www.un.org/en/coronavirus/COVID-19 -photo-essay-we%E2%80%99re-all-together, accessed August 19, 2022.

4. Adia Benton, "Risky Business: Race, Nonequivalence, and the Humanitarian Politics of Life," *Visual Anthropology* 29, no. 2 (2016): 187–203.

5. *WHO Issues Best Practices for Naming New Human Infectious Diseases*, Geneva: World Health Organization, https://www.who.int/news-room/detail/08 -05-2015-who-issues-best-practices-for-naming-new-human-infectious -diseases, accessed August 19, 2022.

6. Morgan Gstalter, "WHO Official Warns Against Calling It 'Chinese Virus,' Says 'There Is No Blame in This,'" *The Hill*, March 19, 2020.

7. Katie Rogers, Lara Jakes, and Ana Swanson, "Trump Defends Using 'Chinese Virus' Label, Ignoring Growing Criticism," *New York Times*, March 18, 2020.

8. Associated Press, "Pompeo, G-7 Foreign Ministers Spar over 'Wuhan Virus,'" *Politico*, March 25, 2020.

9. Rogers, Jakes, and Swanson, "Trump Defends Using 'Chinese Virus' Label, Ignoring Growing Criticism"; and "President Trump Calls Coronavirus 'Kung Flu,'" BBC, June 24, 2020.

10. Jingqui Ren and Joe Feagin, "Face Mask Symbolism in Anti-Asian Hate Crimes," *Ethnic & Racial Studies* 44, no. 5 (2021): 746–58.

11. Natalie Escobar, "When Xenophobia Spreads Like a Virus," *Code Switch*, NPR, March 4, 2020, podcast, 25:12.

12. Ibid.

13. "Stop AAPI Hate Report: 3.19.20–5.13.20," San Francisco: Stop AAPI Hate, April 2021.

14. *Crime Data Explorer*, United States Federal Bureau of Investigation, https://crime-data-explorer.fr.cloud.gov/pages/explorer/crime/hate-crime, accessed August 19, 2022.

15. "Fact Sheet: Anti-Asian Prejudice March 2021," Center for the Study of Hate & Extremism, California State University, San Bernardino, March 2021.

16. Amanuel Elias et al., "Racism and Nationalism During and Beyond the COVID-19 Pandemic," *Ethnic and Racial Studies* 44, no. 5 (2021): 783–93.

17. Neil G. Ruiz, Khadijah Edwards, and Mark Hugo Lopez, "One-Third of Asian Americans Fear Threats, Physical Attacks and Most Say Violence Against Them Is Rising," Washington, DC: Pew Research Center, April 2021.

18. Human Rights Watch, *COVID-19 Fueling Anti-Asian Racism and Xenophobia Worldwide: National Action Plans Needed to Counter Intolerance*, New York: Human Rights Watch, May 2020.

19. Ibid.

20. Ibid.

21. "The COVID-19 Crisis Is Fueling More Racist Discourse Towards Migrant Workers in the Gulf," Migrant-Rights.org, April 5, 2020.

22. Human Rights Watch, *COVID-19 Fueling Anti-Asian Racism and Xenophobia Worldwide*.

23. Salem Solomon, "Coronavirus Brings 'Sinophobia' to Africa," *VOA News*, March 4, 2020.

24. Zinzi D. Bailey et al., "Structural Racism and Health Inequities in the USA: Evidence and Interventions," *The Lancet* 389, no. 10077 (2017): 1453–63.

25. "Life Expectancy in the U.S. Increased Between 2000–2019, but Wide-

spread Gaps Between Racial and Ethnic Groups Exist," U.S. National Institutes of Health, June 22, 2022.

26. Merlin Chowkwanyun, "What Is a 'Racial Health Disparity'? Five Analytic Traditions," *Journal of Health Politics, Policy and Law* 47, no. 2 (2022): 131–58.

27. Annice Kim et al., "Coverage and Framing of Racial and Ethnic Health Disparities in US Newspapers, 1996–2005," *American Journal of Public Health* 100, no. S1 (2010): S224–31.

28. Latoya Hill, Samantha Artiga, and Sweta Haldar, "Key Facts on Health and Health Care by Race and Ethnicity," Kaiser Family Foundation, March 15, 2023.

29. Latoya Hill and Samantha Artiga, "COVID-19 Cases and Deaths by Race/Ethnicity: Current Data and Changes over Time," Kaiser Family Fund, February 22, 2022.

30. Arline Geronimus et al., "'Weathering' and Age Patterns of Allostatic Load Scores Among Blacks and Whites in the United States," *American Journal of Public Health* 96, no. 5 (2006): 826–33; Arline Geronimus, "The Weathering Hypothesis and the Health of African-American Women and Infants: Evidence and Speculations," *Ethnicity & Disease* (2006): 207–21.

31. Matthew Desmond, *Poverty, By America* (New York: Crown, 2023).

32. Andrew Cuomo (@NYGovCuomo), "This virus is the great equalizer," Twitter, March 31, 2020, 12:13 p.m.

33. Zadie Smith, *Intimations* (New York: Penguin, 2020), p. 15.

34. Kimiko de Freytas-Tamura, Winnie Hu, and Lindsey Rogers Cook, "'It's the Death Towers': How the Bronx Became New York's Virus Hot Spot," *New York Times*, May 26, 2020.

35. Juliana Maantay, "Asthma and Air Pollution in the Bronx: Methodological and Data Considerations in Using GIS for Environmental Justice and Health Research," *Health & Place* 13, no. 1 (2007): 32–56.

36. Sue A. Kaplan et al., "The Perception of Stress and Its Impact on Health in Poor Communities," *Journal of Community Health* 38, no. 1 (2013): 142–49.

37. Amanda Dunker and Elisabeth Ryden Benjamin, "How Structural Inequalities in New York's Health Care System Exacerbate Health Disparities During the COVID-19 Pandemic: A Call for Equitable Reform," Community Service Society of New York, June 4, 2020.

38. *Recent Trends and Impact of COVID-19 in the Bronx*, New York: Office of the Comptroller, June 2021.

39. The COVID Tracking Project at *The Atlantic* (online), *New York: All Race & Ethnicity Data*, https://covidtracking.com/data/state/new-york/race-ethnicity, accessed August 19, 2022.

40. Usama Bilal et al., "Spatial Inequities in COVID-19 Testing, Positivity, Confirmed Cases, and Mortality in 3 US Cities: An Ecological Study," *Annals of Internal Medicine* 174, no. 7 (2021): 936–44.

41. See, among others, Douglas Massey and Nancy Denton, *American Apartheid: Segregation and the Making of the Underclass* (Cambridge: Harvard University Press, 1998); Patrick Sharkey, *Stuck in Place: Urban Neighborhoods and the End of Progress Toward Racial Equity* (Chicago: University of Chicago Press, 2013); and Richard Rothstein, *The Color of Law: A Forgotten History of How Our Government Segregated America* (New York: W. W. Norton, 2017).

42. Samrachana Adhikari et al., "Assessment of Community-Level Disparities in Coronavirus Disease 2019 (COVID-19) Infections and Deaths in Large US Metropolitan Areas," *JAMA Network Open* 3, no. 7 (2020): e2016938.

43. Katherine Mackey et al., "Racial and Ethnic Disparities in COVID-19–Related Infections, Hospitalizations, and Deaths: A Systematic Review," *Annals of Internal Medicine* 174, no. 3 (2021): 362–73.

44. David Greene, "Sen. Bill Cassidy on His State's Racial Disparities in Coronavirus Deaths," *NPR Morning Edition*, April 7, 2020, podcast, 07:26.

45. Ibid.

46. Mackey et al., "Racial and Ethnic Disparities in COVID-19–Related Infections, Hospitalizations, and Deaths."

47. Eduardo Bonilla-Silva, "Color-Blind Racism in Pandemic Times," *Sociology of Race and Ethnicity* 8, no. 3 (2022): 343–54.

48. Ibram X. Kendi, "Stop Blaming Black People for Dying of the Coronavirus," *The Atlantic*, April 14, 2020.

49. Zinzi D. Bailey et al., "Structural Racism and Health Inequities in the USA: Evidence and Interventions," *The Lancet* 389, no. 10077 (2017): 1453–63.

50. Dalton Conley, *Being Black, Living in the Red: Race, Wealth, and Social Policy in America* (Berkeley: University of California Press, 2010); Jamila Michener, "George Floyd's Killing Was Just the Spark. Here's What Really Made the Protests Explode," *Washington Post*, June 11, 2020.

51. Fabiola Cineas, "Senators Are Demanding a Solution to Police Stopping Black Men for Wearing—and Not Wearing—Masks," *Vox*, April 22, 2020.

52. Larry Buchanan, Quoctrung Bui, and Jugal K. Patel, "Black Lives Matter May Be the Largest Movement in U.S. History," *New York Times*, July 3, 2020.

53. *Tracking COVID-19 Through Race-Based Data*, Canada: Ontario Health, Government of Ontario, August 2021.

54. Kate H. Choi et al., "Studying the Social Determinants of COVID-19 in a Data Vacuum," *Canadian Review of Sociology/Revue Canadienne de Sociologie* 58, no. 2, 2021: 146–64.

55. John Paul Tasker, "More Racially Diverse Areas Reported Much Higher Numbers of COVID-19 Deaths: StatsCan," CBC News Canada, March 10, 2021.

56. Allison L. Skinner-Dorkenoo et al., "Highlighting COVID-19 Racial Disparities Can Reduce Support for Safety Precautions Among White US Residents," *Social Science & Medicine* 301 (2022): 114951.

57. *COVID-19 Disinformation Briefing No.1*, London: Institute for Strategic Dialogue, March 27, 2020.

58. David Klepper and Lori Hinnant, "Far-Right Using COVID-19 Theories to Grow Reach, Study Shows," Associated Press/PBS News, December 17, 2021.

59. *COVID-19 Disinformation Briefing No.1*, Institute for Strategic Dialogue.

60. Janell Ross, "Coronavirus Outbreak Revives Dangerous Race Myths and Pseudoscience," NBC News, March 19, 2020.

61. Ciarán O'Connor, *The Conspiracy Consortium Examining Discussions of COVID-19 Among Right-Wing Extremist Telegram Channels*, London: Institute for Strategic Dialogue, 2021.

62. Nomaan Merchant, "U.S. Accuses Zero Hedge of Spreading Russian Propaganda," Associated Press/Bloomberg, February 15, 2022.

63. O'Connor, *The Conspiracy Consortium Examining Discussions of COVID-19 Among Right-Wing Extremist Telegram Channels*.

64. Klepper and Hinnant, "Far-Right Using COVID-19 Theories to Grow Reach, Study Shows."

65. Jason Wilson, "The Rightwing Groups Behind Wave of Protests Against COVID-19 Restrictions," *The Guardian*, April 17, 2020.

66. Alex Newhouse, Adel Arletta, and Leela McClintock, *Proud Boys Amplify Anti-Vax and Coronavirus Disinformation Following Support for Anti-Quarantine Protests*, Middlebury College Center on Terrorism, Extremism, and Counterterrorism.

67. Rebecca White, "Group Claims Responsibility for Taking Down COVID-19 Crosses at City Hall," (Spokane) *Spokesman-Review*, May 18, 2020.

68. Associated Press, "Trump Tells Proud Boys: 'Stand Back and Stand By,'" YouTube video, 01:29, September 30, 2020.

CHAPTER THIRTEEN "TRAVELS FAR" (THANKACHAN MATHAI)

1. The Organization of Staff Analysts Union, *MTA Memorandum: Frequently Asked Questions Regarding COVID-19*, New York City: Metropolitan Transit Authority, March 2020.

2. Gabrielle Fonrouge and David Meyer, "Subway Conductor First Known MTA Worker to Die from Coronavirus," *New York Post*, March 26, 2020.

3. Georgette Roberts, "Cortlandt Street Subway Station Reopens 17 Years After 9/11," *New York Post*, September 8, 2018.

4. Christina Goldbaum, "41 Transit Workers Dead: Crisis Takes Staggering Toll on Subways," *New York Times*, April 8, 2020.

5. Ibid.

6. Christina Goldbaum, "N.Y.C.'s Subway, a 24/7 Mainstay, Will Close for Overnight Disinfection," *New York Times*, April 30, 2020; Annie Correal, "What the 'Invisible' People Cleaning the Subway Want Riders to Know," *New York Times*, March 26, 2021.

7. Robyn Gershon, *Impact of COVID-19 Pandemic on NYC Transit Workers: Pilot Study Findings,* New York: New York University School of Global Public Health, October 2020; "Remembering the Colleagues We Lost to COVID-19," Metropolitan Transit Authority, January 2021.

8. Sandra Bloodworth requested that I include the following statement to credit her MTA colleagues who worked on Travels Far: "A memorial to pay tribute to MTA's fallen workers was requested by MTA Chairman and CEO Patrick Foye, and Agency Presidents Sarah Feinberg (Interim, NYCT), Catherine Rinaldi (MNR), and Phillip Eng (LIRR). Beyond her role as artist, Sandra Bloodworth provided the creative leadership on TRAVELS FAR, with technical contributions from MTA Arts & Design staff, Cheryl Hageman and Victoria Statsenko. Monica Murray with Andrew Wilcox, co-led the agency interface with the NYC Transit Family Liaison Unit in conducting the family engagement. Graphics and digital support was provided by Connie dePalma, Gene Ribeiro, Gary Jenkins, and Jessie Mislavsky with web design by Hannah Birch. Many others across the MTA worked to bring TRAVELS FAR to fruition."

9. "TRAVELS FAR" (2020) © Tracy K. Smith, commissioned by Metropolitan Transportation Agency for TRAVELS FAR, a Memorial Honoring our Colleagues Lost to COVID-19.

10. @BarackObama, "Here's an example of the incredible risks and burdens that our essential workers have been facing. And even as we move toward vaccinating our population, we all need to remain vigilant until we've beaten this pandemic," Twitter, January 26, 2021, 6:31 a.m.

11. Chana Joffe-Walt, "Goodbye Mr. Facey," *This American Life,* Episode 738, May 28, 2021.

12. Emily Drooby, "MTA Memorial 'Travels Far' Honors NYC Transit Employees Lost to COVID-19," Net TV New York, February 2021.

CHAPTER FOURTEEN **HOME ALONE**

1. Ezra Klein, "Coronavirus Will Also Cause a Loneliness Epidemic," *Vox,* March 12, 2020.

2. Eric Klinenberg, *Going Solo* (New York: Penguin, 2012).

3. Julianne Holt-Lunstad, "The Double Pandemic of Social Isolation and COVID-19: Cross-Sector Policy Must Address Both," *Health Affairs,* June 22, 2020.

4. Feifei Bu, Andrew Steptoe, and Daisy Fancourt, "Loneliness During a Strict Lockdown: Trajectories and Predictors During the COVID-19 Pandemic in 38,217 United Kingdom Adults," *Social Science & Medicine* 265 (2020): 113521.

5. Martina Luchetti et al., "The Trajectory of Loneliness in Response to COVID-19," *American Psychologist* 75, no. 7 (2020): 897–908.

6. Thomas Hansen et al., "Locked and Lonely? A Longitudinal Assessment

of Loneliness Before and During the COVID-19 Pandemic in Norway," *Scandinavian Journal of Public Health* 49, no. 7 (2021): 766–73.

7. Helen Landmann and Anette Rohmann, "When Loneliness Dimensions Drift Apart: Emotional, Social and Physical Loneliness During the COVID-19 Lockdown and Its Associations with Age, Personality, Stress and Well-being," *International Journal of Psychology* 57, no. 1 (2022): 63–72.

8. The people we interviewed ranged in age from 20 to 86 (20–44 = 28, 45–64 = 17, 65+ = 10). Just under two thirds (34) were women. Twenty-two interviewees were white, 11 were Black, six were Hispanic/Latino, six were South or Southeast Asian, four were East Asian, and six were multiracial. Seven had lost their job due to COVID, three had been furloughed at the time of the interview, and six were essential workers. The vast majority were living alone in the pandemic because they had been living alone before the outbreak hit New York City, but several found themselves alone during the pandemic because one or more of their roommates left the city. A few participants were living alone after experiencing the death of a partner or family member prior to the pandemic, and one participant lost their partner to COVID-19 within the first few weeks of the outbreak.

Due to restrictions on in-person recruitment and research at the time of the study, we recruited participants primarily through listservs of community-based organizations and neighborhood Facebook Groups, which exist for most New York City neighborhoods. We posted information about the study in five to eight neighborhoods for each borough, posting in more groups for boroughs with higher populations. When selecting which groups to post in, we chose neighborhoods of varying demographic compositions in order to ensure a racially and economically diverse sample. Recruiting participants via Facebook neighborhood groups is not ideal, as members of these groups by definition have sought out some level of social connection. However, given the challenges of in-person recruitment during the first wave of the pandemic, recruitment via social media was the safest approach for both the research team and participants.

9. John Cacioppo and William Patrick, *Loneliness: Human Nature and the Need for Social Connection* (New York: W. W. Norton, 2008).

10. Gregory Pratt et al., "As Illinois Sees Largest Daily Increase in Coronavirus Cases, Chicago Mayor Lori Lightfoot Bans Contact Sports; Closes Popular City Parks, Beaches and Trails," *Chicago Tribune*, March 26, 2020.

11. Tom Stienstra, "Bay Area Parks During Coronavirus: What's Open, Closed This Week," *San Francisco Chronicle*, April 8, 2020; Dyer Oxley, "Seattle Parks Will Close Under Order of Mayor Durkan," KUOW, April 9, 2020.

12. Corey Kilgannon, "Summer Is Coming. Don't Count on N.Y.C.'s Beaches for Relief," *New York Times*, May 16, 2006; Anna Sanders, "NYC Outdoor Pools Closed for Summer 2020 Due to Coronavirus Pandemic, Beaches Likely Shut Down Too," New York *Daily News*, April 16, 2020.

CHAPTER FIFTEEN GROWING UP

1. Glen Elder Jr., *Children of the Great Depression: Social Change in Life Experience;* 25th Anniversary Edition (Chicago: University of Chicago Press, 1974).
2. See Richard Setterstein et al., "Understanding the Effects of COVID-19 Through a Life Course Lens," *Advances in Life Course Research* 45 (2020); and Dennis Tamesberger and Johan Bacher, "COVID-19 Crisis: How to Avoid a 'Lost Generation,'" *Intereconomics* 55 (2020): 232–38.
3. F. Glowacz and E. Schmits, "Psychological Distress During the COVID-19 Lockdown: The Young Adults Most at Risk," *Psychiatry Research* 293 (2020): 113486; Autumn Kujawa et al., "Exposure to COVID-19 Pandemic Stress: Associations with Depression and Anxiety in Emerging Adults in the United States," *Depression and Anxiety* 37, no. 12 (2020): 1280–88; Anjel Vahratian et al., "Symptoms of Anxiety or Depressive Disorder and Use of Mental Health Care Among Adults During the COVID-19 Pandemic—United States," August 2020–February 2021, *MMWR Morbidity Mortality Weekly Report* 70 (2021): 490–94.
4. Participants in this study were promised anonymity, and I use pseudonyms for them here.
5. Francesca Fiori et al., "Employment Insecurity and Mental Health During the Economic Recession: An Analysis of the Young Adult Labour Force in Italy," *Social Science & Medicine* 153 (2016): 90–98.
6. Richard Fry and Amanda Barosso, "Amid Coronavirus Outbreak Nearly Three-in-Ten Young People Are Neither Working nor in School," Pew Research Center, July 29, 2020; J. Gao et al., "Mental Health Problems and Social Media Exposure During COVID-19 Outbreak," *PLOS ONE* 15, no. 4 (2020).
7. Kate Power, "The COVID-19 Pandemic Has Increased the Care Burden of Women and Families," *Sustainability: Science, Practice and Policy* 16, no. 1 (2020): 67–73.
8. Changwon Son et al., "Effects of COVID-19 on College Students' Mental Health in the United States: Interview Survey Study," *Journal of Medical Internet Research* 22, no. 9 (2020): e21279; Alyssa Lederer et al., "More Than Inconvenienced: The Unique Needs of U.S. College Students During the COVID-19 Pandemic," *Health Education & Behavior* 48, no. 1 (2020): 14–19; Madeline St. Amour, "Survey: Pandemic Negativity Affected Grades This Fall," *Inside Higher Ed,* January 5, 2021.
9. Lederer et al., "More Than Inconvenienced: The Unique Needs of U.S. College Students During the COVID-19 Pandemic."
10. Sumitra Pokhrel and Roshan Chhetri, "A Literature Review on Impact of COVID-19 Pandemic on Teaching and Learning," *Higher Education for the Future* 8, no. 1 (2021): 133–41.

11. Caitlin Zaloom, *Indebted: How Families Make College Work at Any Cost* (Princeton: Princeton University Press, 2019); Jacob Hacker, *The Great Risk Shift: The New Economic Insecurity and the Decline of the American Dream;* 2nd edition (New York: Oxford University Press, 2019).

12. Kelly Reilly, "Applying to College Was Never Easy for Most Students. The Pandemic Made It Nearly Impossible," *Time*, March 31, 2021.

13. Jeffrey Arnett, "Emerging Adulthood: A Theory of Development from the Late Teens Through the Twenties," *American Psychologist* 55, no. 5 (2000): 469–80.

14. Michael Rosenfeld, *The Age of Independence: Interracial Unions, Same-Sex Unions, and the Changing American Family* (Cambridge: Harvard University Press, 2009).

15. Neil Gleason et al., "The Impact of the COVID-19 Pandemic on Sexual Behaviors: Findings from a National Survey in the United States," *The Journal of Sexual Medicine* 18, no. 11 (2021): 1851–62.

16. Mark Czeisler et al., "Mental Health, Substance Use, and Suicidal Ideation During the COVID-19 Pandemic—United States, June 24–30, 2020," *Morbidity and Mortality Weekly Report* 69, no. 32 (2020): 1049; Christine Lee, Jennifer Cadigan, and Isaac Rhew, "Increases in Loneliness Among Young Adults During the COVID-19 Pandemic and Association with Increases in Mental Health Problems," *Journal of Adolescent Health* 67, no. 5 (2020): 714–17; Cindy Liu et al., "Factors Associated with Depression, Anxiety, and PTSD Symptomatology During the COVID-19 Pandemic: Clinical Implications for US Young Adult Mental Health," *Psychiatry Research* 290 (2020): 113172; Vahratian et al., "Symptoms of Anxiety or Depressive Disorder and Use of Mental Health Care Among Adults During the COVID-19 Pandemic—United States," 490–94.

17. Arlie Hochschild with Anne Machung, *The Second Shift: Working Families and the Revolution at Home* (New York: Viking Penguin, 1989); Kate Power, "The COVID-19 Pandemic Has Increased the Care Burden of Women and Families," *Sustainability: Science, Practice and Policy* 16, no. 1 (2020): 67–73.

18. Elder, *Children of the Great Depression;* Suzanne Mettler, *Soldiers to Citizens: The G.I. Bill and the Making of the Greatest Generation* (New York: Oxford University Press, 2005); Mattias Lundberg and Alice Wuermli, *Children and Youth in Crisis: Protecting and Promoting Human Development in Times of Economic Shocks* (Washington, DC: World Bank Publications, 2012).

19. Lilly Shanahan et al., "Emotional Distress in Young Adults During the COVID-19 Pandemic: Evidence of Risk and Resilience from a Longitudinal Cohort Study," *Psychological Medicine* 52, no. 5 (2022): 824–33.

20. Jeffrey Arnett, *Emerging Adulthood: The Winding Road from the Late Teens Through the Twenties* (New York: Oxford University Press, 2004).

21. Elder, *Children of the Great Depression.*

22. Stanley Cohen, *States of Denial* (Cambridge: Blackwell, 2001).

CHAPTER SIXTEEN AMERICAN ANOMIE

1. Brittany Kriegstein and Larry McShane, "'He Did Not Deserve to Die': Heartbroken Family of New Dad Killed by Stolen Truck Driver Left to Weep and Wonder Why," New York *Daily News*, July 1, 2020.
2. "Bronx Resident Charged in Hit-and-Run Box Truck Crash That Killed Man and Damaged Numerous Vehicles," Press Release from District Attorney Melinda Katz, New York: Queens District Attorney, 2020.
3. Kriegstein and McShane, "'He Did Not Deserve to Die.'"
4. Brad Boserup, Mark McKenney, and Adel Elkbuli, "Alarming Trends in US Domestic Violence During the COVID-19 Pandemic," *The American Journal of Emergency Medicine* 38, no. 12 (2020): 2753–55; Kenneth A. Dodge et al., "Impact of the COVID-19 Pandemic on Substance Use Among Adults Without Children, Parents, and Adolescents," *Addictive Behaviors Reports* 14 (2021).
5. Martin Savidge and Maria Cartaya, "Americans Bought Guns in Record Numbers in 2020 During a Year of Unrest—and the Surge Is Continuing," CNN, March 14, 2021.
6. Peter Nickeas and Priya Krishnakuma, "'It's a Disturbing Trend.' Cities See Large Increases in Carjackings During Pandemic," CNN, January 23, 2022; FBI National Press Office, *Hate Crime Statistics, 2020*, Washington, DC: Federal Bureau of Investigation, 2021.
7. "Attorney General Schmitt Warns of Medical Supply Chain Price Gouging," Missouri: Office of the Attorney General, March 16, 2020.
8. Tonya Riley, "The Cybersecurity 202: Cybercrime Skyrocketed as Workplaces Went Virtual in 2020, New Report Finds," *Washington Post*, February 22, 2021.
9. Simon Romero, "Pedestrian Deaths Spike in U.S. as Reckless Driving Surges," *New York Times*, February 14, 2022.
10. Olga Khazan, "Why People Are Acting So Weird," *The Atlantic*, March 30, 2022.
11. Franklin Zimring and Gordon Hawkins, *Crime Is Not the Problem: Lethal Violence in America* (New York: Oxford University Press, 1999).
12. John Gramlich, "What We Know About the Increase in U.S. Murders in 2020," Pew Research Center, October 27, 2021.
13. United Kingdom Office for National Statistics, *Homicide in England and Wales: Year Ending March 2021*, Wales: Office for National Statistics, February 2022.
14. "Australia Murder/Homicide Rate 1990–2022," *Macrotrends*, https://www.macrotrends.net/countries/AUS/australia/murder-homicide-rate; "Number of Homicide Cases in Taiwan from 2010 to 2020," *Statista*, 2021, https://www.statista.com/statistics/937681/taiwan-number-of-homicide-cases/; "Hong Kong Murder/Homicide Rate 1990-2022," *Macrotrends*, https://www.macrotrends.net/countries/HKG/hong-kong/murder-homicide-rate.

15. Wallis Snowdon, "Homicide Rate in Canada Surges—Driven by Gun Violence in Alberta and N.S. Mass Shooting," CBC News Canada, November 25, 2021.

16. "Rate of Homicide in South Korea from 2010 to 2020," *Statista*, January 2022, https://www.statista.com/statistics/1232149/south-korea-homicide-rate/.

17. David Leonhardt, "Vehicle Crashes, Surging," *New York Times*, February 15, 2022.

18. *The Impact of Lockdown on Reported Road Casualties Great Britain, Final Results: 2020*, United Kingdom Office for National Statistics, September 2021.

19. Lee Hyo-jin, "Korea Sees Largest Decrease Rate in Traffic Accident Casualties Due to COVID-19," *Korea Times*, July 9, 2022.

20. *Traffic Report 2020*, Hong Kong: Hong Kong Police Force, Traffic Branch Headquarters, 2020.

21. *Canadian Motor Vehicle Traffic Collision Statistics: 2020*, Ottawa: Transport Canada, 2020.

22. Australian Associated Press, "Australia's Road Toll Falls Only Slightly Despite Coronavirus Lockdowns," *The Guardian*, December 31, 2020.

23. Richard Slotkin, *Regeneration Through Violence: The Mythology of the American Frontier, 1600–1860* (Norman: University of Oklahoma Press, 2000).

24. Richard Nisbett, "Violence and U.S. Regional Culture," *American Psychologist* 48, no. 4 (1993): 441–49.

25. Marshall Meyer, "COVID Lockdowns, Social Distancing, and Fatal Car Crashes: More Deaths on Hobbesian Highways?," *Cambridge Journal of Evidence-Based Policing* 4, no. 3 (2020): 238–59.

26. Claude S. Fischer, "Paradoxes of American Individualism," *Sociological Forum* 23, no. 2 (2008): 363–72.

27. Alexis de Tocqueville, *Democracy in America: And Two Essays on America* (London: Penguin, 1838; 2003); Robert Bellah et al, *Habits of the Heart: Individualism and Commitment in American Life* (Berkeley: University of California Press, 1985).

28. Fischer, "Paradoxes of American Individualism."

29. Philip Bump, "Most Republicans See Democrats Not as Political Opponents but as Enemies," *Washington Post*, February 10, 2021.

30. Ruth Ben-Ghiat, *Strongmen: Mussolini to the Present* (New York: W. W. Norton, 2020).

31. *Vox* compiled a long list of incidents where Trump advocated violence against his adversaries and supported white supremacists or other extremist groups. See Fabiola Cineas, "Donald Trump Is the Accelerant," *Vox*, January 9, 2021.

32. David Graham, "Trump Brags About Groping Women," *The Atlantic*, October 7, 2016.

33. Christopher Morrison et al., "Assaults on Days of Campaign Rallies During the 2016 US Presidential Election," *Epidemiology* 29, no. 4 (2018): 490–93.

34. Cineas, "Donald Trump Is the Accelerant."

35. United States Congress, Senate, *Domestic Terrorism Prevention Act of 2019*, S.894, 116th Congress, 1st Session. Introduced in Senate March 27, 2019.
36. *The Year in Hate and Extremism 2020*, Alabama: Southern Poverty Law Center, 2021, p. 2.
37. "Donald Trump Coronavirus Briefing Transcript April 3: New CDC Face Mask Recommendations," *Rev*, April 3, 2020.
38. Luke Mogelson, "The Militias Against Masks," *The New Yorker*, August 17, 2020.
39. Government of Australia, Prime Minister of Australia, *Press Conference—Australian Parliament House, Act*, April 2, 2020.
40. Parliament of Australia, House of Representatives, *Ministerial Statements—COVID-19*, August 4, 2020.
41. Kathleen Harris, "Go Home and Stay Home, Trudeau Tells Canadians as Government Warns of COVID-19 Enforcement Measures," CBC News Canada, March 23, 2020.
42. Government of the United Kingdom, Office of the Prime Minister, *Prime Minister's Statement on Coronavirus (COVID-19): 23 March 2020*.
43. Harvey Molotch and Marilyn Lester, "News as Purposive Behavior: On the Strategic Use of Routine Events, Accidents, and Scandals," *American Sociological Review* 39, no. 1 (1974): 101–12; Shanto Iyengar and Donald Kinder, *News That Matters: Agenda-Setting and Priming in a Television Age* (Chicago: University of Chicago Press, 1987); Shanto Iyengar and Adam Simon, "News Coverage of the Gulf Crisis and Public Opinion: A Study of Agenda-Setting, Priming, and Framing," *Communication Research* 20, no. 3 (1993): 365–83.
44. Paul Rutledge, "Trump, COVID-19, and the War on Expertise," *The American Review of Public Administration* 50, no. 6–7 (2020): 505–11.
45. See Steven Webster, *American Rage: How Anger Shapes Our Politics* (New York: Cambridge University Press, 2020).
46. Nina Eliasoph, *Avoiding Politics: How Americans Produce Apathy in Everyday Life* (New York: Cambridge University Press, 1998).

EPILOGUE

1. Dominic Tierney, "What Does It Mean That Trump Is 'Leader of the Free World'?," *The Atlantic*, January 24, 2017.
2. See, for instance: Stephen Pettigrew, "The Racial Gap in Wait Times: Why Minority Precincts Are Underserved by Local Election Officials," *Political Science Quarterly* 132, no. 3 (2017): 527–47; Keith Chen et al., "Racial Disparities in Voting Wait Times: Evidence from Smartphone Data," *The Review of Economics and Statistics* (2019): 1–27; and Stephen Ansolabehere and Nathaniel Persily, "Vote Fraud in the Eye of the Beholder: The Role of Public Opinion in the Challenge to Voter Identification Requirements," *Harvard Law Review* 121 (2007): 1737.

3. See Greg Grandin, *Empire's Workshop: Latin America, the United States, and the Rise of the New Imperialism* (New York: Metropolitan Books, 2006).
4. Katie Gluck, "Biden, Facing Voters in a 2020 Rarity, Attacks Trump from a Battleground State," *New York Times*, September 17, 2020.
5. Jorge Fitz-Gibbon, "Trump Says Democrats 'Want to Take Away Your Freedom' in Twitter Video," *New York Post*, September 29, 2019.
6. Tal Axelrod, "A Timeline of Donald Trump's Election Denial Claims, Which Republican Politicians Increasingly Embrace," ABC News, September 8, 2022.
7. Jake Bittle, "Louis DeJoy: Is Trump's New Post Office Chief Trying to Rig the Election?," *The Guardian*, August 17, 2020.
8. United States House of Representatives, House Committee on Oversight and Reform, *Hearing: Protecting the Timely Delivery of Mail, Medicine, and Mail-in Ballots*, August 24, 2020.
9. Sam Levine and Alvin Chang, "Revealed: Evidence Shows Huge Mail Slowdowns After Trump Ally Took Over," *The Guardian*, September 21, 2020.
10. About 550,000 people said they wanted to vote but did not due to concerns about COVID. See United States Census Bureau, *Presidential Election Voting and Registration Tables Now Available*, April 29, 2021.
11. Annie Karni and Maggie Haberman, "Fox's Arizona Call for Biden Flipped the Mood at Trump Headquarters," *New York Times*, November 4, 2020.
12. Ted Johnson and Dominic Patten, "The Moment When Networks Called the Presidential Race for Joe Biden," *Deadline*, November 7, 2020.
13. Donald Trump (@realDonaldTrump), "I WON THIS ELECTION, BY A LOT!," Twitter, November 7, 2020, 10:36 p.m., Wikimedia Commons, https://upload.wikimedia.org/wikipedia/commons/6/6a/Trump_tweet_-_I_won_this_election.png and https://www.npr.org/sections/live-updates-2020-election-results/2020/11/07/932062684/far-from-over-trump-refuses-to-concede-as-ap-others-call-election-for-biden, accessed November 11, 2022.
14. Maggie Haberman, *Confidence Man: The Making of Donald Trump and the Breaking of America* (New York: Penguin, 2022).
15. Tim Elfrink, "After Electoral College Backs Biden, Trump Continues Falsely Insisting He Won: 'This Fake Election Can No Longer Stand,'" *Washington Post*, December 15, 2020.
16. National Health Commission of the People's Republic of China, Chinese Center for Disease Control and Prevention, *Tracking the Epidemic (2020): National Health Commission Update on December 31, 2020*.
17. Haidong Wang et al., "Estimating Excess Mortality Due to the COVID-19 Pandemic: A Systematic Analysis of COVID-19-Related Mortality, 2020–21," *The Lancet* 399, no. 10334 (2022): 151336; David Adam, "The Pandemic's True Death Toll: Millions More Than Official Counts," *Nature*, January 18, 2022.

18. Zhongjie Li et al., "Active Case Finding with Case Management: The Key to Tackling the COVID-19 Pandemic," *The Lancet* 396, no. 10243 (2020): 63–70.

19. Keith Bradsher, Chang Che, and Amy Chang Chien, "China Eases 'Zero Covid' Restrictions in Victory for Protestors," *New York Times*, December 7, 2022; Vivian Wang, "A Protest? A Vigil? In Beijing, Anxious Crowds are Unsure How Far to Go," *New York Times*, November 28, 2022.

20. "China's True Death Toll Estimated to Be in Hundreds of Thousands," Bloomberg, January 16, 2023.

21. "China Says COVID Deaths Top 12,600 and More Than One Billion Infected," Bloomberg, January 22, 2023; James Glanz, Mara Hvistendahl, and Agnes Chang, "How Deadly Was China's Covid Wave?," *New York Times*, February 15, 2023.

22. Matt Woodley, "Australian Death Rate in 2020 Lowest on Record: AIHW," The Royal Australian College of General Practitioners, News GP, June 9, 2022.

23. "Coronavirus: Arrests at Australia Anti-Lockdown Protests," BBC News, September 5, 2020.

24. Conor Friedersdorf, "Australia Traded Away Too Much Liberty," *The Atlantic*, September 2, 2021.

25. Kathy Katella, "5 Things to Know About the Delta Variant," *Yale Medicine*, March 1, 2022.

26. Nazrul Islam, Vladimir M. Shkolnikov, and Rolando J. Acostal, "Excess Deaths Associated with COVID-19 Pandemic in 2020: Age and Sex Disaggregated Time Series Analysis in 29 High Income Countries," *BMJ* 373, no. 1137 (2021).

27. *Prime Minister's Statement on Coronavirus (COVID-19): 19 December 2020*, Prime Minister's Office, December 19, 2020.

28. Ibid.

29. "COVID-19 Vaccine: First Person Receives Pfizer Jab in UK," BBC News, December 8, 2020.

30. Yasmeen Abutaleb, Laurie McGinley, and Carolyn Y. Johnson, "How the 'Deep State' Scientists Vilified by Trump Helped Him Deliver an Unprecedented Achievement," *Washington Post*, December 14, 2020.

31. Katherine Ellen Foley, "Trump White House Exerted Pressure on FDA for COVID-19 Emergency Use Authorizations, House Report Finds," *Politico*, August 24, 2022.

32. *Donald J. Trump, 45th President of the United States. Tweets of December 14, 2020*, University of California, Santa Barbara, American Presidency Project.

33. Annie Karni and Maggie Haberman, "Trump Delays a Plan to Fast Track Vaccines for White House Staff Members," *New York Times*, December 13, 2020.

34. Abutaleb, McGinley, and Johnson, "How the 'Deep State' Scientists Vilified by Trump Helped Him Deliver an Unprecedented Achievement."

NOTES 423

35. Jenna Romaine, "Alarming Number of Americans Think Vaccines Contain Microchips to Control People," *The Hill*, July 19, 2021.
36. U.S. Senate Committee on Homeland Security & Governmental Affairs, *Testimony of Pierre Kory, MD Homeland Security Committee Meeting: Focus on Early Treatment of COVID-19*, December 8, 2020.
37. Sheryl Gay Stolberg, "Anti-Vaccine Doctor Has Been Invited to Testify Before Senate Committee," *New York Times*, December 6, 2020.
38. Steven Lloyd Wilson and Charles Wiysonge, "Social Media and Vaccine Hesitancy," *BMJ Global Health* 5, no. 10 (2020).
39. Reuters Staff, "Fact Check: Unfounded Claim That 50 Million Americans Would Die from COVID-19 Vaccine," Reuters, June 23, 2020.
40. In late November, 18 percent of Americans surveyed by Pew Research said they would "definitely" not get vaccinated, and 21 percent said they "probably" would not. See Cary Funk and Alec Tyson, "Intent to Get a COVID-19 Vaccine Rises to 60% as Confidence in Research and Development Process Increases," Washington, DC: Pew Research Center, December 3, 2020; and Warren Cornwall, "Just 50% of Americans Plan to Get a COVID-19 Vaccine. Here's How to Win Over the Rest," *Science*, June 30, 2020.
41. Mark Harrison, "Disease, Diplomacy and International Commerce: The Origins of International Sanitary Regulation in the Nineteenth Century," *Journal of Global History* 1 (2006): 197–217.
42. Jeanne Abrams, *Revolutionary Medicine: The Founding Fathers and Mothers in Sickness and in Health* (New York: New York University Press, 2013).
43. Charles-Edward Winslow, "The Evolution and Significance of the Modern Public Health Campaign," *Journal of Public Health Policy*, South Burlington, VT, 1923.
44. Institute of Medicine, *The Future of Public Health* (Washington, DC: National Academies Press, 1988).
45. Harrison, "Disease, Diplomacy and International Commerce."
46. Alfred Crosby, *America's Forgotten Pandemic: The Influenza of 1918*, 2nd edition (Cambridge: Cambridge University Press, 1989; 2003), p. 10.
47. Ibid., p. 312.
48. Norman Howard-Jones, "International Public Health Between the Two World Wars—The Organizational Problems," *History of International Public Health* 3, Geneva: World Health Organization, 1978.
49. Crosby, *America's Forgotten Pandemic*, p. 323.
50. Ibid., p. 315.
51. Stephen Collier and Andrew Lakoff, *The Government of Emergency: Vital Systems, Expertise, and the Politics of Security* (Princeton: Princeton University Press, 2021).
52. Titan Alon et al., "This Time It's Different: The Role of Women's Employment in a Pandemic Recession," National Bureau of Economic Research, No. w27660, 2020.
53. "The Pandemic's True Death Toll," *The Economist*, May 21, 2023; Char-

lie Giattino et al., "Excess Mortality During the Coronavirus Pandemic (COVID-19)," Our World in Data, May 2023; Jennifer Kates and Josh Michaud, "Ten Numbers to Mark Three Years of COVID-19," Kaiser Family Foundation, March 6, 2023.

54. Matt McGough et al., "Premature Mortality During COVID-19 in the U.S. and Peer Countries," Kaiser Family Foundation, April 24, 2023.
55. Adam Tooze, *Shocked: How Covid Shook the World's Economy* (New York: Viking, 2021), p. 22.
56. Centre for the Future of Democracy, *The Great Reset Public Opinion, Populism, and the Pandemic*, Cambridge: University of Cambridge, January 2022, p. 16.
57. Matthew Gentzkow, "Did COVID-19 Bring Americans Together?," *Tech Policy*, October 6, 2021; Levi Boxell et al., "Affective Polarization Did Not Increase During the Coronavirus Pandemic," National Bureau of Economic Research, Working Paper no. 28036 (2020).
58. "While Many Say Their Country's Coronavirus Response Has Been Good, Publics Are Divided over COVID-19's Impact on National Unity," Pew Research Center, September 10, 2020.
59. Claude S. Fischer, "Paradoxes of American Individualism," *Sociological Forum* 23, no. 2 (2008): 363–72.
60. Philip Bump, "Democrats Have Joined Republicans in Calling Their Opponents 'Enemies,'" *Washington Post*, August 1, 2022.
61. As Camus put it, "But what does it mean, the plague? It's life, after all." Albert Camus, *The Plague* (New York: Alfred A. Knopf, 1948).
62. Crosby, *America's Forgotten Pandemic*.
63. Atul Gawande, "The Aftermath of a Pandemic Requires as Much Focus as the Start," *New York Times*, March 16, 2023.
64. David Wallace-Wells, "Apparently the Pandemic Emergency Is Over," *New York Times*, May 6, 2023.
65. Dan Treglia et al., "Parental and Other Caregiver Loss Due to COVID-19 in the United States: Prevalence by Race, State, Relationship, and Child Age," *Journal of Community Health* 48, no. 3 (2022): 1–8; Liz Donovan and Fazil Khan, "The Pandemic Robbed Thousands of NYC Children of Parents. Many Aren't Getting the Help They Need," *The City*, January 26, 2023.
66. Bret Stephens, "The Mask Mandates Did Nothing. Will Any Lessons Be Learned," *New York Times*, February 21, 2023; Ron DeSantis, *The Courage to Be Free* (New York: HarperCollins, 2023).
67. Arundhati Roy, "The Pandemic Is a Portal," *Financial Times*, April 3, 2020.

APPENDIX A NOTE ON THE RESEARCH

1. Haidong Wang et al., "Estimating Excess Mortality Due to the COVID-19 Pandemic: A Systematic Analysis of COVID-19-Related Mortality, 2020–21," *The Lancet* 399, no. 10334 (2022): 1513–36.

2. George Calhoun, "Part 1: Beijing Is Intentionally Underreporting China's Covid Death Rate," *Forbes*, January 2, 2022.

3. Richard Luscombe, "Florida Governor Under Fire over Claims State Is 'Cooking the Books' on COVID-19," *The Guardian*, June 26, 2020; J. David Goodman, Jesse McKinley, and Danny Hakim, "Cuomo Aides Spent Months Hiding Nursing Home Death Toll," *New York Times*, April 28, 2021.

4. Sheryl Gay Stolberg, "Trump Administration Strips C.D.C. of Control of Coronavirus Data," *New York Times*, July 14, 2020.

5. C. Wright Mills, *The Sociological Imagination* (New York: Oxford University Press, 1959), p. 226.

6. Robert Park, "The City: Suggestions for the Investigation of Human Behavior in the City Environment," *American Journal of Sociology* 20, no. 5 (1015): 577–612.

INDEX

ILLUSTRATION CREDITS

37 Patrick Chang

89 Photo used with permission of Sophia Zayas

137 Eric Klinenberg

172 Vanessa Ryan

218 Patrick Chang

221 New York City Health Department, NYU Furman Center

233 New York City Department of Health and Mental Hygiene; analysis by Jocelyn Drummond of NYU.

256 Robert Hamada

288 Marc A Hermann/MTA. TRAVELS FAR (2020) © MTA Arts & Design. A Memorial Honoring MTA Workers Lost to COVID-19. Sandra Bloodworth, Artist; Tracy K. Smith, Poet; Chris Thompson, composer.

289 TRAVELS FAR (2020) © MTA Arts & Design. A Memorial Honoring MTA Workers Lost to COVID-19. Sandra Bloodworth, Artist; Tracy K. Smith, Poet; Chris Thompson, composer.

291 TRAVELS FAR (2020) © MTA Arts & Design. A Memorial Honoring MTA Workers Lost to COVID-19. Sandra Bloodworth, Artist; Tracy K. Smith, Poet; Chris Thompson, composer.

A NOTE ABOUT THE AUTHOR

Eric Klinenberg is the Helen Gould Shepard Professor in the Social Sciences and director of the Institute for Public Knowledge at New York University. He is the coauthor of the #1 *New York Times* best seller *Modern Romance* and author of *Palaces for the People, Going Solo, Heat Wave,* and *Fighting for Air.* He has contributed to *The New Yorker, The New York Times Magazine, Rolling Stone, Wired,* and *This American Life.* He lives in New York City.

A NOTE ON THE TYPE

This book was set in Janson, a typeface long thought to have been made by the Dutchman Anton Janson, who was a practicing typefounder in Leipzig during the years 1668–1687. However, it has been conclusively demonstrated that these types are actually the work of Nicholas Kis (1650–1702), a Hungarian, who most probably learned his trade from the master Dutch typefounder Dirk Voskens. The type is an excellent example of the influential and sturdy Dutch types that prevailed in England up to the time William Caslon (1692–1766) developed his own incomparable designs from them.

Composed by North Market Street Graphics,
Lancaster, Pennsylvania

Printed and bound by Berryville Graphics,
Berryville, Virginia

Designed by Soonyoung Kwon